THE
MONTH-BY-MONTH
BABY BOOK

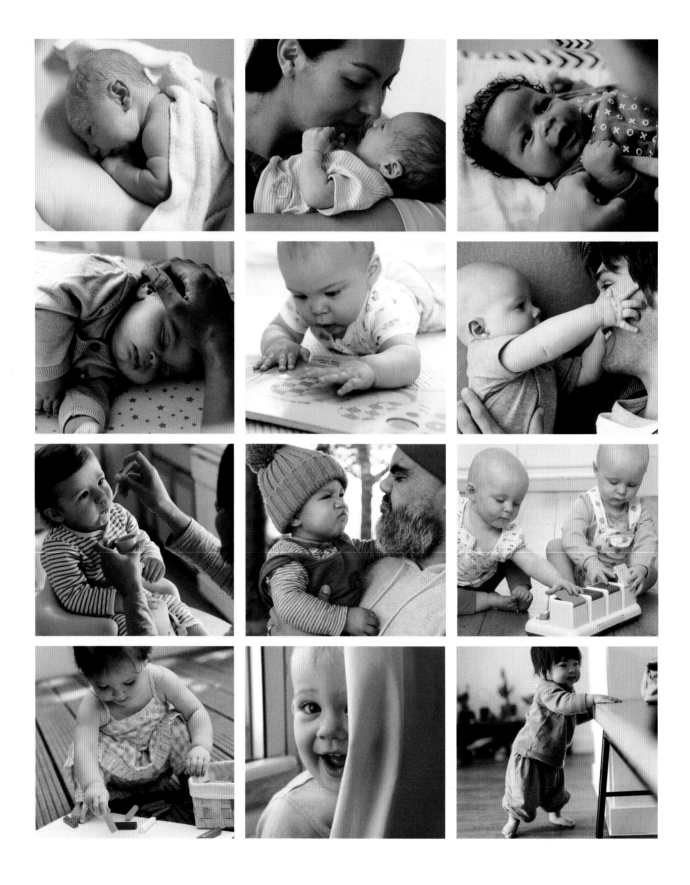

THE
MONTH-BY-MONTH
BABY BOOK

In-depth, monthly advice on your baby's growth, care, and development in the first year

Contents

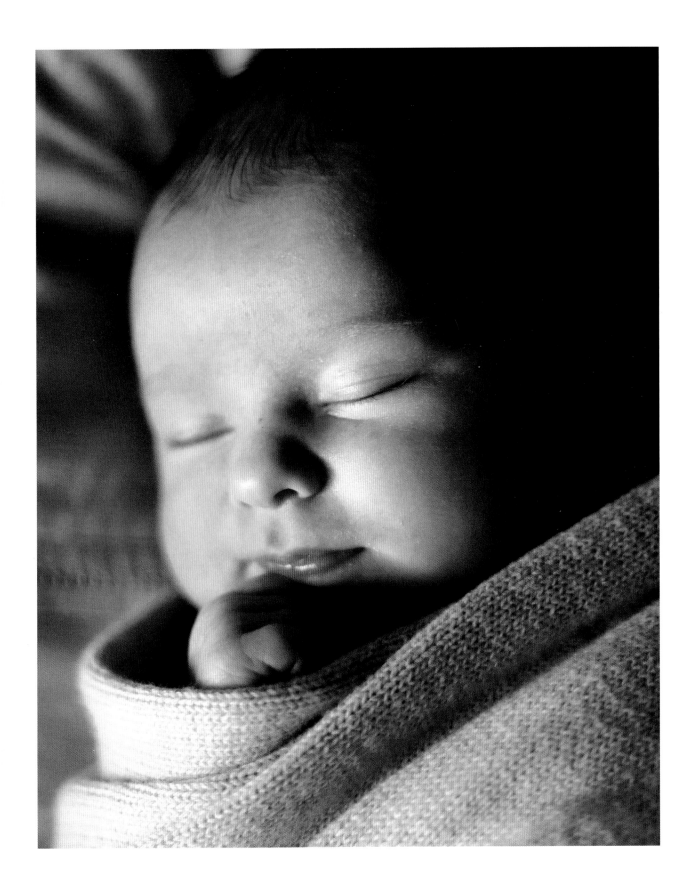

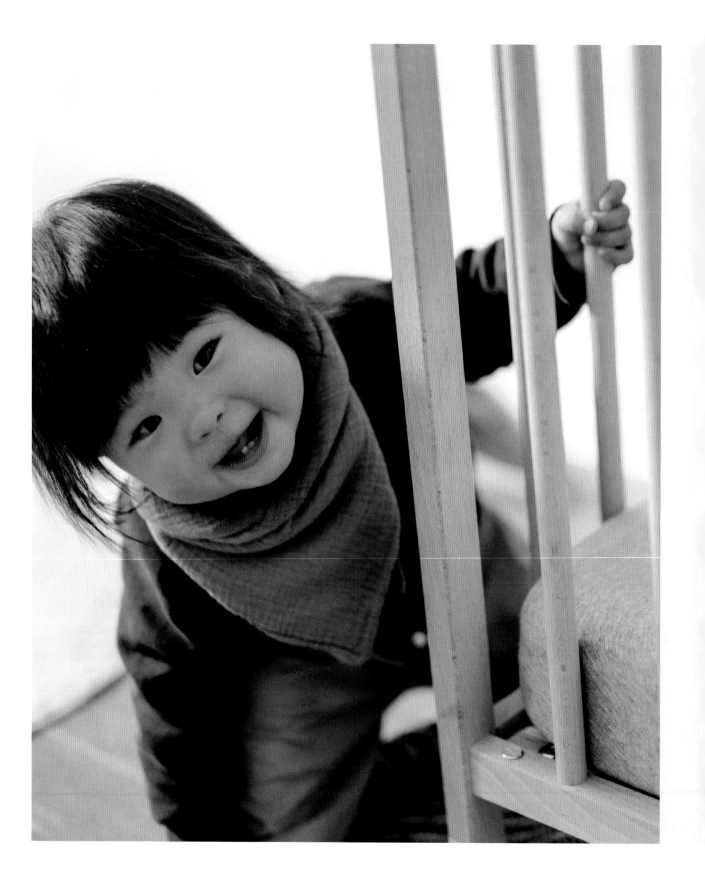

Your baby's health

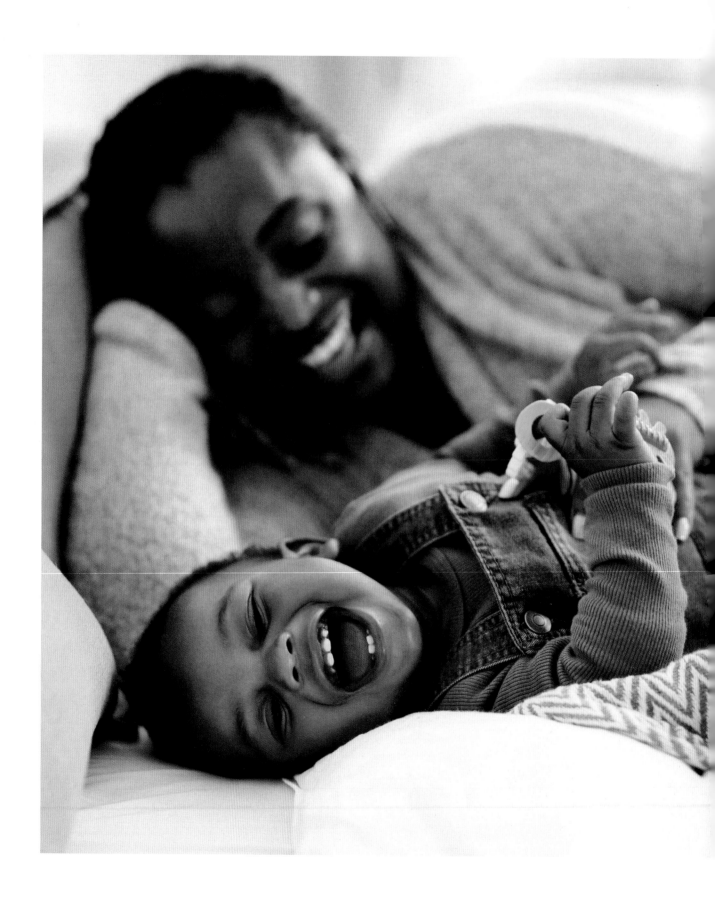

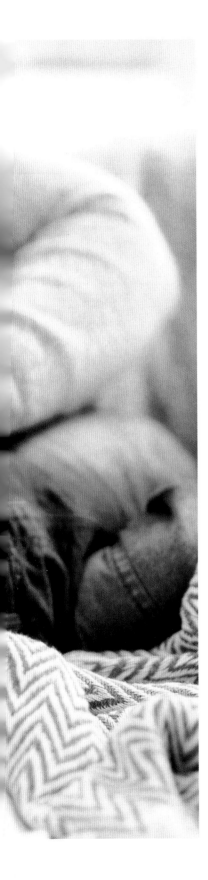

Introduction

In these days of advanced technology when so much can be achieved at the touch of a screen, there is still nothing to compare with the miracle of a new baby. For new parents, the reality of having created this little being is life-changing; their baby's future is in their hands. The sense of achievement and responsibility is immense and will change parents' perspectives forever.

By adulthood most of us have learned what is required to get a job, run a home, and have a social life. The one area most first-time parents have not learned about is how to bring up a baby. Once, families would hand down child-rearing skills, for better or worse. These days, families may be scattered across countries or continents; grandparents may be working. Parents cannot always take family support for granted. At the same time, research and medical care have improved child health dramatically and advanced our knowledge of how best to raise babies. Parents want to have real input into how their child develops, because they have a vision of the kind of person they hope their child will grow up to be.

The first year of a baby's life is the time of most rapid growth and development. Parents see their baby changing almost day by day. They will be filled with wonder and pride but may be overwhelmed by how much they need to learn. At this time, more than at any other age, they need reliable, balanced, and reassuring information about what to expect and what to do for their baby.

In *The Month-by-Month Baby Book*, parents will find a comprehensive guide to each step of their baby's first year of life. There is specialized advice on each stage of their baby's growth and development, with current evidence-based guidelines on breast- and bottle-feeding, starting solid food, sleeping, health screening, and immunizations. Common problems and worries are discussed, with friendly, reassuring help. A detailed medical section provides an accessible reference to common illnesses and first aid. Supportive information is given for parents, from breastfeeding and postpartum care for mothers, to work options, childcare, family networks, and maintaining parents' identities and relationships.

The book is written for all parents and caregivers involved in raising children. The aim is to make this first year a happy, rewarding, and confident start to the rest of the whole family's life together.

Dr. Ilona Bendefy

YOUR
NEW BABY

Once your baby is born, you'll find that life takes on a new momentum as you grapple with all the first-time experiences that caring for a growing baby involves. The first days—and weeks—can pass in a bit of a blur, so this chapter gives you the kind of background information that's so useful to know from the beginning. From bonding and parenting approaches to your rights and benefits, to feeding your baby, choosing diapers, and buying equipment, it's essential preparation for parenthood.

Being a parent

IT'S A LIFELONG AND, AT TIMES, DEMANDING JOB—BUT THE REWARDS ARE AMAZING.
You have anticipated this moment for the past nine months, if not longer. Now that your baby has arrived, you have someone else to love and care for, someone for whom you must create a safe, nurturing environment, and whose needs come before your own.

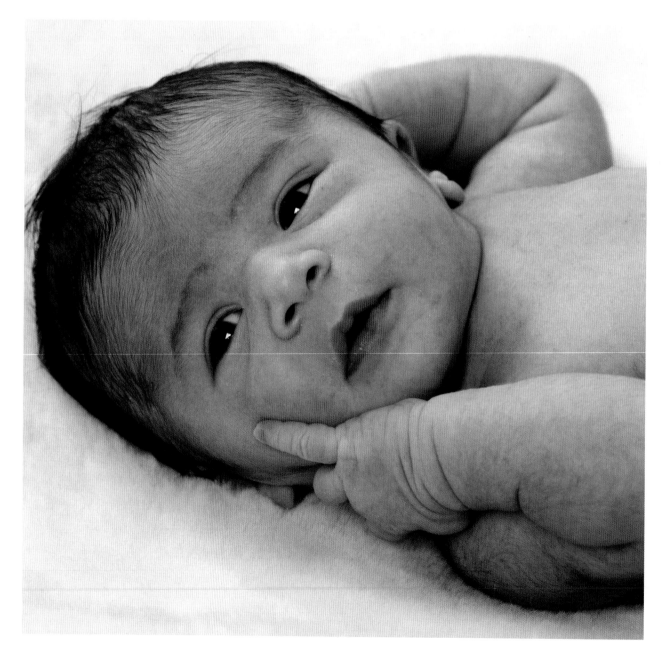

Adjusting to parenthood

Your baby is roughly as long as your elbow to your fingertips, yet is able to turn your whole world on its head. Welcome to parenthood!

Although you may have already made practical adjustments to your life—put a crib in your bedroom, dedicated a drawer to diapers and another to sleep sacks and so on—the reality of living with and having complete responsibility for your baby can come as a bit of a shock.

Time difference

The most dramatic change you will notice at first is how your time is no longer your own—both day and night. Particularly in the early weeks, your baby will need almost constant care—waking for feedings when you would rather sleep, and chances are baby will need a diaper change just as you sit down with a cup of coffee. This is physically and emotionally exhausting. However, even at your most tired, be assured that this is just a phase.

As you get to know your baby and start to feel more confident as a parent, you should find that life settles down

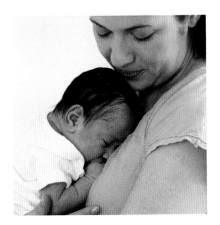

Duty of care You might be surprised at how fiercely protective of your baby you feel—that's your parental instinct kicking in.

into a more predictable pattern. That's not to say that you'll be back to eight hours' sleep a night any time soon, but after about three months, your baby will probably be sleeping longer at night and less during the day. By 12 months, most babies sleep for around 10–12 hours at night and have a couple of naps during the day.

Trusting your instincts

Becoming a parent is the most exciting and fulfilling experience imaginable—but along with the highs comes an entirely new realm of fears and worries. Is my baby feeding too much or too little? Am I playing with them enough? Is my baby ill? Are they developing normally? Trust your instincts and never be afraid to share your concerns and ask for help. It's worthwhile to remember that no matter how much well-meaning advice you receive, you are the best authority on your baby. Nature has an amazing knack of tuning you in to your baby's needs—and if you don't know the answer right away, you'll soon figure it out. If you can't, then seek advice.

Talk to your partner, too. Talking about your hopes, fears, and concerns divides the burden. Even if you don't find the answers, reaffirming you are in this together is an essential part of coping with the demands of parenting.

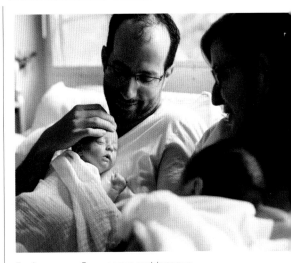

Two's company Every parent could use two pairs of hands, but with twins, sharing the care is even more of a necessity.

The responsibility of a new life in duplicate (or multiple) can be overwhelming. Both you and your partner will need lots of support from family and friends. Try to concentrate solely on your babies, and forget about housework or doing much else for at least the first three months. Delegate making meals and running the home to your partner and family, and spend this precious time getting to know your twins and focusing on the best ways to juggle their needs.

Becoming a family

As soon as you have a baby, you become a family. This changes the dynamics of your relationship with your partner and your relatives.

You and your partner

Before your baby came along, your spare time could be dedicated to one another. If you have individual hobbies, each of you could pursue them without feeling tied to home. However, as soon as you have a baby, your time for each other, and for individual pursuits, is much less of a priority. None of this matters, of course, because your baby is the center of your world, but inevitably there will come a moment when the full realization dawns that life has changed for you, particularly as a couple.

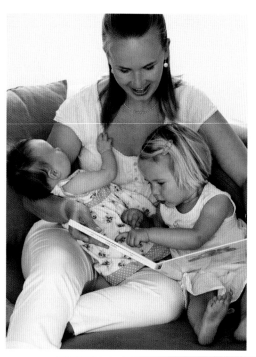

Sibling rivalry Giving your toddler time and attention will help with accepting the new arrival more readily and lessen feelings of jealousy.

Remind each other every so often that you are in this together. You will be tired and fretful, you may even be snappy or tearful, making it more important than ever that you actively lean on one another for support. Keep talking and try to make time for each other—even if it is just 20 minutes to sit down and eat a meal together—every day. Reassure yourselves that the fatigue of the early days passes soon enough, and that this is the beginning of a journey in which every step you take together in the common goal of doing the best for your baby (even when they're old enough to make their own decisions) is a step that brings you closer together and reaffirms the strength of your relationship.

One common point of tension in the early months is when a new work-life balance begins as parental leave ends for one or both of you. A stay-at-home parent may feel that they have lost some of their independence, while little has changed in the life of the parent who is back in the workplace. They may feel that the burden of responsibility for the family's day-to-day welfare falls too heavily on their shoulders. On the other hand, the parent who is working may feel left out or alienated, and that their contribution as the breadwinner separates them from the fun part of being a parent.

In fact, you both have crucial roles for the family's well-being and it is important that you love, support, and respect one another for the choices you have made. When the weekend comes, try to give the primary care giver even just a few hours' time out, while the working parent immerses him- or herself in family life.

Both of you juggling work and childcare puts its own strain on your relationship. In this case, you both need to share as many of the household tasks as you can, and be ready to ask each other for help when you need it. Try not to make assumptions about what the other is going to take on and which tasks fall to you, since this often leads to misunderstandings. Make lists or notes every morning if it helps, keep talking, and be prepared to be flexible.

Brothers and sisters

If you already have other children, the arrival of a new baby will cause a shift in their lives, too. It is extremely rare that any family completely escapes some form of sibling rivalry along the way (be prepared that it may not happen right away). If you can show each other and all your children love and respect, siblings are much more likely to show love and respect toward one another, even if they squabble at some point about having to share you. Involving all your children with the baby care is important, and so is making time for each child individually—and that goes for step-children or children from a previous relationship, too.

In time, siblings become a support network for you and your baby, providing help for you, and unconditional love for your baby, well into adulthood.

Step-children

A new baby provides step-children with an unmistakable reminder that one of their parents has moved on beyond their original family. Some step-children see the new sibling as the glue that bonds the whole family—old and new—together, and welcome the new life gladly, but others feel resentful. Give step-siblings as much opportunity as possible to play and help with the new baby. Try to avoid terms such as "half brother" or "half sister," which create a distance. Instead, talk about how much the baby is going to love having a big brother or sister.

If your step-child doesn't live with you, keep to the same visiting schedule, and plan activities that you all can enjoy together on those days. Reassure your step-child that your love for him or her won't ever change.

Extended family

You have become parents, but your parents, your in-laws, and your siblings have become grandparents and aunts and uncles, too. Welcoming your wider family into your baby's life, and ensuring they have regular contact, gives baby the opportunity to have a distinct sense of family identity their place in the world. Today, we are often scattered from our own parents or siblings, and it may not always be easy to spend time together. If this is true for you, consider inviting your parents or in-laws to stay every so often, or going to stay with them. It may be a little daunting taking your baby to stay with relatives, but there are positive gains to be made. Grandparents who see a lot of their grandchildren and are actively involved in their care share a much closer bond than those who become acquainted on the occasional fleeting visit. And the love you all have for your child gives you a

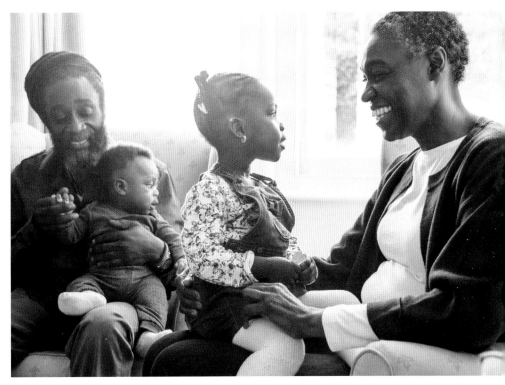

Family ties Involving your family in your baby's life will not only gain you much-needed practical help, but will also allow your child to build close and lasting relationships.

common link that can bring you closer.

For week-to-week contact, join a social networking site through which you can contact relatives and share photos; or download a social chat program, and invest in a webcam—even if you are at opposite ends of the country, or the world, your baby can still grow up with a sense of family connections. Finally, babies love to look at faces so show photographs of relatives, pointing at them and naming them one by one. This is a great way of providing your baby with a sense of his wider family.

SINGLE PARENTING

It takes only two—you and your baby—to make a family and you can provide your baby with everything they need, from food to clothing and especially love. You are also the person who best knows your baby, so your instincts will ensure that you make no more mistakes than any other parent. Being a single parent does not mean that you are alone. If you feel isolated, pick up the phone and talk to someone—a friend, a doctor, or a family member—to share how you feel. Or consider joining a local or online parents' support group to seek advice and encouragement from other parents that may share your feelings. During the first few weeks, be prepared to ask for help from willing friends and family; you may even want to consider staying with someone while you adjust to being a parent.

Parenting approaches

There are no hard-and-fast rules when it comes to good parenting practice. Your own approach to parenting will emerge in time.

Before you had your baby you may have had some fixed ideas about the right and wrong ways to bring up a baby. The reality is that as you settle into your new role, some of the ideas about parenting you thought were nonnegotiable suddenly become less important, while others move up the agenda. Beyond the fundamental requirements to love, nurture, respond to, feed, and clothe your baby, there is so much to learn as you go along. It is essential to talk to your partner about how you will raise your baby and how, in the years to come, you will set expectations for behavior.

One thing is certain—as your baby becomes a toddler, they will soon learn if one of you is a soft touch and one the disciplinarian, and whether or not they can play one of you off against the other. Presenting a united front and giving a clear, consistent message is the key to success, whatever approach to parenting you decide to take.

Reflecting you

Your approach to parenting will inevitably, in part, reflect the ways in which your parents brought you up. In addition, it will demonstrate your own culture and values, and your faith if you have one. It will also reflect your personality: if you tend to be laid back, it's more likely that your parenting style will be laid back; if you are a list-maker and organizer, the chances are that your approach will be more routine based. No approach is definitive, but you need to be comfortable with the one you choose, so that you can stick to it and provide a secure environment in which your baby can develop.

Setting boundaries

A newborn baby does not yet have the mental acuity to understand right from wrong, yes from no, good from bad. But in only a matter of months, they will begin to explore the world by such actions as reaching and grabbing, at which point, gently setting boundaries gives them the opportunity to discover what's around, but also keeps them safe.

Furthermore, as they become more aware, your boundaries will make them feel secure in what is otherwise a baffling melee of sight, sound, taste, touch, and scent. They need you to guide them on appropriate behavior and actions. Setting boundaries isn't about becoming a disciplinarian with a strict rule book. Rather, boundaries provide an important structure for your baby's life, and when it comes to right and wrong, a moral code for their behavior. Ultimately, boundaries make them feel secure.

Introducing discipline

During your baby's first year, there are very few reasons for saying "No." You cannot teach a baby to control their behavior at this age because they unable to do so—the part of their brain that controls social understanding and behavior won't be fully developed for another year or two. So "discipline" at this stage should be about gentle correction or distraction, and saying "No" only when your baby is doing something that is unsafe for them, or for others.

Whatever boundaries you set, it is important to follow the same pattern of correction each time. One useful approach is "repeat, remove, distract." So, you repeat the boundary (for example, "Don't touch the vase, it may break"), then remove the temptation (put the vase away) or remove your baby from the danger, if relevant, and then distract them quickly. The next time baby does the same thing, respond with the same sequence: repeat, remove, distract. Through the consistency of your words and actions, from about nine months, your baby should begin to associate certain commands with certain consequences. This is a vital lesson

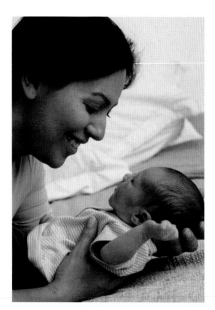

Perfect parent Of course, there's no such thing, but with plenty of love, kindness, and consistency you'll be the best parent there is.

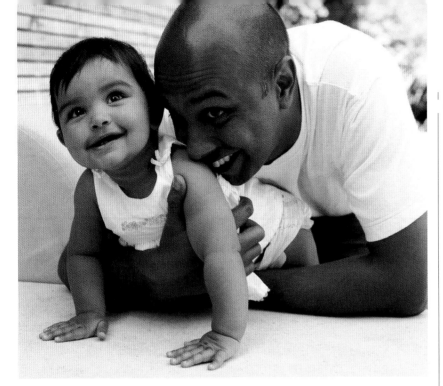

Out of harm's way Once baby is mobile, you'll need to remove them repeatedly from danger. Explain why some things are out of bounds, and distract them by moving on to a safer place or activity.

for the toddler years when all children learn to push boundaries, as they will trust that you mean what you say.

Giving reasons

When you ask your baby not to do something, let them know why in very simple terms: "Don't touch the oven—it's hot, ouch," and mime touching something hot. They won't fully understand, but they'll begin to get the idea during the first year. Getting upset with your baby won't achieve anything. As baby matures, they will listen and respond more readily when you are calm. Get their attention, speak clearly, and show them by acting it out yourself.

ASK A CHILD PSYCHOLOGIST

When does parenting become "pushy" as opposed to "encouraging"? We live in a competitive world and there is a growing trend for parents to fill their children's—even their babies'—time with activities to race them through developmental milestones. However, children will rarely be hurried. Encouraging your child to learn means giving them time to explore the world, and giving them a degree of autonomy to discover what is around them and to discover the principles of cause and effect

(whether that's in actions, language, or sounds). It also means giving lots of praise when they make a new discovery, behave well, or learn to do something for themself. Above all, children learn best through play, when they are happy, relaxed, and able to work at their own pace. If you allow lots of playtime, and read stories and sing songs together, your baby will have all the encouragement needed to develop their mental acuity at a perfect pace, without being pushed to go too fast.

POSITIVE PARENTING

Whatever your values and the specifics of the way in which you want to raise your baby, there are certain fundamentals of parenting that will make your approach more effective and loving, and some methods that are best avoided. Positive parenting is about championing the good in your child. Children thrive on praise, and they also love attention. If they get lots of praise and attention for good behavior, but find that bad behavior is reprimanded or ignored, they soon learn to focus on the good.

Key positive parenting traits
• Give lots of extra praise and attention when your baby does as you've asked.
• Show how proud you are of your baby. Even minor achievements can be celebrated with clapping and cheering. Your baby will love this and soon want to elicit those reactions again.
• Show respect to your baby.
• Be consistent in your rules or expectations and follow through with rewards for positive behavior.
• Show your baby your love by giving them your undivided attention and lots of physical affection.

Parenting traits to avoid
• Even if you feel frustrated, try not to react angrily toward your baby. If you stay calm, your baby will stay calm and be far more likely to respond positively to you.
• It is never appropriate to criticize your baby. As they gets older, focus on behavior ("You did not share your toy"), not on them ("You are selfish").
• Stick to your rules and routines: your baby will feel more secure knowing what's expected.

Parental rights and benefits

Once your child is born, you will have paperwork to fill out, and if you're employed, you may be eligible for paid or unpaid leave.

In the blur of a new baby's arrival, filling out forms can feel like the last thing you want to do. However, there are certain forms that should be submitted before you leave the hospital, and other notifications that should be made within 30 days of the baby's birth. Even though you have other things on your mind right now, it's important to sift through the paperwork and make the necessary phone calls to make everything fall into place.

Registering the birth

Registering your baby's birth with your city or state is required to get your baby a birth certificate. Most hospitals make this process easy for you by supplying you the proper forms to fill out while you're a patient in the maternity ward, and they take the completed forms and submit them to the proper authorities on your behalf. Many hospitals suggest that you submit the birth certificate paperwork before you're discharged, but this may not be required. If you prefer, you may be able to submit the paperwork yourself shortly thereafter. (Rules differ by municipality.) Within a few weeks, you can expect to receive a birth certificate in the mail. If you need additional copies, contact your local Office of Vital Statistics to find out the procedure. There's usually a nominal fee for extra birth certificates. If you'd like to get your child a social security number now, it's easiest to do it through the hospital. There may be a form to fill out requesting a number, and you'll have to supply the social security numbers of both you and your partner. The paperwork will be submitted to the Social Security Administration on your behalf, and within a few weeks, your baby should receive a social security card and number in the mail. There is no fee for this process.

Applying for health insurance

After your baby is born, you need to add them to your family's health insurance plan so they'll be covered. Each health insurance plan is different, but in most cases, you'll have 30 days from the baby's birth to add them to the plan. It's usually as simple as calling the customer service number for your insurance company and alerting them about the birth. They will want to know the baby's name and birth date, and they may send you updated insurance cards, if the names of all covered family members appear on the card. Once you let the insurance company know about your baby, they'll receive coverage and benefits the same way that you do.

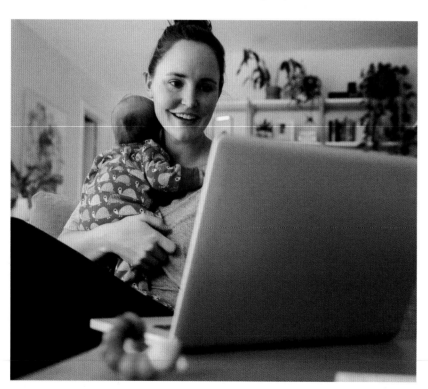

Seeing what help is available You have certain rights and benefits depending on your circumstances so make sure you find out what you're entitled to so that you don't miss out.

Far fewer companies offer paid paternity leave to their male employees than paid maternity leave to their female employees. Some company policies have been adding paternity leave to their list of benefits, but it's a slow-growing trend. If you want to take time off from work to take care of and bond with your baby, you'll most likely have to use saved-up vacation days or sick time to do so. Be sure to check with your supervisor and/or your human resources department to be sure that you can use vacation or sick leave in this manner. Your company may also frown upon taking too much time off up front; it might benefit your career if you take only a week or two off at the beginning, then sprinkle in a few more vacation days over the course of the next several weeks. If you'd prefer a larger chunk of time and your company won't let you use up all of your vacation and sick days, keep in mind that you, too, may be eligible for unpaid paternity leave, in the form of the Family and Medical Leave Act (FMLA). If eligible, you'll be able to take off up to 12 weeks to be at home to get to know your infant. You may be able to switch off with your partner so that your baby has one parent or the other at home for 24 weeks. This will give you the time to figure out what kind of baby care you'd like when both parents return to work.

Is there any support system available for single parents? You may find it difficult to juggle your parenting responsibilities along with everything else, particularly when you've got a newborn who is completely dependent upon you. It's beneficial to take any and all offers of help when you're just starting out; let someone else cook or clean while you feed the baby, or let someone else babysit while you nap or pay the bills. If you live in the same area as your parents or siblings, you may have a network of eager babysitters waiting for you to call for help. If you live far from family, call on some trusted friends. There are some support groups for single parents, so you might meet other people in a similar situation. Single parenthood has become more prevalent in recent decades, so there's no need to feel alone.

Your right to time off work

The US is one of very few countries worldwide that don't offer women guaranteed paid maternity leave. Policies vary at different companies, so it depends on your individual workplace as to whether or not you'll be eligible for paid maternity leave. Even if you are eligible, the percentage of your salary that you'll receive, and the number of weeks you'll receive it, will vary by the company. Your company may also allow you to use sick days or vacation days that you've accumulated to stay home with your baby; again, this policy varies by the company. During your pregnancy, you should have spoken with your supervisor and/or your human resources department to determine your eligibility for paid maternity leave and/or using sick or vacation days. A handful of states, including California, offer paid maternity leave for new parents. This may be partial pay for a few weeks' time. Even if you're not eligible for paid maternity leave, it's very possible that you might be eligible for unpaid maternity leave. Through the Family and Medical Leave Act (FMLA), you can take off from work for up to 12 weeks in a 12-month period and your employer is required to hold your job (or a similar one) for you during that time frame. To qualify, you'll have to have been an employee with your current company for at least 12 months and worked at least 1,250 hours during the past 12-month period. You'll also have to work within 75 miles of an office where 50 or more of your company's employees work. (FMLA does not apply to very small companies.) While you are on FMLA, your employer is required to continue your health insurance coverage at the same rate. If you meet the FMLA criteria, you are eligible, whether you're male or female and whether you work for a private company or state or local government. Some people opt not to use their entire 12-week allotment all at once, instead opting for a few days off here and there, as needed. This is allowed, since no rules require you to take the days off consecutively.

Breastfeeding at work

The Fair Labor Standards Act (FLSA) requires employers to provide adequate breaks for an employee to express milk for a year following the birth of a child. There are 32 states with laws that extend these rights. These laws generally outline ways that employers should accommodate an employee who needs to pump breast milk during business hours—for example, supplying a secluded place near an electrical outlet where the employee can plug in the pump and express milk undisturbed.

PARENTAL RIGHTS AND BENEFITS

Understanding your child

YOU'LL DISCOVER MORE AND MORE ABOUT WHAT MAKES YOUR BABY TICK AS EACH MONTH GOES BY. Your baby has their own unique genetic makeup, of course, but at least some characteristics are inherited from you. In the first year, as they negotiate developmental milestones and develop their own personality, you will gather clues as to what kind of child they will eventually become.

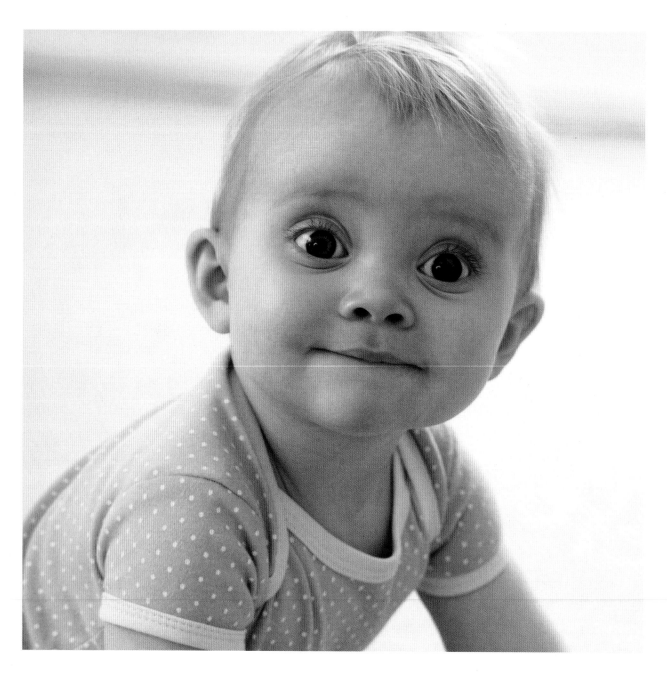

Your child's genes

Friends and family always look to see which parent a baby resembles.
As they grow, you may recognize which traits your baby has inherited.

Passed from parent to child, genes are segments of DNA containing genetic information that determine features or characteristics unique to an individual. A baby's genetic traits are inherited from both parents. Furthermore, a parent's DNA consists of their parents' DNA, which is why some children show likenesses to one or more of their grandparents.

Eye color

Certain physical traits are determined by the presence or absence of a dominant or recessive gene, making some characteristics predictable. For example, if both biological parents have blue eyes, their baby will have blue eyes, because they will have inherited recessive blue genes from both parents. However, if one parent has brown eyes and the other has blue, their own parents' genes will play a role in determining eye color. If one parent's brown eyes are the result of both a brown and a blue gene from their own parents, there is a chance for a blue-eyed baby. However, if one biological parent has two brown genes, even if the other parent has blue genes, the baby will have brown eyes, because they will always inherit one dominant brown-eye gene. Other characteristics that work this way are hair color—dark hair is dominant, while blond or red hair is recessive—and hair type—curly is dominant; straight is recessive.

Polygenic traits

A polygenic trait, such as height, is a characteristic that is determined by a combination of genes, rather than just one. As a guideline, experts say that taking the average of the height of both biological parents and then subtracting 2 in (5 cm) for a female baby and adding 2 in (5 cm) a male baby gives a good idea of adult height. But, genes themselves contain dominant and recessive triggers, called alleles. Even if both biological parents are short, they may still have "tall" (dominant) alleles, it's just these are outnumbered by "short" ones. If a baby inherits genes made up of most or all of a parent's "tall" alleles, and only a few or none of the "short" alleles, he could end up being taller. Polygenic traits are also influenced by environmental factors, such as good or poor nutrition. Other polygenic traits include intelligence and skin color.

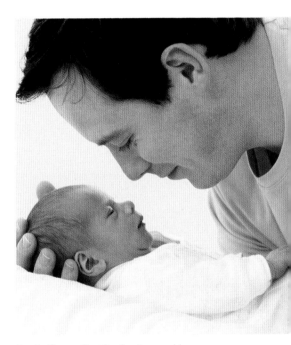

Family likeness Spotting family resemblances is an early preoccupation for everyone who will be invested in a baby's life.

ASK A PEDIATRICIAN

Is my baby likely to be musical like me?
In 2001, geneticists at St. Thomas's Hospital in London, working with the Institute for Deafness in Maryland, published a study of hundreds of twins that supported the notion that musical ability is inherited. Certainly, Johann Sebastian Bach came from a long line of well-respected musicians. So, generally, yes, it is likely that your baby will be musical like you, especially if you encourage innate talent by playing a variety of music and offering instruments to play with. Equally, if you are sporty, you are likely to produce children with the physical build and, say, hand–eye coordination to follow in your footsteps. Inevitably, though, nurture also comes into play. If you are musical, you will naturally encourage your child to love music; if you love sports, you'll encourage them to play sports, which in turn hones their in-built talent.

Your developing child

Your baby's growth in the first year is remarkable. At no other time in human life is development so evident and so rapid.

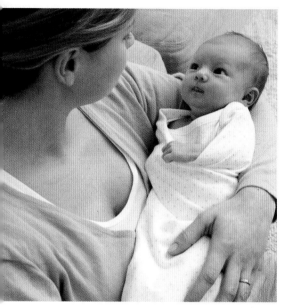

Soft focus At first, your baby must be up close to see your face; by eight months, they'll identify people and objects from across the room.

ASK A CHILD PSYCHOLOGIST

Can I spoil my baby with love? Babies need to feel secure and you and your partner are the people best placed to ensure that happens. Showing your baby love by giving them lots of attention, in the form of playing with them, attending to their needs, being close at all times, and giving them plenty of embraces and kisses does not spoil them—it confirms that they are the center of your world. With a deep sense of security in you, they will develop confidence to explore their world independently. As your baby matures, you can also show love by setting boundaries and limits: giving in to them every time isn't in their best interest; it's more important to show them what is safe and to teach them right from wrong.

Physical milestones

The most striking physical change during your baby's first year is size. By the time they are one, they'll be around 12 in (30 cm) longer than at birth, and about three times as heavy. During that time, muscle tone and physical coordination will develop so that by two months, they'll be able to hold up their head for a few seconds, and by three months, they may be able to roll over. By the time they are 6–7 months, they will have developed enough muscle strength to sit unaided, and from sitting they will learn to crawl (usually by 6–9 months), and then, by a year, they will be able to stand up, possibly unaided, and may even be able to walk.

Fine motor skills will progress from swiping at objects at about three months to holding a small object using a pincer grip at 8–10 months. At around 10 months, they can use a sippy cup and drink with help, and by 12 months can make a mark on paper with a big crayon or piece of chalk.

These major physical milestones are among the most visible, but baby's body is developing in many unseen ways, too. Over the first year, sight will improve from being able to focus only on objects as little as 8–10 in (20–25 cm) away from their face to being able to distinguish depth and distance at a year. Your baby rapidly learns to recognize sounds, so that by only a few months old, babies can identify where a particular sound is coming from and can turn their head toward it.

Early learning milestones

Your baby's brain has "plasticity," which means that the brain is able to create, adapt, and change its neural pathways according to all the new experiences life brings. This plasticity ensures your baby's rapid intellectual development. Within a few days of birth, baby will prefer your face to anyone else's and will recognize your scent. These experiences make baby feel secure.

By six months, baby's language skills will have developed enough that they may recognize their own name when you say it, and by nine months, will understand when you say "no" (although not always comply), and may even be able to look at the correct image of an object in a book if you ask them to find it.

They will begin to make recognizable sounds. At first, at a few months old, they may coo, gurgle, or make strange vowel sounds, but by around 10 months, these may become a discernible "mama" or "dada," although it's unlikely baby will use them discriminately. However, by a year, baby may have managed the first meaningful word—often "dada" when referring to daddy (because babies find the consonant "d" easier to sound out than the "m" sound for mama), although "cat" and "spoon"are often cited as first words, too.

Behavioral and personality milestones

By the end of your baby's first year, you've gone from having a bundle of mystery to a young toddler, who is already showing clear signs of the person they are going to be.

You might be relieved to hear that baby's behavior with regard to sleeping will gradually improve month by month, as their stomach grows to hold enough food to prevent waking up for feedings. By the time baby is one year old, they should be sleeping through the night, going to bed at around seven o'clock, and waking about 12 hours later.

At first, baby will show preferences for certain people—parents, primary caregivers, and siblings—and by six months old, may become wary of strangers. When baby is six months old, they will begin to display distinct personality traits, such as the sort of things they find amusing and the things that make them frustrated. They may throw away toys when they become upset with them, or cry in anger.

By eight months old, baby will object to you taking away a toy and believes that everything belongs to them. They'll still be anxious if they must leave you, but will be interested in other babies and "chat" with adults they are close to. He wants to please

FULFILLING POTENTIAL

We are all born with a built-in genetic blueprint that gives us our relative strengths and weaknesses, and determines certain character traits. However, most psychologists now accept that although a baby might be genetically predisposed to being better at some activities than others, the way in which they are brought up, and environmental factors (such as the value of nutrition) also influence developing skills. Bring out the best in your baby by playing with and reading to them and letting them explore the world (safely). When on solids, give the full spectrum of nutrients, and above all provide a loving, secure environment to give them confidence to reach their full potential. That way, you can nurture whatever gifts nature has bestowed.

you and will thrive on your love and affection.

Girls and boys

All children develop at different rates, regardless of their gender. However, there are certain aspects of early learning that seem to favor girls over boys, or vice versa. For example, studies show that girls learn to understand language and talk more quickly and they have more honed fine motor skills (girls will write sooner, for example). On the other hand, boys tend to be more physical and their gross motor skills are often ahead of girls, certainly by the time they reach toddler age.

One study at Cambridge University indicated that boys understand the laws of motion more quickly than girls—for example, they understand the speed and direction of a rolling ball sooner than girls tend to. Girls tend to be more wary; boys more fearless. Needless to say, things inevitably even themselves out, and whether nature or nurture results in stereotypical behavior for girls and boys is still the subject of much debate.

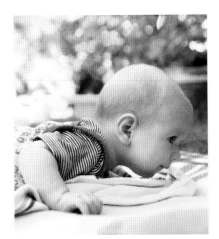

Head control After a couple of months, babies' neck muscles are strong enough to allow them to lift their heads.

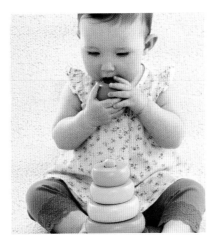

Sitting upright comfortably At around six months old most babies can sit up unaided, and interact with their toys.

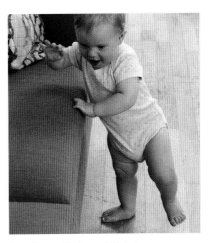

Standing up By the end of their first year, most can stand with a little support.

Baby basics

GETTING TO KNOW THE BASICS OF BABY CARE WILL HELP PREPARE YOU FOR THE FIRST WEEKS. There's an enormous amount to take in immediately after your baby is born, so the more you can learn beforehand about feeding your baby, putting them down to sleep, changing them, and keeping them clean, the more confident and in control you're likely to feel.

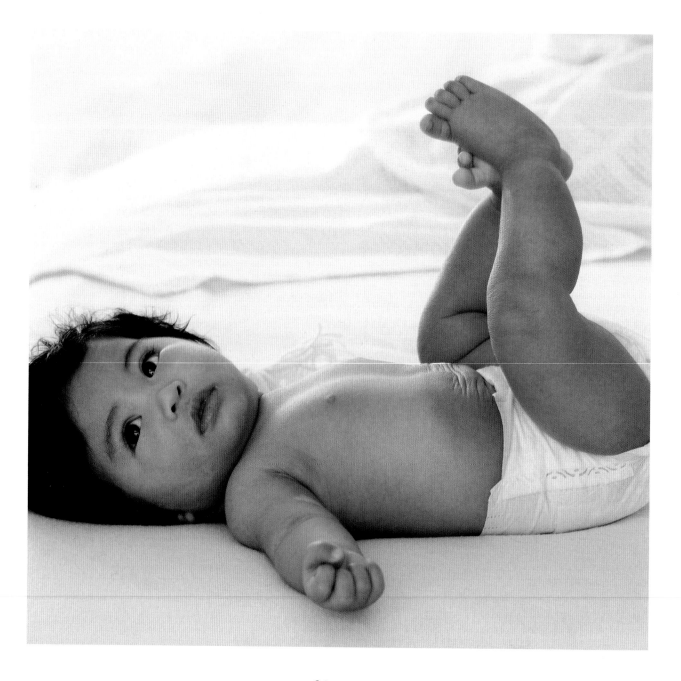

Feeding your baby

For the first year, milk will form your baby's main diet, providing the nutrients needed for optimum growth and development.

Whether you choose to breastfeed or bottle-feed, it's completely normal and understandable to be a little nervous about feeding. Knowing what to expect can make the process easier, more successful, and relaxing.

Why breastfeed?

Breastfeeding is the best way to ensure that your baby gets all the nutrients needed, and there is a host of health benefits (see box, right). The composition of your breast milk will change to meet the needs of your growing baby. It includes healthy fats (including essential fatty acids—EFAs) that are necessary for healthy growth and optimum development (particularly in the brain), and the calcium it contains is better utilized by babies than that in formula.

Breast milk contains hormones and growth factors that encourage healthy weight gain and development. It also reduces your baby's risk of acquiring diabetes and both childhood and adult obesity, as well as protecting against allergies, asthma, and eczema. Most importantly, perhaps, breastfeeding reduces your baby's risk of crib death or sudden infant death syndrome, (SIDS, see p.31), improves bonding, and, according to new research, promotes the development of your baby's facial structure, aiding speech and vision.

In some literature, breastfeeding is considered to be the "fourth trimester" in terms of your baby's brain growth and development. You'll also be passing on your antibodies through your breast milk, which can help keep baby well until their immune system matures.

Research has found that breastfed babies have fewer incidences of vomiting and diarrhea, and are protected against gastroenteritis, as well as ear infections, respiratory illnesses, pneumonia, bronchitis, kidney infections, and septicemia (blood poisoning). There is also a reduced risk of chronic constipation, colic, and other tummy disorders.

Breast milk contains compounds that are known to destroy bacteria such as E. coli and salmonella that would make your baby unwell. There are other health benefits for your baby, including a reduced risk of heart disease, obesity, and iron-deficiency anemia. For more guidance see pp.26–27.

Benefits for you

Not only is breastfeeding good for your baby, but it's also the healthiest choice for you. It reduces your risk of breast and ovarian cancer and of osteoporosis. There's also growing evidence to suggest that parents who breastfeed may be lowering their risk of having a heart attack, heart disease, or stroke. Breastfeeding uses up around 500 calories per day, so it can promote postpartum weight loss, as well as delay the return of menstruation. Last, but not least, breastfeeding is very convenient—there are no bottles to wash or sterilize, nothing to prepare, and no equipment to carry around.

YOUR BABY'S FIRST YEAR

In most cases, your baby will have a milk-only diet until around six months old. Whether you choose bottle- or breast-feeding, baby will need an increasing amount of milk over the coming months, and milk should be the mainstay of their diet throughout the first year (see p.184).

Starting solids normally begins at around six months (see pp.236–237), when your baby will start on very liquid purees—usually baby rice mixed with a little of their usual milk—and pureed fruits and vegetables. Once these foods are accepted, a range of others can be introduced—particularly those that are rich in iron and protein, such as meat, fish, and eggs. The texture of foods should change as quickly as your baby finds acceptable, from purees to mashed to lumpy and then chopped foods. By the end of the year, your baby should be enjoying three meals a day.

Throughout this book, we'll guide you through the stages of starting solids, helping you make the right choices for your baby at the right times. You may decide to choose "baby-led" eating, in which your baby is started on whole foods, rather than purees, at their own pace (see p.217 and pp.236–237).

How breastfeeding works

It's a natural process based on supply and demand—letting your baby nurse will trigger your breasts to make more milk to satisfy.

During pregnancy, your body begins to prepare for breastfeeding. Your areola becomes darker (which some people believe helps your baby to see it and encourages feeding), tiny bumps around your areola grow bigger and more noticeable (known as Montgomery's tubercles, these secrete oil that lubricates your nipples to prevent drying, cracking, and infections while feeding), and your placenta stimulates the release of hormones that make milk production possible.

Women are born with milk ducts (a series of channels that transport milk through the breasts) and during pregnancy, these begin to prepare for feeding. The milk glands expand dramatically so that by the end of pregnancy, each breast may be up to 1 lb 5 oz (600 g) heavier!

The lactation system, inside breasts, is somewhat like a small tree, with milk glands forming clusters like grapes high up in the breast. These make milk. This milk travels down from the glands through the milk ducts, which widen beneath the areola to form milk "sinuses." These empty into about 20 little openings in your nipple, which release milk when they are stimulated by baby's sucking.

This sucking sends a message to the pituitary gland to release oxytocin, a hormone that makes you feel calm and loving, and prompts milk-producing cells to empty their milk into the ducts. This is known as the "let-down" reflex, and it can also be triggered when you hear your baby cry (and sometimes other babies!), or even simply think about your baby.

Once the milk is let down, your baby's gums compress the sinuses where the milk begins to pool. If baby sucks on your nipple rather than the whole areola, only a little milk can be drawn out and you may experience some discomfort. This is why it is essential to get your baby's "latch" correct from the outset (see opposite).

Your baby's sucking also stimulates nerves in the nipple that send messages to the pituitary gland in your brain to secrete the hormone prolactin. This hormone is responsible for ensuring that your milk is continually produced according to your baby's needs. The more milk that is removed from your breasts, the more milk your body makes to replace it, so even expressing milk can help keep up your supply if you are unable to breastfeed immediately.

Colostrum

From about 15–16 weeks of pregnancy, your breasts begin to produce colostrum, which is your baby's first milk. This is a very nutritious, deep-yellow liquid containing high levels of protein, carbohydrates, healthy fat, and antibodies. It is very easy to digest, and just a few teaspoons will provide hugely concentrated nutrition for your baby, and keep them hydrated before your milk "comes in." Colostrum has a laxative effect on your baby, helping them pass early stools (meconium), which is important for the excretion of excess bilirubin,

BREASTFEEDING

• Breastfeeding will be much more successful when you are relaxed, so find a comfortable place to sit down and put your feet up.

• Breastfeeding parents will need (often instant) access to their breasts, so loose-fitting, comfortable clothing that unzips or unbuttons easily is essential. You'll also need a nursing bra that you can open and close with one hand.

• Your baby will feed until they've had enough. If they doze off after a few moments, gently wake them by burping them or stroking their cheek.

• Check that your entire areola is in baby's mouth; baby will stimulate the release—and resupply—of your milk by pressing on the milk sinuses (see right). If they're only hitting a few, you could end up with blocked ducts (see p.59), sore nipples, and a hungry baby!

• Don't worry about whether they are getting enough. Your baby's weight gain will be monitored over the first few weeks of life, and as long as they put on weight, have plenty of wet diapers (see pp.44–45), and seem alert when they are awake, all will be fine.

• Try not to give up! Breastfeeding can take a little while to settle into a comfortable experience, but it does become easier over the first few weeks. Try to remember that you are doing what's best for your baby.

which may otherwise cause jaundice (see p.372).

Consistency of breast milk

When your milk comes in two to three days after your baby's birth (although sometimes a little later, if you've had a cesarean), your breasts will feel engorged and perhaps even a little painful. Each time your baby suckles, they will receive two types of milk. The first milk out of the breast is known as "foremilk," which is thinner in consistency and slightly bluish white in color. This hydrates your baby and satisfies their thirst. Next, they will receive "hindmilk," which is

the thicker, more nutrient-dense, and calorific milk that provides everything your baby needs for growth, development, and energy. It's important to empty your breast completely at each sitting to ensure that your baby gets both types of milk. If baby gets only a little of your hindmilk, they may be hungry soon afterward and need another feeding.

Feeding on demand

Feeding your baby whenever they are hungry will encourage your breasts to produce the milk needed. While it can be tempting to put your baby on a schedule, they may be left

| ASK A BREASTFEEDING EXPERT |

Is it worth breastfeeding for just a few days? Yes! Breast milk is the perfect first food and will give your baby a great start to life. Colostrum, the first milk you produce, is rich in protein and vitamins to support your baby's growth and development, and contains a vital antibody called sIgA. This antibody plays a crucial role in building your baby's immune system, lining their gut and respiratory systems and protecting your baby from illness. Breastfeeding has significant health benefits to you, too, lowering the risk of breast cancer, ovarian cancer, and cardiovascular disease.

LATCH YOUR BABY ON TO YOUR BREAST

Gently stroking your baby's cheek or the corner of their mouth will stimulate the rooting reflex, and they will naturally open their mouth to seek out food. The next step is to ensure baby is correctly latched on to your breast. Getting this right can make breastfeeding more comfortable and efficient.

When your baby opens their mouth wide, bring them to your breast—not the other way around! Their tongue should be

down and forward, and your nipple should be aimed at the roof of their mouth as you draw them on to your breast. When baby is properly latched on, all of the nipple and some of the breast tissue should be in their mouth. Your baby is correctly positioned if their tummy is to yours—tummy-to-tummy. Their lower lip will be rolled out and their chin will be against your breast. Their lower arm may be tucked beneath you, and their upper

arm may reach around to hold your breast. Their nose should be free of your breast so baby can breathe.

If your baby is correctly latched on, you should hear only a low-pitched swallowing noise—not a clicking or smacking noise—and you should see baby's jaw moving, a sign they are feeding successfully. Your breasts may be tender at first; trying a few different positions can improve comfort (see p.58).

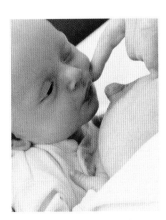

Rooting reflex Help your baby root for your nipple by stroking the cheek closest to it. Baby will purse with their lips, ready to suck.

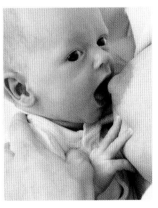

Get it right Make sure your baby's tongue is down and forward, and your nipple is aimed at the roof of their mouth before they latch on.

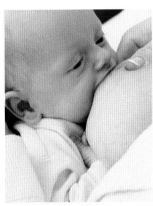

Latch on Make sure your baby takes the nipple and a good proportion of the areola into their mouth for a good latch.

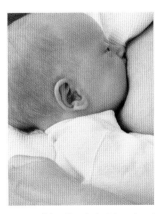

Best position Your baby's head and body must be in a straight line so they can swallow easily, and their chin should touch your breast.

bewildered and hungry, and your breasts will fail to meet demand (see p.58). A good feed normally lasts about 20 to 30 minutes, but a young baby will probably want to nurse every couple of hours, so you might feel as if you're feeding around the clock. If baby is falling asleep on the breast, or losing concentration and looking around, it may be that they aren't very hungry, and you'll be better off trying again later.

Getting support

Breastfeeding is not always easy in the beginning, and you may require the support of your ob/gyn, your baby's pediatrician, or a lactation consultant to help to get established, or go to a mothers' group. You'll need support from your partner, too. You'll be spending very long hours feeding your baby, and until you are able to express a little milk that can be fed to your baby via a bottle (see box, below), your partner won't be very involved. Your partner will need to understand that you are breastfeeding to give your baby the best possible start in life. Studies have shown that family and friends play an important role in the decisions that new moms make about feeding. Parents who are supported feel more confident and tend to breastfeed longer.

EXPRESSING BREAST MILK

Once your milk supply is established—at around a month or six weeks after the birth—you can begin to express a little milk. This will not only buy you some freedom, allowing your partner or someone else to feed baby from time to time, but it will also provide you with a store of frozen milk that can be used if or when you go back to work.

Not everyone finds expressing easy, and you may need to experiment with different pumps (for example, manual, battery-operated, or electric) or do it by hand (see p.83) to produce enough milk. If you're nursing eight times a day, 3 fl oz

(90 ml) is usually adequate for a single feeding, so don't worry if you don't manage to extract much at first. Relaxing somewhere near your baby can make the process more successful, and you may find that if your baby regularly feeds from only one breast in a sitting, you can simultaneously express from the other.

If your baby is born prematurely, they may not be able to feed at the breast initially, in which case you will be helped to express and get your milk supply established, ready for when your baby is physically able to feed themselves.

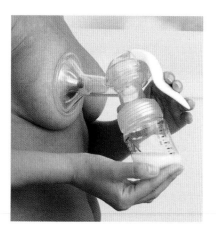 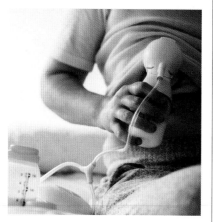

Manual pump Hand or manual pumps are affordable, lightweight, quiet, and easy to use—you simply operate the plunger to express milk (left). **Electric pump** This pump is automatic, so generally quicker and better if you need to express milk quite frequently (right).

ASK A BREASTFEEDING EXPERT

Is there any reason why I won't be able to breastfeed? Most women can breastfeed, and provide sufficient milk to meet their babies' needs. Even women with small breasts or inverted nipples can successfully nurse, so try not to worry. Some women have concerns in advance that it will be too difficult, but with the support of a pediatrician, lactation specialist, and your partner, you may find breastfeeding a truly rewarding experience.

There are some cases when breastfeeding may not be possible. These include taking some types of medication, which would be unsafe for your baby, or suffering from a breast infection or disease, such as cancer. Very, very rarely, some women don't generate enough milk for their babies, although current support makes this less likely. Women who have had a breast reduction may find feeding difficult (although not always impossible); similarly, your baby may be unable to breastfeed because they are premature, too small, have a problem sucking, or have birth defects in their mouth, such as cleft palate, or digestive problems, in which case you may want to express milk (see box, left).

Bottle-feeding

If you can't or do not want to breastfeed, or plan to do so for a short period of time, you'll need to master the art of bottle-feeding.

Parents who cannot, or choose not to breastfeed should not feel guilty. There is a very good range of formulas on the market that will encourage healthy growth and development, and it's perfectly possible to make bottle-feeding sessions warm, nurturing, and positive (see p.59).

Bottle-feeding equipment

You'll need six to eight bottles, nipples, and caps, a bottle-brush for cleaning, a sterilizer (optional), a measuring cup, formula, and bottled water or a pot to boil water, which is then cooled to make up the feed. There are many bottles and nipples available, and you can buy anything from colic bottles and self-sterilizing, to "natural" and slow- or fast-flow nipples. You may need to experiment when your baby is born, to see what works best for them.

Nipples should be slow-flowing for new babies, and gradually become "faster" as they get a little older. Silicone nipples are more durable; however, latex tends to be closer to the sensation of a nipple. Choose from a traditional bell shape, an "orthodontic" nipple that manufacturers claim most resembles a nipple, or a flatter nipple that is particularly easy for young babies to manage.

Choosing formula

Choose a formula that is appropriate for your baby's age. Most formulas contain roughly the same beneficial ingredients, but you may want to look for one that contains probiotics to encourage digestive health, and omega oils, which aid brain development. You can make formula from a powder or a liquid, or buy it ready made. Breast milk contains two types of protein: whey and casein. The balance in breast milk is in favor of whey, with a 60:40 ratio (60 percent whey, and 40 percent casein). It is a good idea, therefore, to look for a formula with this same ratio intact. Formulas that have a greater percentage of casein tend to be harder for your baby to digest. Formula is designed to provide your baby with the right amounts of essential nutrients. It is balanced to ensure that it is easily digestible, and meets your baby's needs for both fluid and food. It is, therefore, extremely important to follow the manufacturer's mixing instructions to the letter.

Your first bottle-feeding

Bring your own choice of ready-made infant formula to the hospital. No one formula is better than another. Pediatricians recommend choosing first instant formula (whey-based). Your nurses or midwife will be able to show you the best positions for bottle-feeding (see p.59). Feed your baby responsively rather than adhering to strict timings. Feed little and often, around ½–1 fl oz (15–30 ml) each feed, and do not force your baby to finish a bottle.

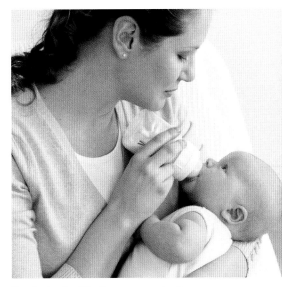

Comforting feed Making eye contact with your baby while you bottle-feed helps promote bonding and makes them feel secure.

ASK AN EXPERT

Do I need to sterilize all my baby's feeding equipment? Washing bottles carefully is important because every trace of milk needs to be removed. While many experts feel it isn't necessary in places with safe drinking water, you may choose to sterilize your baby's feeding equipment as well. There are several methods to choose from: You can use high heat, such as steam, or a chemical cold-water treatment that is designed to kill any germs. There is a wide variety of sterilizers available, including those that work in the microwave. It's also fine to use your dishwasher, as long as your machine reaches a temperature of at least 176°F (80°C) or more, which is necessary to kill any harmful bacteria or viruses. This will help your baby avoid germs that cause illness.

Sleeping arrangements

Your baby will spend a lot of time asleep in the coming months, so you want them to be comfortable and safe while they're sleeping.

There is a wealth of options when it comes to choosing your baby's first bed, and you can spend a lot of money on features that may not be necessary. For example, although a rocking cradle might look like a good way to settle down at night, your baby may get used to being rocked to sleep, and find the transition to a crib or bed more difficult. Whatever your budget, the most important considerations are safety and comfort.

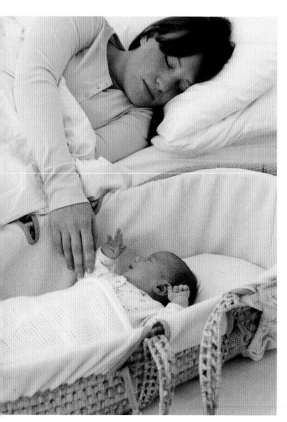

Portable bassinet A lightweight bassinet is ideal as you can move it around and keep your baby close while they sleep.

Little beds

After having been tightly confined in your uterus for months, your baby is likely to settle down better and feel more secure in a snug environment. For this reason, their "first" bed should be small enough to feel cozy and comfortable. Experts now recommend that your baby sleeps in the same room as their caregivers for the first six months of life, so a "portable" bed, such as a bassinet, is a practical choice. (Just be aware that you should avoid putting your baby's bassinet directly on an underheated floor since this puts your baby at risk of overheating.)

Cradles and cribs are less mobile, which can be a disadvantage in the early days, but many parents like something sturdier. This first bed will probably only last a few months, so it isn't usually worthwhile spending a lot! If you buy used, it's recommended that you buy a new mattress, to help lower the risk of Sudden Infant Death Syndrome (SIDS) (see box, right), and be sure that any used crib meets the current standards of the US Consumer Product Safety Commission (cpsc.gov).

If you go for a full-size crib, there are certain features that will help ensure your baby's safety and help you get the most for your money (see p.108). Mattresses can be made of foam, natural, or hollow fibers, and must fit the crib snugly so there are no gaps in which a baby could get trapped. The mattress cover should be easy to clean. You can put a bassinet (without the legs) inside a crib when your baby is small, which helps ease the transition to a big crib later.

ASK A DOCTOR

I'd like my baby to sleep in our bed, but is it safe? There is a great deal of controversy over whether or not it's safe to co-sleep, so really, it's up to you to weigh up the arguments and decide what's best for you and your family. The latest guidance strongly advises that your baby is most safe when they sleep in their own separate sleep space, such as a bassinet. It is now estimated that around 50 percent of sudden infant death syndrome (SIDS) deaths occur while co-sleeping, many of which relate to high-risk circumstances.

A parent who is a deep sleeper, is intoxicated, taking medication that induces deep sleep, or who smokes, should not co-sleep. It is recommended that you do not co-sleep if your baby was born prematurely or very small (weighing less than 5½lb/2.5kg) at birth, or if any other children, siblings, or pets will share the bed, too. It is also not recommended to use a sleeping nest or pod in your adult bed as there is an increased risk of suffocation. To protect your baby, you may wish to invest in a sleeping nest or a low bassinet with a removable side that can be placed beside your bed.

Regardless of whether you intend to co-sleep or not, you may still find yourself falling asleep after a feed or while comforting your baby at night. It is therefore important to ensure your bed and bedding are always as safe as possible and that you consider any risks before every sleep.

SUDDEN INFANT DEATH SYNDROME (SIDS)

Sudden Infant Death Syndrome (SIDS or "crib death") is the unexplained death of a baby. It occurs most often in babies under four months, but can occur up to the age of one. The cause is still largely unknown, but a lot of research has gone into identifying risk factors and the measures that can be taken to prevent it.

Remember that crib death is rare, so don't let yourself worry about it so much that you stop enjoying your baby's first few months of life. However, follow the advice below to reduce the risk as much as possible:

• Use baby sleeping sacks, swaddles, or place baby's feet at the bottom of the crib, then securely tuck a blanket under three sides of the mattress, placing the top edge no higher than the chest.

• Keep your baby in a crib in a room with you for the first six months.

• Keep your baby's head uncovered to prevent the baby from getting too hot.

• Don't smoke in pregnancy and don't let anyone smoke in the same room—or house—as your baby.

• Never fall asleep with your baby on a sofa or armchair.

• Avoid overheating by keeping the room temperature at approximately 64.4°F (18°C).

• Never allow your baby to sleep with a hot-water bottle; electric blanket; next to a vent, heater, or fire; or in direct sunshine.

• Avoid sleeping with your baby if they were premature (born before 37 weeks) or weighed less than 5½ lb (2.5 kg) at birth (see opposite), or if you or your partner are smokers (even if you never smoke in the house), feel very tired, or have recently drunk alcohol or taken medication or drugs that make you sleep heavily. Official guidelines advise that you do not co-sleep with a baby under any circumstances.

• Breastfeeding your baby reduces the risk of crib death.

• A pacifier can cut the risk of SIDS in half.

However don't use one for a breastfed baby under four weeks, and only use it when your baby is going to sleep.

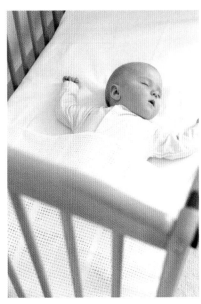

Safe sleeping To reduce the risk of SIDS, your baby should sleep on their back with their feet at the foot of the bed.

Your baby's bedding

You will need two or three mattress protectors, three fitted sheets, a mattress pad, and a waterproof mattress protector, but nothing more. Newborns and infants shouldn't be put into cribs with loose top sheets or blankets, quilts, or comforters, pillows, or even bumper pads, since they all pose a risk of suffocation. If they go over your sleeping baby's nose or mouth, baby won't have the coordination or inclination to push them off. To keep your baby warm, consider purchasing a baby sleeping sack, or wrap them in a tight swaddle. If you insist upon putting your baby under a blanket on cold nights, for their own safety, place your baby's feet at the bottom of the crib, then securely tuck the blanket under the mattress on three sides and place the top of the blanket no higher than their chest.

What temperature?

It is important to keep the temperature of your baby's bedroom on the cool side. Not only will they sleep better, but also they will have far less risk of overheating—something that has been linked to SIDS. A room temperature of 60.8–68°F (16–20°C) is ideal. As a general rule, if the room temperature is 60.8°F (16°C), your baby will need a sheet and three layers of blanket, or a 2.5 tog sleeping sack plus a blanket. The warmer the room is, the fewer layers they'll need.

Early routines

Many babies feel more secure when they sleep in the same place for naps and at night. Creating a familiar environment that baby associates with sleep will help them settle down more easily—and sleep longer. Create a sleep corner in your bedroom, or move their bed around so you can keep an eye on them during the day. Some parents prefer to use a regular "bed" at night, and use a portable crib for their baby's naps. This has the advantage of helping your baby differentiate between shorter daytime sleeps and longer nighttime sleeps.

This also allows for a bit more flexibility, because it means that your baby can enjoy their nap wherever you happen to be.

All about diapers

Your baby will be in diapers for at least a couple of years, so choosing the type of diaper that best suits your lifestyle is important.

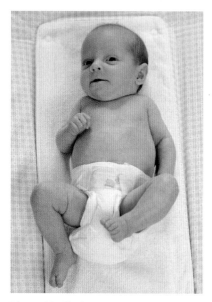

Disposable diapers Disposables are very convenient and absorbent, but can be costly.

CHANGING PLACES

Although you may have created a lovely set-up on the changing table in your baby's bedroom, this may not always be practical. Babies often need fairly "instant" changes, particularly in the middle of a feed, or in the event of a sudden explosion at the bottom end! You may find it useful to keep a diaper bag handy or to set up mini changing stations in rooms where you plan to feed your baby, near their bed, and where you'll spend time playing. Fill a basket with diapers, wipes, barrier cream, diaper sacks, and/or a plastic bag or tub to contain reusables, and a fold up changing mat. Check the stations every evening, so that you can keep them fresh, tidy, and fully stocked!

There are two main types of diapers: disposables and reusables, both of which have their advantages and disadvantages. Many parents choose to use a combination of the two—disposables when they are out and about and on vacation, and sometimes even at night, because they tend to be more absorbent, and reusables the rest of the time. Figure out a system that's best for you. There's not much point in feeling virtuous about doing your part for the environment if your stress load hits the ceiling and you end up using an environmentally unfriendly tumble dryer to try to get through a pile of laundry. If you do choose disposable, biodegradable disposables are an environmentally kind choice to consider.

If your baby is prone to diaper rashes, their skin may respond better to disposables. If your budget is tight and your organizational skills are immaculate, reusables may be right for you. There is no right way. It's a question of balance and practicality.

Disposable diapers

These are undoubtedly more convenient and there appear to be fewer cases of diaper rash, fewer leaks, and fewer changes necessary with disposables. They are, however, much more expensive, produce a high level of waste, and must be disposed of properly. The majority contain human-made chemicals, too.

Your baby will go through approximately 5,000 disposable diapers from birth to potty training,

and this can have a pretty dramatic effect on the environment. Go for disposables that do not contain any bleaching agents, which are a major source of pollution during manufacture and decomposition.

Diapers that are better for your baby's bottom and the environment are those that don't contain gels, perfumes, dyes, and/or latex. Those that are at least 50 percent biodegradable can help reduce the growing problem with landfills, and diapers that use sustainable materials, that are chlorine-free, and that use less plastic packaging will also make an impact.

If you go with disposables, keep in mind that you'll need an average of 8–12 diapers per day, so make sure you stock up! Ask your doctor to assess the probable size and weight of your baby, so that you don't end up buying a lot of diapers that will instantly be too small. It's best to buy one or two packages of newborn disposables, and then see if baby is ready to move up. "Bikini diapers," which fold down, will help keep the umbilical cord free from irritation. Most parents purchase diaper sacks (biodegradable), to efficiently dispose of diapers at home and out of the house. (See also "How to change a disposable diaper, p.44).

Reusable diapers

Reusables produce less waste and use fewer raw materials in their manufacture. Your baby will also be wearing soft, natural fibers next to the skin. However, washing reusables can waste a lot of water, and requires cleansing agents. It can also be very time consuming, unless you can afford a laundry service. Your baby will also need to be changed more often, since reusables tend to be less absorbent.

There are two main types of reusables. Two-part diapers consist of a diaper and a wrap. Diapers can be traditional terrycloth, which will require pins or clips, a folded diaper (known as a pre-fold, and which also requires a fastener), or a shaped diaper. On top, you will place a wrap designed to keep the moisture in and prevent leaking. Wraps can take the form of a pull-up pant, or wrap around with fastenings (often Velcro).

All-in-one diapers combine the inner diaper and the "wrap" in a single waterproof garment. These diapers look a little more like disposables, and are normally self-fastening. Some moms find them harder to wash and thoroughly dry; they also tend to leak. You'll also need disposable diaper liners, which provide a barrier between the fabric and your baby's skin, and make it easier to lift out and dispose of poop. Booster pads can be useful at night to provide greater absorbency. If you choose pre-folds or terrycloth, you'll need diaper pins or clips. Plastic diaper clips are a great alternative to pins, not only because they are easier to fasten, but because they'll prevent accidental

pricking. Finally, you'll need a large bucket with a lid to store dirty diapers, and a plastic carrier to transport dirty diapers when you are out and about.

Reusables also come in "sizes" according to the weight of your baby, and you'll need to purchase about 20 diapers and three or four wraps to begin with. Don't buy too many; your baby will grow and move on to the next size more quickly than you expect. Equally, however, you don't want to be left with only one clean diaper and a pile of unwashed, dirty diapers! Although they can require a hefty investment every few months, reusables should prove to be cheaper in the long run.

CHANGE A REUSABLE DIAPER

Gone are the days when we had to rely on terrycloth or cotton diaper squares that had to be folded and pinned—no easy task with a small, fractious baby to change. Today's reusables come in a variety of styles and colors, and often use easy-to-manage clips or Velcro tabs to make fastening them quick and efficient. Set up a clean, dry area in a warm room

to change your baby—on a changing table is ideal—and gather all the supplies you need: a clean diaper; cotton pads, and water or baby wipes; a diaper bucket or bag to store the dirty diaper; and some emollient cream if your baby is prone to diaper rash.

If you are using "flushable liners," be aware that many sewage systems cannot

handle them, and they will need to be disposed of with the regular trash; if you are using reusable liners, you will need to shake or rinse off any excess feces before putting the liner in the diaper bucket to be washed.

When you put the clean diaper on, make sure that it fits snugly, but it should not be too tight or it might pinch the skin.

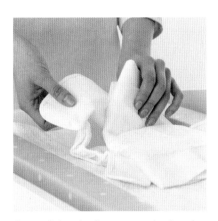

Get ready Lay the diaper out on the changing mat, place the lining on top, then move it to one side while removing the dirty diaper.

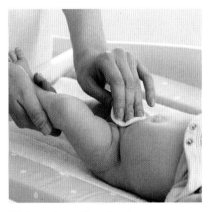

Wash your baby Clean the diaper area thoroughly with cotton pads and water or a baby wipe.

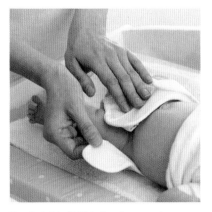

Comfortable fit Slide the diaper under the baby's bottom, fold the outer edge over, and fasten the tabs or snaps.

Essential equipment

Although a visit to the store may suggest otherwise, you don't need a huge pile of new gadgets and equipment—just some key items.

Feeding equipment

Breastfeeding doesn't require any special equipment to start off with. However, there are a few items that make nursing easier and more comfortable and are necessary for expressing milk (see p.28). Bottle-feeding does require a few essentials to keep your baby safe and healthy.

Breastfeeding
- 3–4 good-quality nursing bras that you can open with one hand.
- Breast pads for leaks.
- Breast shells to catch those leaks.
- Nipple cream for sore or chapped nipples; choose a lanolin-based one that can stay on your breast while your baby is feeding.
- A pump, if you want to express, and 2–3 feeding bottles (with caps and nipples) to store your expressed milk. Some people use special freezer bags designed for breast milk.

- A U-shaped feeding pillow to stay comfortable during long feedings.

Bottle-feeding
- 6–8 bottles; smaller bottles are more appropriate for newborns and babies who do not consume much milk at one sitting. You'll need caps and nipples, too.
- Cleaning equipment and a bottle brush.
- A teapot—you might want a quick and regular source of fresh, boiled water for making up bottles.
- A designated measuring cup, spoon, and knife.

In the bedroom
- A bassinet, crib, or cradle, which will keep your baby secure in the early days. They are soon outgrown, so if your budget is tight, go for a full-size crib, which should comfortably fit your child during the first 18 to 24 months of their life.

- A full-size crib that meets the new standard from the US Consumer Products Safety Commission.
- Bedding (see p.31).
- A changing table. Any hard surface at hip height will work, including the top of a sturdy chest of drawers. If you are purchasing a new chest of drawers, look for one with a lip to prevent your baby from rolling off.
- A changing mat—go for one that is easily washed and comfortable; you may want a few fold-up spares for your mini changing stations.
- A baby monitor; a two-way monitor is ideal, so you can hear your baby and baby can hear you!
- Diapers and the other elements of a changing station (see p.32).
- A bouncy chair that can be moved—remember baby shouldn't sleep in it.
- A nightlight, to help with those late-night feedings, or a light that will keep the room dim enough to see

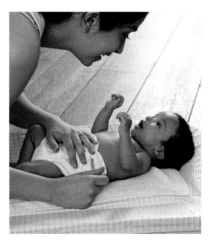

Changing mat Keep a couple of mats in strategic locations around the home, and at least one foldable mat to fit in your diaper bag.

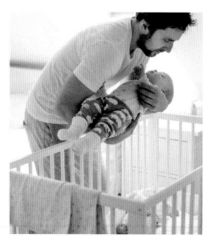

Crib Your baby's crib is an important purchase, so do your research beforehand to help you make the right choice.

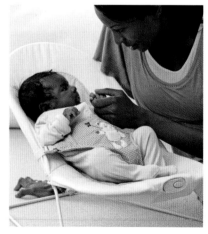

Bouncy chair This compact, portable seat is a comfortable and safe place for your baby to enjoy calm time or practice moving their legs.

your baby, but discourages them from fully waking.

- Large chest of drawers or baskets for storage.
- A diaper bucket for reusables, or a container for disposables.
- If you are planning to co-sleep, you may want to invest in a baby nest or bed divider (see p.30).

Out and about

- A rear-facing car seat is required for all infants, with an easy-to-manage five-point harness. Second-hand car seats are not recommended for safety reasons. Your car seat may come as part of a travel system, which can include various fittings, including a stroller and portable crib that fit onto one base.
- A front carrier for transporting your baby or keeping them calm when you need your hands free. Choose one with wide shoulder straps to protect your back. Be careful with babies under four months old in front carriers; these can be a suffocation hazard for infants with weak neck muscles.
- A carriage or stroller. Newborn babies need to lie flat, and a traditional carriage with a flat base provides a perfect secure environment. Most strollers can be adjusted to lie flat, so are suitable from birth, and the seat can be raised so your baby can sit up when older. There are many different types, but make sure the one you choose has a five-point harness and a double-locking folding mechanism; is easy to fold and erect; comfortable for your height; and suits your lifestyle. If you do more shopping than jogging, storage space may be more useful than a reinforced suspension. Your baby's first stroller should be rear-facing—that is, facing you.
- A diaper bag. Ideal for transporting all your baby's paraphernalia; some come with detachable changing mats. Plenty of pockets means you can

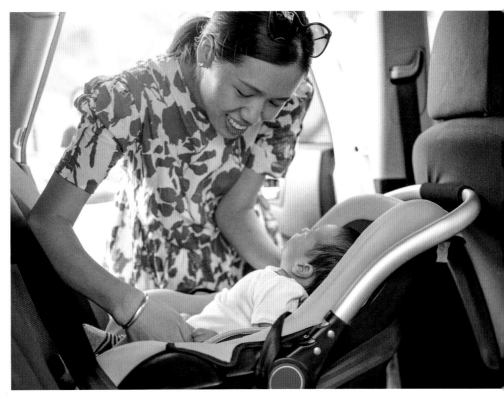

On the move To keep your baby safe while they're traveling in the car, it's important that you find the right car seat for them—one based on their height and weight.

keep bottles, diapers, and clean clothes separate.

Staying clean

- Wipes—choose water-based wipes with no fragrance or other chemicals; biodegradable are best.
- Small, thin washcloths for reaching those tiny folds and crevices, or cotton pads (cotton balls sometimes leave skin-irritating fluff behind).
- An all-in-one bath and shampoo product designed for babies. You'll only need a little, so investing in a good, natural product is probably worthwhile.
- Burp cloths, which can be used to mop up spit-up, leaks, and drool, and protect your clothes when burping and feeding.
- Washable bibs that will slip over or fasten behind your baby's neck easily.

These are helpful to protect baby's clothing during feedings.

- A baby bath—although this is not essential. It's perfectly acceptable to wash your baby in a full-size bath or even the kitchen sink. Invest in a nonslip mat if you use the tub, and line the sink with an old sheet or dish towel to keep baby comfortable. If you purchase a baby bath, make sure it is sturdy and you can easily fill and drain it.
- A thermometer, if you aren't confident about assessing the temperature of your baby's bath water.
- 2–4 towels—preferably hooded, which will keep your baby's head warm and dry while you use the body of the towel to dry them off. You'll probably use two when you bathe (see p.57), and the others may well be in the wash!
- A bowl for sponge baths (see p.45).

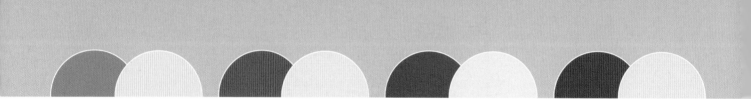

YOUR BABY
0-3 MONTHS

YOUR BABY
4-6 MONTHS

YOUR BABY
7-9 MONTHS

YOUR BABY
10-12 MONTHS

YOUR BABY
MONTH BY MONTH

Your baby's first year whizzes by so fast, yet every single day is a new adventure for you and your child, punctuated by triumphs and tears, amazing developments, and the occasional setback. There's also so much to learn, so this chapter acts as your companion, day by precious day, pointing out the highlights and pitfalls you are likely to encounter along the way. From feeding and sleeping to crawling and communicating (and staying sane as a parent, too), it's a unique and illuminating insight into an unforgettable 12 months.

Your baby from
birth to 3 months

BIRTH

0

MONTH

1

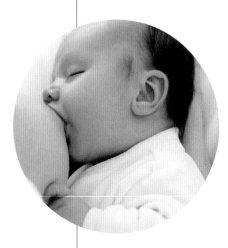

Your baby is fully dependent, but their **senses function well**— they'll know the smell and voices of their parents.

MONTH 1: ESTABLISH A SLEEPING ROUTINE

Initially, your baby will sleep up to 18 hours a day, decreasing to about 15 hours by three months. However, it's unlikely that they'll sleep through the night.

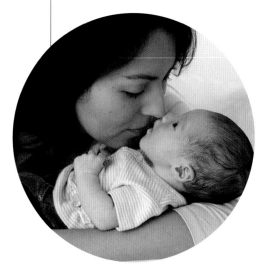

NEWBORN: WITHIN DAYS YOUR BABY WILL RECOGNIZE YOU

Your baby's early vision is fuzzy, but they can focus on your face if it's within a 12 in (30 cm) range. From one week old, your baby will recognize your face. By six weeks, they can see up to 24 in (60 cm) away.

Physical contact Being held and touched makes your baby feel secure.

> " From a helpless newborn to a smiling baby with a mind of their own, your baby's development is astonishing. "

MONTH

2

MONTH

3

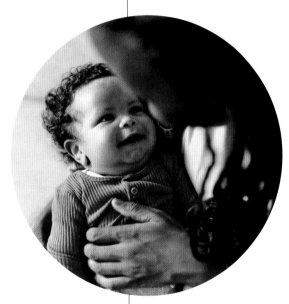

Self-expression
Your baby can now make use of a range of facial expressions to tell you how they feel, or what they need.

MONTH 2: PLACE YOUR BABY UNDER A BABY GYM

By now, your baby may have discovered their hands, but they won't yet recognize them as their own. Your baby will start to swipe at objects within their reach, and try to bat them away.

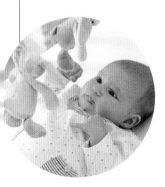

Your baby will **reach out** to swipe at objects within their reach.

MONTH 3: KEEP TRACK OF YOUR BABY'S WEIGHT

Your baby's weight gain is probably fairly steady now, but it's still reassuring to get them weighed at the baby clinic every so often. Although every baby is different, most gain an average of approximately 4–7fl oz (120–200 g) each week until they are about six months old.

The first seven days

SOME BABIES ARE BORN WITH A FULL HEAD OF HAIR WHILE OTHERS ARE NEARLY BALD. Skin-to-skin contact with your baby immediately after birth as well as in the weeks and months to come helps you form a close bond. Such contact also stabilizes your baby's heart and breathing rates and helps baby maintain a normal body temperature.

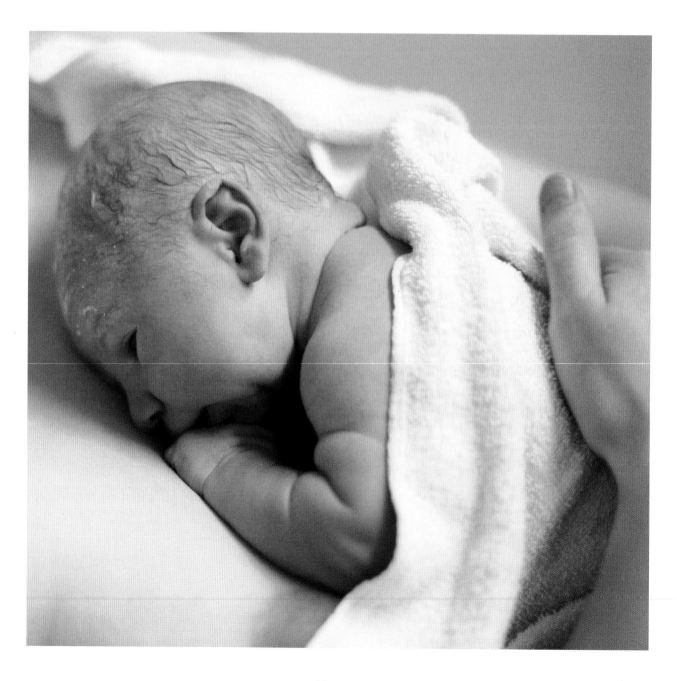

After your baby's birth

While you gaze in wonder at your new baby, your doctor or midwife will check that all is well. Then you'll be able to say hello properly.

After nine long months of pregnancy, today you can finally hold your baby in your arms for the first time. You may experience an overwhelming rush of emotions, ranging from tearfulness, pride, and intense love, to exhaustion and elation. You may also feel somewhat daunted by the prospect of caring for such a tiny, fragile human being, and nervous about their health and well-being. Labor takes an enormous physical and emotional toll, and you will need time to rest and recover after the birth.

Your baby's appearance

Don't be surprised if your newborn looks nothing like you had imagined. They may be covered in a white, waxy substance known as vernix, which has protected their skin in the amniotic fluid, and they may be streaked with blood from the birth canal. If baby had a bowel movement during labor,

their skin, hair, and nails may be stained with a blackish, tar-like substance called meconium that forms the first bowel movements. If your baby is premature, they may also have a covering of fine hair, known as lanugo.

Your baby's genitals may be enlarged and their head may look squashed or elongated, because babies' skulls change shape to negotiate the birth canal. Their nose may be flattened and their eyes might be puffy or even sealed shut. If you do glimpse baby's eyes, they'll probably be blue or gray. All babies have blue eyes in the uterus, which are lighter or darker depending on their ethnic origin. The irises develop their final color between six months and three years after birth.

Many newborns have birthmarks, such as stork marks on the eyelids or nape of the neck that fade over time.

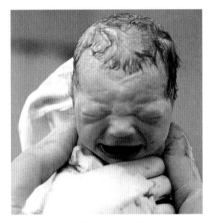

First impressions Newborn babies often look somewhat squashed and wrinkly, but within a day or two their appearance smooths out.

BREASTFEED AFTER BIRTH

Even if you don't plan to breastfeed after this, offering your baby their first feeding within an hour of birth ensures that baby receives colostrum, your early milk, which contains high levels of nutrients, antibodies, and other health benefits (see pp.26–27). It also reduces your risk of heavy bleeding after birth and stimulates mild contractions that help your uterus shrink back to normal size.

Your nurse will help you into position and your baby may root around to find your breast and begin nursing. Encourage baby by lying them next to you under your arm to nurse easily. Their mouth should open wide and take in the whole areola. This is known as latching on (see p.27).

THE APGAR TEST

At 1 and 5 minutes after your baby is born, a medical professional will assess your baby's appearance (skin color), pulse (heart rate), grimace response (reflexes), activity (muscle tone), and respiration (breathing and effort), then will provide a score between zero and two for each criterion. These scores are all added together to calculate your baby's APGAR

score. Most babies are born with an APGAR score of around 7, with very few babies receiving a 10. The main purpose of the APGAR score is to act as a useful tool for medical professionals to check to see if your baby requires any additional medical care or special attention.

You and your new arrival

As your baby begins to acclimate to their new environment,
your doctor will check to see that you are recovering well.

After the exertion of giving birth, you'll probably feel sticky, sweaty, and in need of a shower. You may also want to use the bathroom. The first time you urinate it can sting, especially if you've had stitches, so it can help to take a cup with you, fill it with warm water, and pour it over the area as you urinate.

Your body after the birth

It's a good idea to replenish your depleted energy reserves—a cool drink and a snack should taste delicious right now.

The doctor or labor nurse will

AFTER A CESAREAN

A cesarean section is major surgery, so you need to give your body time to recover. It is normal to feel shaky, tired, tearful, drowsy, and nauseous after the surgery, and you will be given medication to help you deal with any pain. If your cesarean was unplanned, you may feel the need to talk through why it was necessary with your doctor. Your body will be somewhat compromised by the incision, so your nurse and/or doctor will advise you on how to breastfeed comfortably, use the bathroom, roll out of bed, and lift your baby without causing damage to the incision. Medical staff will encourage you to become mobile, which will prevent clots from forming in your legs. But try to rest as much as you can.

check your pulse and blood pressure to ensure they are returning to normal. Your uterus will be gently palpated to observe if it is well-contracted, vaginal blood loss will be checked to ensure it is not excessive, and your perineum will be examined to assess whether or not any cuts or tears need stitching. Your temperature will also be taken. It is normal to experience a slightly raised temperature after the birth, but if it remains high, or begins to rise, this can be a sign of infection. Your urine may be tested to make sure your kidneys are working normally and you'll be asked to confirm that you've urinated. It's normal to experience continued vaginal blood loss, known as lochia, after birth. The bleeding is usually heavier than during a normal period and small blood clots are common for the first few days. You'll need maternity pads to deal with the flow—you should not use tampons because they could cause infection.

Your baby after the birth

During the first 72 hours, in addition to the APGAR score (see p.41), a pediatrician, midwife, or neonatal nurse will check that your baby is well and will check your baby for signs of jaundice, infection of the umbilical cord or eyes, and thrush in the baby's mouth. Your baby may become increasingly alert during the hours following the birth, opening their eyes frequently and gazing at

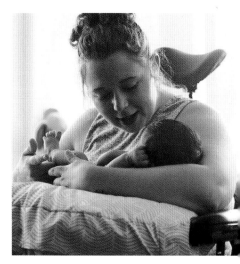

The first hours Now you can spend time getting to know your brand-new baby, bonding and admiring every precious little feature as you hold baby in your arms.

your face. You may notice your baby has some mild spots or a rash. After months curled up in the confines of your womb, your baby's arms and legs will be bent but will straighten out over the coming weeks. Your baby will probably respond to the sound of your voice and exhibit some reflexes (see p.47). They may cry, sleep, or look around at their new environment, although they won't see much beyond about 12 in (30 cm).

The golden hour

The hour immediately after your baby's birth is known as the golden hour because it is an important time for the attachment process between mother and baby. New moms experience changes in brain chemistry immediately after birth that increase their desire for nurturing. Holding your baby naked, skin-to-skin, at this stage has been shown to promote bonding, calm your baby, increase baby's resistance to infection, and get breastfeeding off to a good start.

Try not to worry if you miss out on this first hour of bonding, perhaps because your baby requires medical attention right after birth. Obviously, it's much more important that they receive the care they need first. You can make up for any lost time later by giving them "Kangaroo care" (see p.54).

On the maternity ward

How long you stay in the hospital after giving birth depends on a few things. If you had an uncomplicated vaginal delivery, and your newborn is healthy and breastfeeding or bottle-feeding, you may well be discharged and be able to go home the following day. Before you are discharged, your medical team will do a postpartum check to monitor your vital signs such as pulse, temperature, and blood pressure, as well as check that your uterus is starting to contract to normal size and position and that you can urinate with no problem.

However, if you have had a long or difficult birth, undergone a cesarean, or have concerns about your baby's health, you may have a slightly longer stay in the hospital. If you have had a cesarean, providing you are well enough, are able to walk to the bathroom, urinate without the need for a catheter, and can eat and drink without vomiting, you may be able to leave the hospital between 36 and 48 hours after the birth.

If you do need to stay in the hospital, use the opportunity to rest and ask for help with feeding, or any aspect of caring for your baby, from the experienced staff on hand. Having answers to your questions may help to build your confidence in caring for your baby once you are back home.

NEWBORN CHECKUPS

An examination will be done by a hospital pediatrician before you return home, or within 72 hours by your own pediatrician or midwife if you have had a home birth. Your baby will be weighed and measured from the top of their head to their heel and around the head. The measurements are plotted on a chart to show your baby's size in relation to that of other babies. Their stomach will be palpated to check the organs. The opening of their anus will be examined and, if your baby is a boy, the doctor will look at his penis and check that his testicles have descended into the scrotum. Your baby's eyes will also be checked for cataracts and they will be given a hearing screening test. If this doesn't take place in the hospital, it will be arranged by your own pediatrician.

Once your baby has passed all the checkups on their scheduled discharge day, (most babies do without any problems), they will be allowed to go home. Assuming all is well, their next checkup will take place later in the week (see pp.92–93).

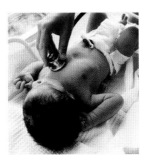

Heart and lungs The doctor uses a stethoscope to listen to your baby's heartbeat and to check that the lungs sound healthy and free of fluid.

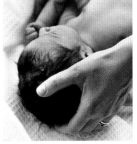

Head shape The head is carefully examined and the fontanels (soft areas between the skull bones) are checked for irregularities.

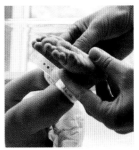

Feet and hands The palms and soles of the feet are checked, all the toes and fingers are counted, and reflexes are tested.

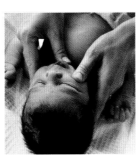

Mouth and palate The mouth is examined to check that the roof (palate) is normal, and that the tongue can move freely.

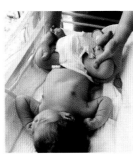

Hips The legs are opened wide and bent upward to check the stability of joints and look for "clicky" hips or other signs of dislocation.

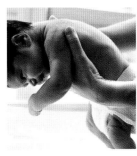

Spine Your baby will be held up so that the spine can be examined to check that it is straight and there is no sign of abnormality.

Early care

Your initial efforts to feed, change, and calm your baby may feel a bit clumsy, but don't worry—you'll soon be up to speed.

Learning to feed your baby

If you are breastfeeding, try not to worry if your first sessions haven't gone perfectly well. Over the next day or two, your baby's attempts to nurse may be a little erratic, especially in the first 24 hours after birth, when they're resting. Just let baby nurse when they want to, and don't expect any kind of pattern to emerge. For the next two to three days, your breasts will be producing mainly colostrum. This is a highly concentrated deep yellow liquid that is rich in antibodies, immunity boosters, and proteins that help nurture and protect your baby from illness. Your breasts probably won't feel very different at this stage because the amount of colostrum your baby needs is very small—they can't fit more than a few teaspoonfuls at a time into their tiny tummy.

Your baby doesn't need a lot of milk now, but let them nurse whenever they need to; this will stimulate the production of mature milk over the next day or so, and help prevent your breasts from feeling overly full and engorged when the milk does come in.

Keep going with skin-to-skin contact and encouraging your baby to latch-on well—this will make breastfeeding more comfortable for both of you.

If you are bottle-feeding, your baby will also want the bottle little and often, so offer a bottle every two to three hours. Let baby feed for as long as they want to—if baby's had enough of the bottle, don't push them to drink more.

HOW TO CHANGE A DISPOSABLE DIAPER

It's important to change your baby's diaper regularly because urine, combined with the bacteria in feces, can make their bottom very sore. Diaper changing takes a bit of practice if you've never done it before, but you'll soon be up to speed on the best ways to keep diapers straight and secure (especially after a few leaks).Gather all the equipment you need beforehand to make the change as quick and easy as possible. If your baby doesn't particularly like being changed, and objects to a cold plastic changing mat, try placing a towel over it to make them feel a bit more comfortable.

When cleaning your baby's bottom, remember to wipe from front to back if your baby is a girl, away from the vagina. This minimizes the risk of infection. If you're changing a boy, keep his penis covered with a clean cloth or diaper so you don't get caught by an unexpected sprinkle!

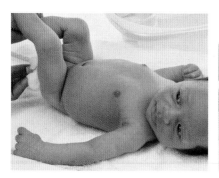

Clean the bottom Holding your baby's ankles, lift their bottom, and gently clean with a damp cotton pad.

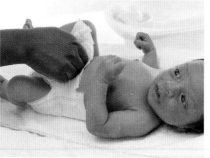

Position the diaper Slide the opened-out diaper under the bottom so the back of the diaper (with the tabs) lines up with the waist.

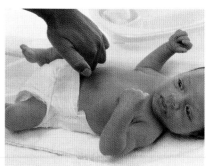

Secure tabs Fasten the tabs over the front flap. Fold the flap down ensuring the cord stump is not restricted, then check the fit.

Your baby's diapers

Your newborn can have as many as 8 to 10 bowel movements in every 24 hours, so you will need to change their diaper frequently to keep them comfortable and prevent diaper rash. A bowel movement often happens right after feeding, but if it doesn't, don't worry: as long as baby has at least one movement per day, they're probably fine. For the first couple days after birth, baby will pass meconium, a black, tarry substance that filled the bowels when baby was in the uterus. You can't see if your baby's diaper is wet, but you can tell by its weight. If the diaper is heavier than a clean one when you change it, this indicates that baby is well-hydrated.

Staying clean

You don't even need to think about bathing your baby yet. Some experts recommend not giving baby a full bath until the umbilical stump has completely fallen off, and that could take several weeks. For the time being, it's much easier to give a sponge bath (see box, right). Check that the warm water in the bowl you're using doesn't become cold before you're done, or your baby won't be happy.

Skin-to-skin contact

If you haven't had the opportunity for much skin-to-skin contact so far, you can indulge yourself and your baby now that you've had a little more chance to recover after the birth. This can help to improve the way baby latches on during breastfeeding which in turn boosts your milk supply.

The optimum time for this type of contact is when baby is feeding. If you are breastfeeding, open your baby's sleep suit or lift up their undershirt, and let their tummy press against yours. If it's not too cold, your baby can wear just a diaper. Drape a light blanket or sheet over them to protect

HOW TO GIVE A SPONGE BATH

Sponge bathing is a good alternative to a full bath for a young baby and to keep an older baby clean between baths. It simply involves gently wiping them from head to toe, paying attention to all those little dimply folds and creases in-between. It's important to do this every day because if dirt, fluff, or milk is allowed to accumulate, it can make your baby's sensitive skin feel irritated and sore. It also prevents skin infections.

Gather all you need before you start: a bowl of lukewarm water; a washcloth or cotton pads; a towel; clean diaper; diaper cream, if needed; and fresh clothes, if necessary. Keeping your baby's undershirt on to start, gently clean their face, under the chin, neck, hands and feet, and diaper area. Finally, remove the undershirt and clean baby's tummy, paying attention to the cord stump (see p.51) and under the arms, where dirt is often trapped.

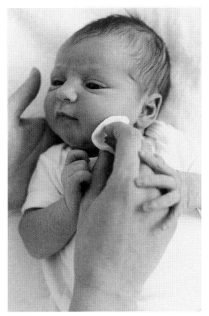
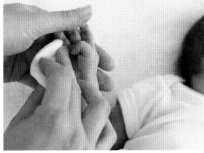
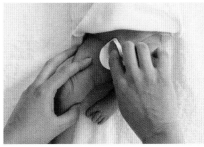

Face and neck Clean your baby's face and neck; use a fresh pad for each eye, and then wipe over and behind (but not inside) each ear (left). **Hands and feet** Wipe baby's hands and feet, being careful to clean between all the fingers and toes (top right). **Diaper area** Clean your baby's bottom and thigh creases, changing cotton pads frequently (bottom right).

them from drafts. Many women who experience difficulties with breast-feeding in the early days notice that they have more success when there is skin-to-skin contact with their baby.

If you are bottle-feeding, lift up or open your own top to allow skin-to-skin contact. It will promote bonding and help your baby feel secure.

Partners can also remove their

shirts and go skin-to-skin to establish their own warm relationship.

When your baby is a little older, you or your partner may want to bathe with them to achieve skin-to-skin contact, which is particularly helpful if baby is frightened by the bath. When baby is difficult to calm, holding their skin close to yours may be all they need to settle down.

Finding your way

Taking care of your new baby may be confusing at first and you may not know what is needed from you—try to relax and go with the flow.

As you settle your baby to their new environment. You'll probably be most comfortable keeping them next to you most of the time and, in fact, experts recommend that baby sleeps in your room for the first 6 months. Although it's tempting to hold baby constantly, it's important to set them down so you can get some rest, too. Even the easiest labor is physically and emotionally exhausting, and it will take some time

for you to feel like yourself again. Your baby will let you know when you're needed, and you'll soon be able to discern between cries. In the early days, baby will sleep a great deal, and wake when hungry—or when they want the comfort of being held.

Going home

If you are in the hospital, you will be discharged when the doctors are

confident that both you and your baby are well, and that you are comfortable with the care you need to give. When you are discharged from the hospital, you'll need to settle your baby in the car seat for the trip home. If you're being driven, you may find it easier to sit in the back seat with them.

A doctor will examine you before you're discharged, and then you won't be seen again for 6 weeks. Your baby, however, will be seen later in the week by their pediatrician (see pp.50–51). They were probably examined by a staff pediatrician at the hospital, so this may be their first meeting.

Feeding

You will continue to produce colostrum, which is your baby's ideal first food. Exactly how much milk your baby needs varies, but on average, a two-day-old baby will probably take just under 3 teaspoons (14 ml) at each feeding. You can expect feeding to take 40 minutes or longer at the moment. If your nipples are starting to feel sore, or breast-feeding is at all painful, it's likely that your baby isn't latching on correctly. Try to ensure that you get all your areola into their mouth, and adjust position so their tummy is against yours (see p.27). If you do experience discomfort, ask for help from your pediatrician, or a lactation (breast-feeding) consultant. Nipple cream can help ease discomfort: find a brand that can be left on while nursing. Pat

HOW TO HOLD YOUR NEWBORN

You may feel a little daunted at the prospect of holding your tiny baby, but it will soon become instinctive. Your baby is not as fragile as you think, but it is important to handle baby gently in order to keep them feeling snug, secure, and safe. Hold them firmly in case baby throws their body backward. Babies are born

with a "startle" reflex (see box, opposite), and will thrust their arms outward if you do not support their neck and head.

A newborn's neck muscles are fairly weak, and dangling limbs will make them uncomfortable, so hold their entire body by cradling them close to you.

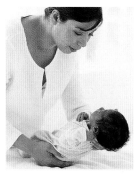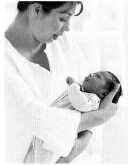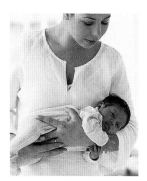

Pick baby up Slide one hand under your baby's neck to support the head, place the other hand beneath the bottom, and lift gently (left). **Support the head** Rest your baby's head in the palm of your hand, keeping it raised slightly higher than the body (middle). **Face-down hold** Support your baby on one arm with their head near the crook of your elbow and slide your other arm between their legs so that both hands are supporting baby's stomach (right).

Your baby is born with more than 70 reflexes, which are nature's way of protecting from harm and promoting survival. Most of these disappear in six months. The main reflexes are:
• **Moro or startle reflex** If the neck or head are unsupported, your baby will thrust out their arms.
• **Grasp reflex** This reflex is also known as the Palmar grasp. If you place your finger in the palm of your baby's hand, their fingers will instinctively curl around it and grip onto it tightly.
• **Sucking reflex** Your baby sucks when something is placed in their mouth; this ensures baby will get nourishment.
• **Rooting reflex** If you stroke your baby's cheek, it will make them turn toward you, looking for food.
• **Stepping reflex** If you hold your baby upright on a flat, hard surface, they will "walk" by placing one foot in front of the other as you support their weight.

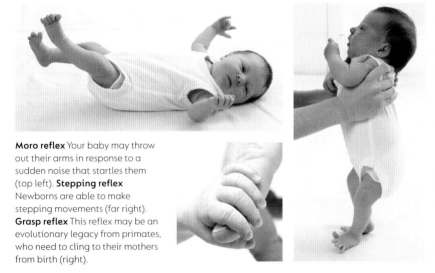

Moro reflex Your baby may throw out their arms in response to a sudden noise that startles them (top left). **Stepping reflex** Newborns are able to make stepping movements (far right). **Grasp reflex** This reflex may be an evolutionary legacy from primates, who need to cling to their mothers from birth (right).

your nipples dry before rubbing a pea-size amount on to each nipple.

If you are bottle-feeding, your baby may take a few more teaspoons (30 ml) at each feeding. Bottle-feeding tends to be quicker, but not always. Your formula-fed baby will probably feed for between 20 and 40 minutes.

Weight loss

It is normal for newborn babies to lose weight during the first week after birth. Breastfed babies tend to lose 7–10 percent of their birth weight; bottle-fed babies lose an average of 5 percent.

Most regain this weight by 10–14 days old. If your baby is feeding well, is urinating, having bowel movements, and appears healthy, there shouldn't be anything to worry about.

Diaper contents

Baby will continue to pass meconium, which can be very sticky and difficult to clean! Warm water and a drop of baby bath can help clean up the worst of it, but try to use only water on baby's genitals. Urine should be pale or straw colored; if it becomes dark or smelly, talk to your pediatrician.

My baby sounds very snuffly when they sleep, and is constantly snorting and hiccuping. Is this normal? Babies can be very noisy sleepers, and you can expect to hear grunts, groans, little mewling sounds, short cries, and even snorts and hiccups. Your baby may also appear to stop breathing for up to 15 seconds, which is known as "periodic breathing" and can occur until your baby is 6 months old. There may be a buildup of mucus in the respiratory system, including the nose, after the birth, which may cause baby to snuffle, cough, and snort to clear it. This normally passes by the time baby is 4 to 6 weeks old. If the nose seems blocked and baby is struggling to feed, talk to your pediatrician; your baby may have a cold or other infection, and may need saline nose drops to help clear their nose (see p.376).

How should I care for my baby's genitals? Your baby's genitals may appear swollen for a couple of weeks after the birth, which is caused by pregnancy hormones in their system. The genitals are very delicate and will need to be carefully cleaned with warm water for a few weeks after the birth; after this, you can use a little of your baby's pH-neutral baby bath to keep the area scrupulously clean. Always clean from front to back in baby girls; lift a baby boy's penis and scrotum to clean around them, and be careful not to pull back the foreskin. If your baby has been circumcised, your pediatrician will advise you on the best way to keep the area clean. It's normal for there to be a little discharge in the early days, but if it is smelly or yellow, you should report it to your pediatrician.

Adjusting to your new role

You've now been a parent for 72—mostly waking—hours. It's hard to manage when you're tired, so try to rest whenever you can.

Although your baby may seem impossibly tiny and fragile, they are growing stronger every day and will be alert for longer periods of time. Their needs are straightforward at this stage, and regular feeding, changing, and time in your reassuring presence will help them feel secure and content.

New babies often cry a lot in the early days, partly in response to the shock of a whole new environment, and also because it is the only way they know how to communicate. This can be very upsetting for new parents, especially when you can't pinpoint what might be wrong. The best thing to do is to work your way through the list of reasons baby might be crying and try to address them (see pp.68–69). Keep in mind that this is probably a phase and as you get to know your baby better you will be able to understand their cries and anticipate their needs much more easily.

It isn't possible to "spoil" a newborn baby, and every time you respond to your baby's cries, you will develop a strong bond with them, encourage trust, and teach them that this new world is a safe place to be. Some babies undoubtedly cry more than others as they let you know that something isn't quite right. If baby doesn't respond to being held, burped, fed, or changed, you can try to reduce stimulation around them, which can help to soothe them.

Find a comfortable place in a dim, quiet room and lay baby on their side.

Rhythmically pat their back until they settle down to sleep. Then remember to place them on their back. It's easy to feel inadequate when you can't get your baby to stop crying, but try to relax and remind yourself that this is what babies do, and it is no reflection of your abilities as a parent.

Getting support

If you feel like you'll never have a shower or a hot cup of coffee again, you are not alone. Babies have a knack for waking and needing attention just when you think you'll get a break. For the first couple of weeks, it's a real help to have another pair of hands available to hold your baby or calm them when they're crying, to allow you a little time to relax, wash, and eat.

If you're exhausted and finding it difficult to handle baby's constant crying, ask your partner or a family member to take over for a couple hours so you can sleep. You'll likely feel much more able to take charge again once you've had real rest.

If baby becomes distressed when you put them down, try carrying them on your chest in a carrier, which will free your hands and soothe them. Time showers, meals, and naps when you have someone around to help; don't feel guilty about not playing hostess. Your helpers will love to spend time with your baby, and help you recover from the birth. Leave a list of jobs on the fridge, so visitors know exactly how they can help around the house.

HOW TO MIX FORMULA

Follow the manufacturer's instructions to the letter. Too much formula powder or liquid can cause your baby to become constipated or thirsty; too little may mean that your baby isn't getting the nutrition they need. First, boil water (to kill any germs) and allow it to cool, or measure out bottled water. Once you've mixed the formula, gently warm your baby's bottle in a pitcher of hot water: a microwave can cause "hot spots," which could burn baby's mouth. It's best to make fresh bottles when you need them. If you need to prepare them in advance, store them in the back of the fridge, below 39°F (4°C), and don't keep them more than 24 hours.

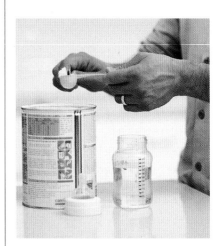

Preparing a bottle of formula Level off each scoopful as you measure out the formula. Add the formula to the cooled, boiled water in a sterilized feeding bottle. Then vigorously shake the bottle so there are no lumps left and the mixture is completely smooth.

I should be over the moon now that my baby is here, so why am I feeling so tearful and emotional? Tearfulness, temporary feelings of inadequacy, exhaustion, and anxiety are experienced by about 60 to 80 percent of all new moms in the days following the birth. Commonly known as the "baby blues," these emotions are thought to be caused by a drop in pregnancy hormones, combined with a surge in the hormones that are produced for breastfeeding.

You may find yourself constantly in tears, irritable, frustrated, and weary, and you may wonder how you will cope. Baby blues can last for a few hours or up to five days, and you may feel inexplicably under the weather. Don't be embarrassed about crying or feeling anxious. Explain how you are feeling to your partner, and say yes to offers of support during this period. If you don't feel any better in a week, talk to your doctor who will assess whether you are developing postpartum depression, for which you may need extra help.

HOW TO BURP YOUR BABY

Most babies take in small amounts of air when feeding. This can become trapped in their intestines, causing pain. Gas can also make your baby feel full, which may prevent them from feeding properly. Burping encourages your baby to release the air trapped in their digestive system, easing any discomfort. You might want to try a little burping session halfway through feeding and again at the end. If your baby isn't bringing up any gas after 5–10 minutes, don't keep trying. It may be that baby doesn't have any to burp up, or it may be released later.

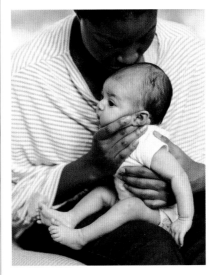

Sit the baby on your lap. Lean them slightly forward, support their head, then gently rub or pat their back until they burp.

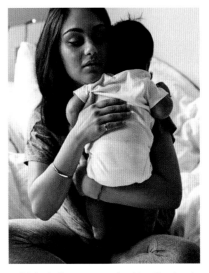

Hold the baby over your shoulder. Gently rub or pat the baby's back until they burp. They may bring up some milk, so place a cloth over your shoulder.

Your baby's milk

Chances are that your milk will "come in" today, which means that your breasts will start producing "transitional" milk, a mixture of colostrum and mature milk that looks yellowish and creamy. Your breasts may become harder and possibly slightly engorged, making it difficult for your baby to latch on. Try to get all of your areola into your baby's mouth (see p.27), and massage your breast downward to release some milk and make it easier for baby to get your nipple in their mouth.

Over the next 10 days or so, less and less colostrum will be produced, so by the time your baby is two weeks old, your breast milk is considered to be "mature." Your body will produce just enough for your baby's needs, so feed them as often as they want to ensure that your supply meets their demand. The more you feed, the more milk you will make. You may find that you are feeding for between 30 and 60 minutes at each session (and sometimes longer), and your baby may drop off to sleep while nursing. Gently nudge baby awake by stroking their cheek. When baby comes off your breast, burp them before getting them down to sleep. Most breastfed babies will nurse between 8 and 12 times in a 24-hour period. If you've had a cesarean, it may take slightly longer for your milk to come in, but keep baby nursing at your breast and report any problems to your doctor.

Life for bottle-feeding parents may be more straightforward at this point because you can see exactly how much milk your baby is getting. You'll still be feeding every 2–3 hours, and your baby will probably need a couple ounces (30–60 ml) at each feeding for the first week or so, or until they weigh 10 lb (4.5 kg).

Getting checked

In the week after birth, you'll venture out to the pediatrician's office for the first time, to make sure your baby is doing well.

You'll have your baby's first appointment at the pediatrician's office in the first week after they're born, which offers you opportunities to ask any questions you may have. If you're breastfeeding you'll be offered support. The pediatrician will also check your baby to ensure they are healthy and well and beginning to put on weight. Report anything that concerns you, no matter how minor it may seem. Being responsible for a new life can be daunting at the best of times, and there may be a simple solution to address any problem.

Advice for mom

If you're breastfeeding and this is your first child, chances are that you're still trying to get the hang of everything. You might be experiencing pain, your baby might not be latching on properly, or your baby might not be gaining enough weight. Don't hesitate to report any problems you may be facing when breastfeeding; it can be very reassuring to get advice and guidance from a professional. Pediatricians often give new moms advice about breastfeeding, and many will offer to watch you breastfeed your baby and advise on your technique, with hands-on suggestions for improving the process. Don't feel uncomfortable lifting your shirt in front of the pediatrician; after all, this is a doctor who's seen it all before, and whose advice can only benefit you and your

baby. If you're still having problems, ask your pediatrician for a referral to a lactation consultant in your area or for the contact information of the local chapter of La Leche League. Both can be invaluable resources for new moms who are trying to figure out the art of breastfeeding while combating sleep deprivation and all of the new responsibilities of motherhood.

Baby checkups

You will be asked lots of questions about your baby's feeding and sleeping patterns, bowel movements, wet diapers, and general happiness, which will provide information about their overall health and well-being. Your baby will be weighed during some visits to monitor their weight and see if they are beginning to gain weight.

Weight gain is often slower in breastfed babies, so don't be alarmed if baby doesn't seem to be filling out as quickly as you'd hoped.

Your doctor will let you know if they are concerned about your baby's weight, and evaluate your breast-feeding technique. In many cases, improving your baby's latch and nursing for long periods in order to build up your milk supply will ensure that your baby gets what they need to put on weight and grow at a good rate.

Your baby will probably be undressed for weighing, and your pediatrician will take a look at any rashes or spots, and offer advice. It's normal for babies to look a little mottled in the early days, but if you have concerns, point them out now. Your baby should be given a full exam, with the pediatrician checking them from head to toe to make sure that everything is all right, since this is probably the first time your pediatrician has met your baby. Your baby's height, weight, and head circumference will be noted in their medical charts and also plotted on percentile graphs to see

---

THE NEWBORN BLOOD SPOT TEST

On day five, and sometimes up to eight days after your baby's birth, you will be offered a blood spot (heel prick) screening. This involves taking a small blood sample (normally around 4 drops) to test for one of nine rare but serious health conditions. These are sickle cell disease, cystic fibrosis, congenital

hypothyroidism, and six inherited metabolic diseases: phenylketonuria (PKU), medium-chain acyl-CoA dehydrogenase deficiency (MCADD), maple syrup urine disease (MSUD), isovaleric acidemia (IVA), glutaric aciduria type 1 (GA1), and homocystinuria (pyridoxine unresponsive) (HCU).

how they're growing compared to other babies and themself over time. You'll see the pediatrician many times during the first few months, so it's important to feel comfortable with them and be able to ask anything that's a concern to you. Be as honest as you can with your pediatrician; there is no shame in admitting that you are struggling to deal with exhaustion or a baby who seems to cry inconsolably. Similarly, don't be afraid to cry or express any anxieties or worries at the doctor's office. Your health practitioners are experienced in all kinds of different scenarios and can offer you invaluable help and advice. If your baby has fallen asleep in the detachable car seat on the drive over to the doctor's office, don't wake them when their name is called; let them sleep while you and the pediatrician discuss other things first; the physical exam can wait until the end of the appointment.

TAKE CARE OF YOUR BABY'S UMBILICAL CORD

It is important to keep your baby's umbilical cord stump clean and dry. It's no longer suggested that alcohol or antiseptic ointments, talc, or liquids be used on it. Instead, plain warm water, with a little baby wash if the area becomes dirty, will do the trick.

Look for "bikini" diapers, which are fastened below the umbilical area to prevent irritation, or you can fold down an ordinary diaper. You can expect the umbilical cord area to look a little mucky in the beginning. However, if it is very red or sore looking, or if there is a smelly discharge, see your doctor, who can rule out infection.

Between 5 and 15 days after your baby's birth, the umbilical cord stump will dry, blacken, and drop off. Underneath there will be a small wound or sore that will heal over the next few days.

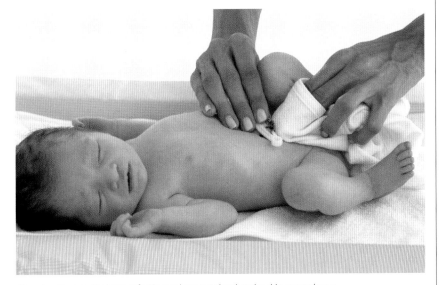

Cleaning the cord To keep infection at bay, gently wipe the skin around your baby's umbilical cord stump with a soft, wet washcloth, then dry the area.

ASK A PEDIATRICIAN

Is my baby suffering from jaundice?
About two-thirds of all full-term babies develop jaundice (see p.372) a few days after birth. Jaundice is caused by buildup in your baby's blood of bilirubin: a natural by-product of red blood cells. Typically jaundice settles down without treatment about 10 days after birth. Make sure the baby gets plenty of sunlight and feed them often to help encourage their body to excrete the bilirubin. Call your doctor if you have concerns about any of the following: the yellow color is visible at the knee or lower, appears darker (changing from lemon yellow to orange yellow), or if the "whites" of the eyes appear yellow; your baby has a fever; your baby has any difficulty eating; your baby is more sleepy than usual; it is hard to wake up your baby; your baby is irritable and is difficult to console; your baby arches their neck or body backward.

I have twins. Will my body be able to produce enough milk to feed them both?
Many new mothers of twins worry that they won't have enough milk to feed two babies. However, breastfeeding works on the principle of supply and demand, so your body will produce milk to the precise requirements of your babies, even during their hungrier periods when they are having a growth spurt.

Should I wake my baby for a feeding?
Most parents are reluctant to wake a sleeping baby, since this may be the only opportunity to get some sleep or catch up on chores; however, your baby does need to be fed frequently (at least every two to three hours) to get enough milk for growth and development, so if they are going longer than this, you might need to wake them up to be fed. If you're breastfeeding, it's also important to put baby to your breast frequently (ideally, about 8 to 12 times in every 24-hour period) in order to build up your milk supply.

Bonding with your baby

Bonding continues throughout your lives as you develop a close, powerful connection with each another.

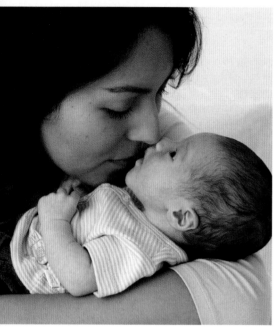

Gentle touch Touching encourages weight gain and reduces fear and anxiety in both of you.

REGISTERING THE BIRTH

At the hospital, you'll receive paperwork for your baby's birth certificate. The hospital will forward the form to your city or state's office of vital statistics. You should receive a copy of the birth certificate in a few weeks. You can request a Social Security number for your baby at the hospital, too. The card will be mailed to your home in several weeks.

Bonding is the development of an intense attachment between parents and their baby. It encourages us to love our babies, feel affection for them, and protect and nourish them. It is what gets us up in the middle of the night to feed them! Bonding also fosters a sense of security and positive self-esteem in your baby. Skin-to-skin contact (see p.45) encourages this process, and can be practiced by all parents of a newborn.

Babies are tactile, sensory beings. Caressing your baby will trigger the release of the hormone oxytocin in them. Increased levels of this hormone are associated with feelings of happiness, relaxation, and security. Not all parents find the process of bonding easy, particularly if the birth was difficult. Be patient, look into baby's eyes, hold them close, and sing and speak to them. They will respond to your smell and touch, and to your voice, which might already be familiar from the womb.

Family bonding

Your partner may have begun bonding with the baby since the very first ultrasound scan, or when they first felt those magical kicks. It's worth noting that partners often spend less time with their baby directly after the birth, and need to be given the chance to develop confidence in handling and changing their precious newborn. Give your partner plenty of opportunities to be alone with their baby and try to stand back so your partner can find their own style. Help if need be, and make sure they have all they needs to change, sponge bathe, and settle baby down to sleep every so often—this way, they'll get to know baby as well as you do and develop that all-important bond.

Bonding with twins

Parents of twins or multiples can find the bonding process more of a challenge because the huge amount of physical energy needed to take care of twins can sap you of the emotional energy you need to bond. Just like bonding with a single baby, it doesn't always happen instantaneously, and so you need to give yourself time to feel strong attachments to your twins.

Be aware if you are developing more of a bond with one baby than the other. This sometimes happens if one baby needs more time and attention. Try to allocate more relaxed and playful time with the baby you feel less bonded to, as this can help to balance your feelings of closeness more evenly between the two of them.

You may also find that you bond more with one baby, while your partner bonds more easily with the other. This can be a practical measure to ensure both babies develop the security they need for their emotional well-being.

Sleeping babies

What a week! Your baby has probably spent most of it sleeping—between feedings—although it certainly may not seem like it!

Most newborns will wake up every two to four hours to be fed. They have tiny tummies and are dependent upon a milk-only diet, which digests very quickly. Your baby will wake when they are hungry and sleep when they are tired, and you cannot force them to do otherwise! It's best to have realistic expectations.

If you are breastfeeding, you can encourage baby to sleep well by making sure they fill their tummy. If possible, baby should drink from both breasts at each feeding. Now that your milk has come in, baby will probably feed on demand for between 5 and 30 minutes at each breast. They should empty one breast before moving to the other to make sure they get the fat-rich hindmilk that comes at the end of a feeding.

Bottle-fed babies tend to sleep a little longer because formula is slower to digest than breast milk.

Day and night

Many babies wake up for longer periods in the early hours, and sleep all day. In the beginning, it's probably easiest to follow baby's lead, sleeping when they sleep. You can start to establish a difference between night and day by keeping things quiet and low key in the run up to bedtime. Try to settle baby down while they are still awake. If they fall asleep at the breast they may have discomfort from gas. Allow them to nurse until sleepy, but burp them and put them to bed before they are totally asleep.

Avoid the temptation to overdress them. If the weather is warm, just a diaper with a blanket may suffice, and add more layers if they seem cold. When baby wakes up at night, feed and change them efficiently, without too much talking.

Most importantly ...

Lack of sleep can make you overly anxious and upset. Not only is this transmitted to your baby, making them irritable, it also makes it difficult for you to get a good, restful sleep. Try to be calm when you put them down to sleep. Remember—this is a temporary phase and you will get your nights back eventually.

HOW TO SWADDLE YOUR BABY

Being wrapped up can help to calm your young baby when overstimulated, and prevent them from being disturbed by their own startle reflex (see p.47), which can cause their body to jerk while they are asleep. Choose a soft cotton sheet to swaddle your baby since heavy blankets can cause them to overheat. The idea is to make them feel secure, rather than to keep warm. Keep arms free unless baby is unsettled, in which case swaddle them loosely with arms tucked in.

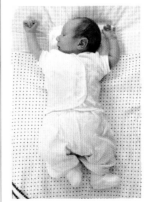 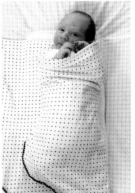 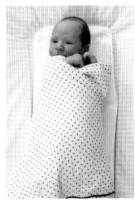

Position your baby Spread out a sheet and fold down a corner to create a long straight edge. Position your baby at top-center (left). **First tuck** Bring across one side of the sheet and tuck it snugly beneath the opposite side. Make sure it's not too tight (middle). **Second tuck** Wrap the other side of the sheet around. Tuck in the edges beneath your baby (right).

Your NICU baby

If your baby was born prematurely or wasn't well at birth, they may have been placed in a neonatal intensive care unit (NICU) or a neonatal unit in order to get the best possible medical help and attention from specialist doctors and nurses.

If your baby needs urgent medical care in the NICU, you may not be able to enjoy skin-to-skin contact or encourage the first feeding immediately after birth. You'll probably feel bereft without your baby and extremely anxious about their well-being, especially if they are in an incubator. However, try not to be alarmed by all the tubes and monitors—the incubator protects your baby from infection, provides oxygen if needed, and monitors their temperature, oxygen levels, heart rate, and lung capacity.

Feeding your baby

If your baby is unable to feed from your breast or a bottle, tubes may be placed in their mouth or nose, or directly into their stomach. It may be possible for you to express your breast milk, so this can be given to your baby through a tube. You will need to begin expressing (see p.28) as soon as possible after the birth, even if your baby isn't yet ready to take the milk. For a baby who is small or unwell, breast milk is the best choice. It is rich in proteins, fats, vitamins, minerals, and antibodies, supporting your baby's immune system, growth and development.

Hospital staff will show you how to express your milk; most units have a special room with comfortable chairs and an electric breast pump specifically for this purpose. You'll need to keep expressing every couple of hours or so to build up your milk supply. Even if you are able to express only a little in the early days, it should make a big difference to your baby's overall health. Your milk will be fed to your baby through a tube, or possibly via a

KANGAROO CARE

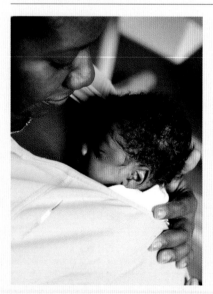

Hold baby close Research has found that babies benefit greatly from being held closely, skin-to-skin.

One of the best ways of promoting the healthy development of a new baby, whether premature or full term, is to practice Kangaroo care. This involves holding them—dressed only in a diaper and probably a hat—against the skin of your chest, between your breasts. Turn their head so their ear is pressed near to your heart, and gather baby up against you so they feel your warmth and love. Kangaroo care allows newborns to experience something like the containment of the uterus while acclimating to the world.

There is a wealth of benefits associated with Kangaroo care. In fact, research has found that, compared with NICU babies who are not held in this way, those that experience Kangaroo care (even for short periods of time every day) experience:
• a more stable heart rate

• more regular breathing (including a 75 percent decreased risk of sleep apnea, which causes babies to stop breathing temporarily during sleep)
• improved oxygen levels in the blood
• a regulated body temperature
• more rapid weight gain and brain development
• decreased crying
• longer periods of being alert
• more successful breastfeeding
• earlier bonding.

A baby's growth rate increases when held in Kangaroo care mainly because they are able to fall into a deep, restful sleep when snuggled against a parent. Sleep allows them to conserve energy for growth and development. Both parents can employ this method of care, and aid the process of bonding.

syringe, bottle, or cup until they are well enough to nurse at your breast.

When you do put your baby to your breast, they may not actually suck, but will enjoy your closeness. If you put a little expressed milk on your nipple, your baby can smell and taste it. A tiny baby will also enjoy catching dribbles of milk in their mouth. Don't expect too much at your first feeding, since premature or sick babies tire easily and need to learn how to suck properly. If your baby is showing definite interest, get some help to make sure they are latching on correctly (see p.27).

Your baby needs you

Although your baby may seem fragile, and you may be worried about holding them with all the equipment around them, it is essential that you offer your baby as much close physical contact as you can. They will recognize your voice and smell and will be comforted by the beating of your heart and your warmth. Holding them as frequently as you can—or, if that is not possible, gently stroking their body in the incubator can vastly improve their well-being. Your regular touch can promote weight gain, encourage healing, and even help them to develop restful sleep patterns. Sing to your baby, talk to them in a calm voice, and reassure them. Research shows that talking to your baby can help to stimulate the developing connections in their brain, yet also makes them feel more relaxed.

Getting involved

While your baby is in the NICU, you may feel overwhelmed, especially if they are in an incubator and attached to tubes and wires. Ask the nurses to explain how the equipment works, and ways you can be involved in your baby's care. You may be able to help with bathing, changing, or feeding,

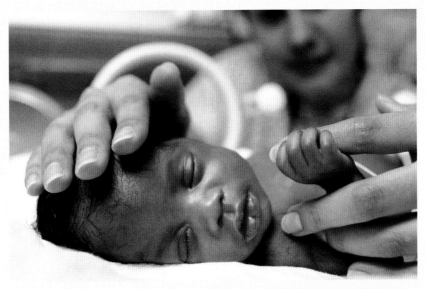

Healing touch It is recommended that you touch and caress your baby, if it is not possible for you to hold them. Spend as much time as possible talking and singing to help them relax.

which will help you become involved in their regular routine.

Look after yourself

Rest often and eat regular, nutritious meals. Get support from family and friends and ask if there is somewhere to stay on hospital grounds, to make it easier to have more time with your baby. Equally, try not to feel guilty if you can't always be with your baby. It's normal to experience guilt, distress, anxiety, and more. Talk to your partner and the health professionals. They are there to support you as well as your baby.

Keep a diary to record your feelings and celebrate milestones, no matter how small. Looking back, you'll see your baby's amazing achievements and find comfort in their progress. Keep a note of questions to ask doctors and nurses and write down the answers so that you can later reflect on them quietly.

HOMEY ATMOSPHERE

Try to interact with your baby as you would if you were taking care of them at home. When you can't be there, decorate the incubator with photos of family; they'll become familiar with your faces and reassured to see you there. You could play soothing music, or create a recording of your voice to be played during your absences, which will comfort baby and help them develop a connection to you.

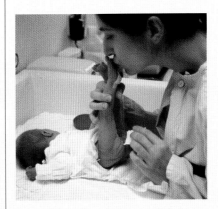

Personal touch Try to forget your clinical surroundings and imagine you're at home.

1 week

DURING EARLY WEEKS, BABIES ARE AWAKE ONLY 10 PERCENT OF THE TIME. Your baby's vision is blurry, though they have recognized you since shortly after birth. When awake, your baby will be fascinated by their new world—and your eyes and your voice.

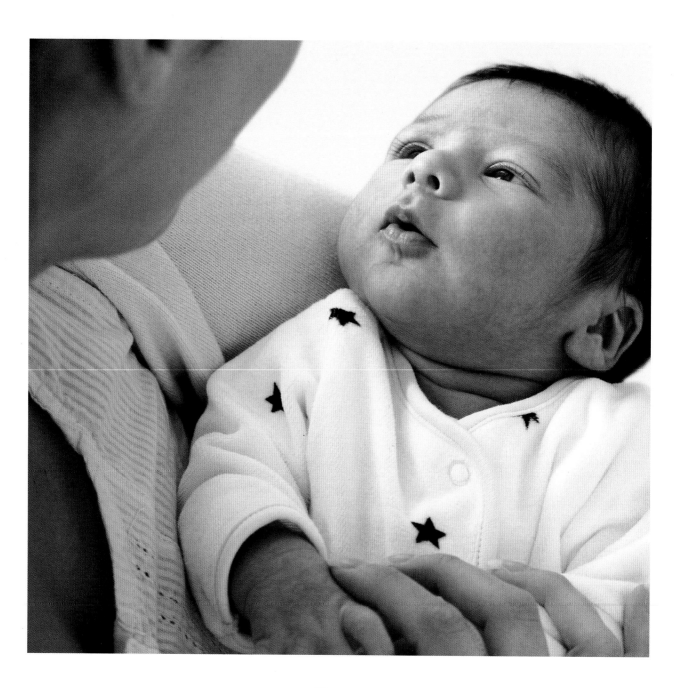

Baby knows you

Your voice and smell have been familiar to your baby since birth, but they now recognize your face and feel secure when they see you.

Although your baby is still too young to focus clearly on your face, they can recognize you and like nothing better than to stare into your eyes. Research has found that babies stare much longer and with greater determination at familiar faces, so you may find them watching you intently. In fact, when they are stimulated and interested, they will stop moving and watch you very carefully. Indulge this passion and look into their eyes. Eye contact is not just essential for the process of bonding, but also acts as an early form of communication between you and your baby. Let them get to know you—position your face around 12 in (30 cm) from theirs—this is the optimum focusing distance for them. Even though your baby won't recognize you yet, they will be drawn to you and want to stare. Your eyes and hairline will offer the most contrast, on which your baby can most easily focus. It won't be very long before they reach up to touch your face.

Forming an attachment

In the early days and weeks after birth, parents and babies are uniquely primed to want to be close to each other. Continuing with skin-to-skin contact will be reassuring for your baby. They may recognize your heartbeat from the uterus, and your smell will comfort them and encourage them to feed. What's more, they are growing familiar with your touch and sense a new confidence in the way you handle them, which helps them feel secure.

GIVE YOUR BABY A BATH

If your pediatrician says you don't have to wait for the umbilical cord to fall off, you might want to give your baby their first bath this week. Lots of infants love the sensation of water, and bath time becomes an enjoyable part of your routine. Make sure the room is warm, and gather a clean towel, fresh diaper, and clothes, so everything is ready. Half-fill a baby bath with lukewarm water, testing it with your elbow (98.6°F/37°C on a thermometer).

ASK A PEDIATRICIAN

Why does my baby cry every time I put them down to sleep? Most babies prefer to be held, particularly in the first week or two when they are adjusting to life outside the uterus. Swaddling (see p.53) can help them feel more secure, or you may want to put them down awake and stroke them until they settle down. Keep in mind that most young babies cry between one and three hours a day—it might be that your baby is tired and needs to unwind with a strong cry.

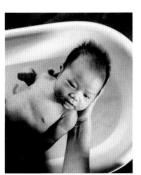

Into the tub Lower your baby into the bathtub, carefully supporting their head, shoulders, and bottom.

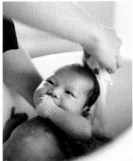

Hair wash Support their head and shoulders, then wet their hair with your hand, a soft washcloth, or sponge.

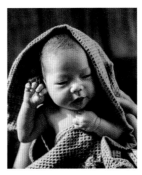

All clean After their bath, wrap your baby up in a soft towel, then gently rub them dry.

Successful feeding

Feeding your baby will be time consuming, but hugely rewarding
as you watch them grow and develop on their milk-only diet.

Breastfeeding

There is no doubt that breastfeeding is an art that takes a little practice—for both you and your baby. Getting latched on correctly can make all the difference when it comes to making sure your baby gets the milk they need. Once you've both mastered latching on, they will nurse more efficiently, competently stimulating your breasts to supply them with just the right amount of milk, and you'll be less likely to experience discomfort.

Latching on incorrectly can make your nipples sore and cause them to crack. It's common to feel "attachment pain" for the first 10 seconds or so, but pain throughout a feeding needs to be checked. If you find you are experiencing problems, don't hesitate to talk to your pediatrician or lactation consultant. It can take at least a few days for your milk supply to meet your baby's demands, and maybe a bit longer for you to feel entirely comfortable and confident with the process. Some parents who don't enjoy breastfeeding at first are happy they persevered once it's going smoothly two to three weeks later.

How long should a feeding take? Don't be tempted to time a feeding. Your baby will nurse for as long as it takes to get the quantity of milk that is right for them. Sometimes they may empty your breast within 10 minutes. On other occasions they may be sleepy and take 20 minutes on each side, or even longer. Don't rush. Sometimes they'll simply nurse for comfort, which is nature's way of increasing your milk supply.

Most newborns feed between 8 and 12 times a day. For the first few weeks, your baby may be on your breast every 90 minutes, although they may manage a break as long as three hours if they've had a good feeding.

Emptying each breast It's best to empty each breast fully before moving to the other, since this ensures your baby gets both the hydrating, thirst-quenching foremilk and the nutritious hindmilk. Emptying each breast fully can also help prevent problems, such as blocked ducts (see box, opposite). If they don't manage both breasts in one sitting, start on the full breast the next time

GET INTO A GOOD POSITION FOR BREASTFEEDING

For your baby to be able to latch on properly, it's important that you are both positioned well. You should be comfortable, with your back well-supported: cushions or pillows may be helpful. There are a number of different positions to try and you'll probably find one or two that suit you best. Cradling your baby at chest level, with their tummy against yours, can be comfortable. A football hold with your baby under your arm is good if your breasts are sore, as it stops your baby pulling on the breast. For night feedings, or after a cesarean, you might find it helpful to feed your baby lying down on your side. Check that baby's head is able to tip back slightly as they nurse. Their chin should touch your breast and they should be able to breathe easily.

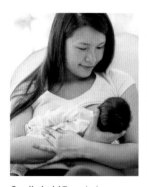

Cradle hold Turn their tummy toward yours, cradling their head in the crook of your arm. Use your forearm as support, then tuck your baby's knees in.

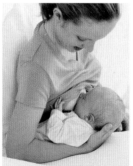

Football hold Tuck your baby's body under your arm, as if holding a football to your chest, and support their neck with your forearm.

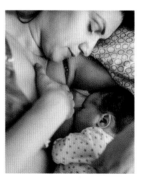

Lying down Lie on your side with your baby facing you and draw them in close to your breast, cradling them with your arm.

BREASTFEED TWINS

You may want to begin breastfeeding your babies one at a time until you feel comfortable with it. If you take this route, the milk stimulation in one breast may cause a let-down reflex in your other breast (known as the "double let down"). Place a sterile container nearby to catch any milk that does leak—you can store this in the freezer for later use.

For simultaneous breastfeeding, keep in mind that, in most cases, one twin is a stronger nurser. Put this baby on your breast first, which allows you to spend more time adjusting the position of your second baby. Your second twin will benefit from the simultaneous let-down reflex without having to work too hard for it. If they are small you may be able to snuggle both of

them in your lap, with their tummies against yours. If this is awkward, try the football hold (see box, opposite), in which their heads are at your breasts and their bodies are nestled against your sides.

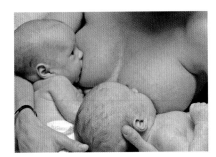

Positioning your twins This mother uses a combination of cradle and football holds. In time, you will find what works best for you.

they feed to make sure that both breasts are eventually emptied. Make a note of the breast on which they last nursed.

Bottle-feeding

It's equally important to be comfortable when you are bottle-feeding, so make sure you are in a comfy chair with your back well-supported, and position yourself so

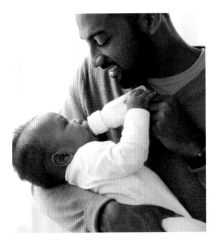

Bottle-feeding position Cradle your baby in a semi-upright position and support the head.

that you can look into your baby's eyes. Just as with breastfeeding, this is a time for bonding, and this will happen more naturally if you imitate a breastfeeding position. Hold your baby close against your chest as you feed them, so they feel comforted. Switch arms regularly to ensure you both are comfortable.

Holding your baby When it's time to feed, stroke their cheek to stimulate the rooting reflex that encourages them to open their mouth. Don't feed your baby when they are lying down— formula can flow into the sinuses or middle ear, causing an infection. Instead, hold them up at a slight angle, and tilt the bottle so that the formula fills the teat and neck of the bottle. A newborn will likely take 2–4 fl oz (60–120 ml) per feed in the first few weeks and may be hungry every 3–4 hours. Follow their lead: babies will not overfeed, so if your baby wants more milk, they may be feeling extra hungry.

In most cases latching on incorrectly is the cause of discomfort during breastfeeding. Adjusting the feeding position can eradicate annoying problems. Other difficulties include:

Sore or cracked nipples Try rubbing breast milk on your nipples after a feeding, and put a cool washcloth or gel pad in your bra to ease discomfort. Emollient nipple cream may help. "Air" your breasts after feedings, and change breast pads frequently.

Leaking It's normal for breasts to leak in the early days. You may leak from one breast while your baby is nursing from the other, and your baby's cries can also stimulate a "let-down reflex." Wear breast pads and nurse your baby often to prevent overflow. Things usually improve within 6–8 weeks.

Blocked ducts Once breastfeeding is established, an oversupply of milk can build up in the breasts, possibly resulting from poor latching on and/or not completely emptying the breasts during feeding. If you have redness or pain in your breast tissue, feed your baby more often to get the milk flowing. If it doesn't improve, inform your doctor.

Mastitis Inflammation or infection of the breast causes red, inflamed areas and symptoms similar to the flu, such as a high temperature. The affected breast may also feel full and tender. Continue nursing your baby frequently, but if you don't feel better within a few hours, call your doctor.

Thrush This can infect the nipples, causing stabbing pains while nursing. Your doctor may prescribe a gel. Your baby may need to be checked, too.

Your baby's weight

At this age, a few ounces matter a lot, especially when you want your tiny baby to start gaining weight steadily.

If you are breastfeeding, your baby's weight is probably a major preoccupation now. When you can't see how much milk your baby is consuming, you're more likely to worry that they're not getting enough to thrive. This is especially the case if your baby lost weight (as is normal) last week and has been slow to regain it. Being told by your doctor that your baby has gained a minimal amount of weight or—worse—none at all, can be enough to send you into a real panic.

There is usually no cause for concern: some babies simply take a little longer than others to start gaining weight. As a rule, once your milk comes in at around three days, your baby should start to gain approximately 1 oz (25 g) a day. Most babies regain their birth weight by two weeks, but some do take a little longer. At this age, weight is less of an issue and your baby's general appearance and well-being are more important indicators of how they're doing: if they are generally alert, waking to be fed, have good skin color and tone, and are having at least 6–8 wet diapers a day, they should be fine.

If your baby seems lethargic, listless, and pale; passes feces less than once a day; or does small, dark feces after they're five days old; their skin becomes more yellow, rather than less, after the first week; or their skin remains wrinkled after the first week, it's a good idea to get some help to make sure they are feeding efficiently. Just keep breastfeeding on demand and they should soon start to achieve steady weight gain.

If you are bottle-feeding, you can also expect your baby to gain about 1 fl oz (25 g) in weight per day from now until they are three months old.

You will need to give your baby about 2–4 fl oz (60–120 ml) of formula six to eight times a day: babies have tiny tummies and can't manage too much more in one sitting. There should always be a little milk left in the bottle at the end of each feeding so you can be sure they've had enough.

TRIM YOUR BABY'S NAILS

Babies' fingernails grow fast, so it's a good idea to clip them to prevent them from snagging the skin. Toenails grow more slowly but they can scratch or occasionally become ingrown. It can be daunting to approach baby's nails with scissors or clippers, but if you use tools made for babies, you're unlikely to hurt them. Cut their nails when they are sleeping or being fed, since they're likely to be calmer. Or you can ask your partner to hold their hands or feet still while you get to work. Don't cut them too short—always leave a little of the white showing. Cut toenails straight across, but fingernails can be slightly rounded.

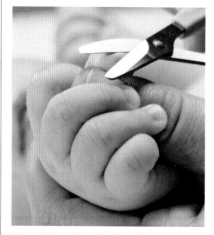

Scissors Use baby nail scissors that have rounded ends to cut your baby's nails.

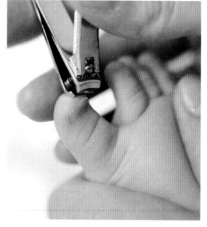

Clippers The small blades of baby nail clippers are ideal for safely trimming tiny toenails.

Going out

If you haven't yet ventured out, you might be going a little stir crazy. Try getting out of the house with your baby now—it will do you good.

Tempting as it is to batten down the hatches and stay indoors with your baby, fresh air and a change of scenery can give you a break from domestic life and lift your mood. Sunshine encourages the production of vitamin D, which you and your baby need for healthy teeth, bones, and restful sleep; vitamin D also helps prevent depression and ease baby blues.

You may not feel up to walking far (or getting dressed for that matter), but even a short stroll to the nearest store or a walk in the local park will help you feel a bit more connected to the outside world and less isolated if you've been ensconced at home with your baby.

If this is your first trip out, time it after a feeding so your baby is relaxed. Dress them for the weather. In general, put them in the same amount of clothing as you, plus an extra layer to keep out the wind. If it's cold, a sleep suit, a warm outer suit, a hat, and a blanket should keep them snug. Their head should feel warm, not hot, to the touch; hands and feet should be a little cooler. Don't forget your keys, cell phone, and bag (fatigue makes you absent-minded), and, above all, enjoy your first outing.

Extra equipment

If you're planning to be out longer than half an hour or so, you will need to take a few essential items with you. Don't leave home without:

• **burp cloths** These are perfect for mopping up—and you can drape one over your shoulder whenever you want to breastfeed discreetly.
• **a diaper bag** with clean diapers, wipes, plastic bags for wet or dirty clothes or diapers, a change of clothes for your baby, diaper cream if you use it, and a portable changing mat.
• **formula and bottles** If you're bottle-feeding, take some prepared containers of formula and sterilized bottles.
• **water and snacks** Take a bottle of water and something to eat in case you feel in need of an energy boost.

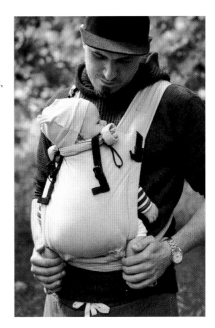

Baby carrier A front carrier pack keeps your baby close and snug.

STRAWBERRY MARKS

Also called hemangiomas, strawberry marks are quite common and nothing to worry about. They often form on the head or neck, but can appear anywhere on a

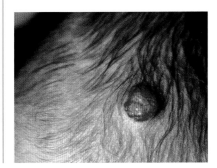

baby's body and may be present at birth or develop in the first few weeks. They may start as a small, bright-red flat area, but usually become raised and look like a strawberry. Strawberry marks grow in size for the first 6 to 12 months, then often shrink and disappear by the age of 7 with no need for medical intervention. Treatment may be necessary if the marks affect your baby's vision or are in an awkward place that impairs feeding or breathing. If concerned, speak to your pediatrician.

Raised swelling A strawberry mark results from an overgrowth of tiny blood vessels.

Taking care of your health

Your focus is on taking care of your baby, but don't neglect your own health. Being fit and well gives you energy to cope as a new parent.

While it can be difficult to find time to put together nutritious meals, it's important to make your diet a priority. Grabbing a sugary snack may keep you going between your baby's feedings, but your energy levels and your overall health will eventually begin to suffer.

Fill the fridge with healthy foods that you can eat on the run: seeds, nuts, fresh fruit and vegetables, hummus, yogurt, smoothies, cheese, eggs, whole-grain toast, and lots of water will keep your blood sugar levels stable, and help you feel calm and relaxed.

It is very important to stay well hydrated. Breastfeeding mothers need about 2.8 quarts (2.7 liters) of fluids per day. This can be 70–80 percent from drinks and another 20–30 percent from food. Smoothies and low-fat milk both count. Because caffeine passes into breast milk, it's best to avoid caffeinated drinks, such as coffee and cola, while you are nursing.

It's perfectly possible to eat well, even when time is tight. A nourishing bowl of soup with a whole-wheat roll can be produced in minutes, as can scrambled eggs on toast.

Try to eat at least five or six servings of fruit and vegetables per day to make sure you get plenty of vitamin C, which your body needs to absorb iron. Iron-rich foods include red meat, dried fruit, fortified breakfast cereals, and legumes.

If friends or family want to cook for you, take advantage of their generosity. There's no shame in accepting help in the kitchen to allow you to concentrate on your new baby and your recovery.

Exercise

It's still early, but you should try to get outdoors when you can for some fresh air and a little gentle exercise. Fatigue caused by a lack of sleep is compounded by a lack of activity. It's good for both you and your baby and the exertion will encourage a more restful night's sleep. Try to build a brisk walk in the park into your routine, or walk to the nearby stores instead of getting into the car.

If you've had a cesarean, you might not feel up to going outside for a walk yet, although a gentle daily stroll (even up and down the block or around the backyard) will help your recovery. Go out for a walk only if you're sure you feel able to. If in any doubt, always check with your doctor first.

ASK A BREASTFEEDING EXPERT

Can I use nipple shields? These are not generally recommended as they may interfere with proper attachment, as well as reduce your milk supply. Nipple shields are also known to increase the risk of skin irritation, blocked ducts, and mastitis.

Is there anything I shouldn't drink? Alcohol can pass through your breast milk, and regular drinking can reduce your milk supply and harm your baby. Restrict your caffeine intake to one cup of coffee a day since caffeine can make babies more irritable and restless. Be careful not to overdo herbal teas. Mint teas, for example, are thought to help soothe babies' gas and colic when drunk by breastfeeding moms. However, they can also have the effect of decreasing milk supply if consumed in large quantities.

Can I smoke while breastfeeding? You could be putting your baby at risk if you do. Nicotine and traces of smoke in your baby's environment can increase the risk of SIDS (see p.31), respiratory problems, ear infections, and behavioral problems.

If you cannot stop smoking or are finding it hard to quit, it's important to not stop breastfeeding, as breastfeeding will still help safeguard your baby from infections and provide vital nourishment that they cannot get from formula. To protect your baby's health, avoid smoking before feeds, as this will limit the amount of nicotine passed into your breast milk and speak to your doctor or health-care practitioner about safe products and support to stop smoking.

You know your baby

Parenthood can be quite daunting, and you may worry about getting it right. Trust that you know your baby best.

If babies came with instruction manuals, the past week and a half might have been easier. But most parents find this steep learning curve difficult, and worry constantly if they are doing the "right thing" for their babies. Your ability to tune in to your baby's needs will guide you in responding to them. Read their signals, and you will be cuddling, cooing, and feeding, changing, and rocking them when they need it.

There is no "right" way to take care of your baby—and your baby is an individual, so what is right for another baby may not be right for yours. Try not to compare your parenting skills with those of other moms either; as you get to know your baby, you will naturally do what is best for them, whether or not your baby manual or friends think differently.

If you are not particularly enjoying taking care of your baby's needs at the moment, try not to worry or think that you are failing as a parent. It's not uncommon for new parents to feel that they are just going through the motions rather than actively treasuring every moment with their new baby. For a small number of parents, resentment can start to build about how much time and energy your baby takes up. If this is happening, seek extra support from family and friends and speak to a health professional about how you feel. You may also be exhausted, so arrange for your partner or a friend to take over to give you time to rest.

Don't push yourself too hard, and try not to panic when things don't go as planned. No two days are ever the same in a household with a young baby, and you'll need to be flexible and sometimes lower your expectations of yourself.

ASK A PEDIATRICIAN

Can I breastfeed when I'm sick? You may not feel up to it, but do continue breastfeeding to keep up your milk supply. Far from passing infection to your baby, you'll provide them with the antibodies you develop against your illness, making it less likely that they'll catch it. Most over-the-counter analgesics are safe while breastfeeding, but check the label or ask your pharmacist before taking anything. Some antibiotics and decongestants, for example, should be avoided. Talk to your doctor about the safety of any medication you take regularly.

CO-BEDDING TWINS

Putting your twins in the same crib is called co-bedding. Don't worry that your twins will overheat or smother each other. Studies show that the risks to your babies are exactly the same if they are in the same crib as they would be if they were sleeping separately.

It is important that you follow the same rules as you would for one baby. For example, make sure that each baby is feet-to-foot in the crib. This means positioning the babies so that they are on their backs either head-to-head,

with their feet at opposite ends of the crib; or side-by-side, with their feet at the same end of the crib.

The side-by-side position poses no greater risks, even if one baby flings an arm over the other. In fact, the babies may comfort each other like this. Keeping your twins in the same crib is also more practical, because having them in the same room as you as long as possible— ideally for six months—reduces the risk of SIDS (see p.31).

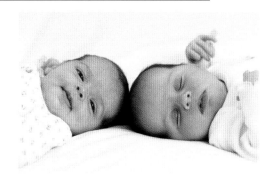

Sharing a crib It is perfectly safe to have your twins sleep in the same crib, either head to head or side by side.

Reflecting on the birth

Many new parents want to share and analyze the birth experience.
Talking about it is healthy, particularly if it didn't go as planned.

Whether you had an unexpectedly quick and easy birth experience, or found yourself using every medical intervention available although you had planned to deliver your baby naturally, you'll probably want to talk about the birth—in detail. Having a baby is a life-changing event and a deeply emotive experience. It's normal to be both proud and unsettled after the birth, and it is equally normal to feel as if you need to make sense of the events.

Some women and their partners feel unhappy with their experience of childbirth and a small number feel traumatized. For women, the birth may have been longer or more painful than anticipated, or complications arose. For partners, being out of control and distressed about their partner's discomfort may have colored their view. You may wish that things had gone as you had hoped they would, or that you had done things differently, or you might wonder why certain procedures or interventions had been necessary. Equally, you may have had a wonderful, positive birth that has left you bubbling with joy and needing to share your encouraging story. However your experience of childbirth unfolded, part of the process of remembering and understanding does involve talking about it—with your partner, your family, the friends you have met in your childbirth classes, and the doctors who are responsible for overseeing your care.

Don't hesitate to talk to medical staff and ask questions if you feel uneasy or uncertain about any element of the birth. Health-care professionals are there to support you and will understand that asking questions is part of coming to terms with your experience. The birth of a baby is amazing, and you will find that most people will be fascinated to hear how your baby came into the world.

Focus on the positive

Whatever your experience, try to focus on the positive elements, and the fact that you have succeeded in creating a new life. While it is perfectly normal to feel some disappointment or even guilt when things didn't go as planned— particularly if it seems that everyone else had a much better experience, or achieved that "natural" birth— you have a healthy baby in your arms, and there could be no better result. Take pride in the wonderful new life you have created.

ASK A DOCTOR

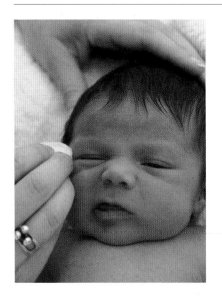

My baby's eyes are sticky. Is this normal? It is very common for newborn babies to suffer from a mild eye infection, which is caused by blood or fluid entering the eyes during the birth. Their eyelashes may appear to be crusty or sticky—or even glued together— after sleeping, and there may be a discharge in the inner corner of the eyes. You can keep their eyes clean by gently wiping off any discharge around them. This condition usually clears up on its own, but if symptoms don't improve in three days, see your doctor.

Cleaning a sticky eye Moisten a cotton pad in cooled boiled water or your own breast milk (which contains antibodies). Wipe inside outward. Use a fresh pad for each eye.

Helping your body heal

Post-delivery, you may feel uncomfortable and sore if you've had stitches or a cesarean. Fortunately, there are ways to encourage healing and to feel better.

Your pelvic floor

If your baby was big or you had serious tears or an assisted birth, your pelvic floor may have become weak and overstretched, causing you to leak urine when you sneeze, cough, or exercise. This stress incontinence usually improves. A weak pelvic floor can also cause a feeling of heaviness in the vaginal area.

You can do something about it by practicing your pelvic floor exercises (known as Kegels) as soon as you feel comfortable to do so (the sooner the better). Start by doing the exercises while you're lying on your back or side, or in the bath. Here's what to do:
• Breathe in, and as you breathe out gently squeeze your pelvic floor muscles up and in, as though trying to stop yourself from urinating, or passing gas.
• Hold for 4 or 5 seconds while you breathe in and out, then relax.
• Repeat 5 times (stop if you feel at all uncomfortable) 5 or 6 times each day. Try to build up to holding a pelvic floor contraction for 10 seconds.

Although it may feel like nothing is happening for the first few days (it can take some time for the muscles to regain enough strength even to move, and for stretched nerves to respond), you will encourage blood supply to the area, promoting healing, and restoring muscle tone. Kegels will also help deal with hemorrhoids.

If you've had a cesarean, Kegels should be slightly easier because your perineum will be less sore. It's still important to do your exercises though, because pregnancy weakens your pelvic floor muscles.

Your lower abdomen

The lower abdomen works with your pelvic floor muscles to help support your back and pelvis. Having strong abdominal muscles can help relieve back pain. Gentle pelvic tilts (see box, below) are an ideal way to start toning the lower abdomen after childbirth.

Quick relief

If your perineum or cesarean incision is tender, apply a cold compress to reduce inflammation and ease pain. Take warm baths or showers to help boost circulation and help healing.

DO A PELVIC TILT

Once you've had the all-clear from your doctor after a vaginal birth, you can use pelvic-tilt exercises to strengthen the lower abdominal area. Lie on your back, knees up and your feet flat on the floor. Place your hands on your stomach so you can feel your muscles tightening. Tighten your stomach muscles and push the arch of your back toward the floor. Squeeze your bottom tight. Hold for a count of six, then relax. If you've had a cesarean, wait 6–8 weeks before working your abdomen. To boost blood flow to the area, suck in your tummy and hold it for a minute or two.

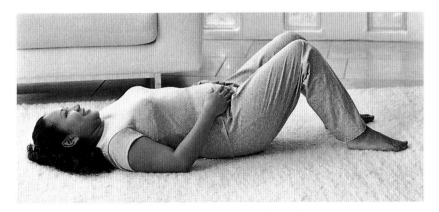

Pelvic tilt Tighten your abdominals and push your lower back into the floor—imagine pulling your belly button in toward your backbone. Try to do three sets of 10, but stop if you feel tired.

Enjoying family life

Adjusting to a new baby can take time for everyone in the family, but maintaining a strong family unit will benefit you all.

Becoming a family is a wonderful event and your life will never be the same again. You may develop a closer bond with your own parents as they settle into the role of grandparents, and spend more time with your extended family. You may have older children, or children from previous relationships, who will need time to adjust to the idea of a new sibling and a different family unit. Your roles may have changed from being simply "partner" to "partner and parent," and

that can alter the way you see and interact with each other. Having a baby offers you an opportunity to build something truly special.

If you have other children, it can be tempting to take turns with your partner to take care of the baby while the other cares for the older children, however, creating opportunities for family time will reap rewards. Whether you sit down together to watch a movie, head out to the park, play board games, or even just spend

some time in the backyard, you will be nourishing the bond that forms the basis of a happy family life.

Spending time together makes every family member feel valued and secure. Even something as simple as cooking or doing the dishes together helps spread the load and makes everyone feel they have a role. Affection, play, communication, and relaxation as a family also improve self-esteem and the family dynamic, and create happy memories, too.

JAUNDICE

This is yellowing of the skin and the whites of the eyes (see p.372). It is common in newborn babies, especially if they are breastfed, and usually resolves itself within two weeks. Prolonged jaundice, however, requires medical attention. About 10 percent of babies are still jaundiced at two weeks old. It is likely to be "breast milk jaundice," but can also be a sign of an underlying condition such as liver disease, particularly if their stools are chalky white. Speak to your doctor: your baby may need to have a blood test.

THE IMPORTANCE OF GRANDPARENTS

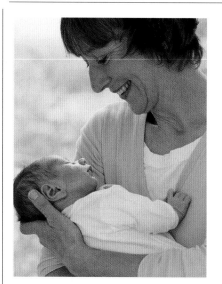

In safe hands Grandparents like to shower lots of love and affection on their newborn grandchildren. This helps build strong bonds between them from the beginning.

Welcoming grandparents into your baby's life is part of celebrating your growing family. You may or may not appreciate their help, depending on your relationship with them. Let them know what you need, and how they can best help you. For example, if they live nearby, your in-laws could cover the cooking while your parents handle the housework. You may also find that having one set of parents around at a time is enough, since too much "help" can in itself be taxing.

Grandparents, aunts, uncles, and siblings are often very willing to give advice. Accept it graciously, but believe in your own parenting skills and instincts. There may be gems of wisdom other members of your family can pass on, so listen, but remember—it's okay to make your own decisions.

Time to engage

Now that your baby is alert and awake longer, playing with them will help to stimulate their senses and improve coordination.

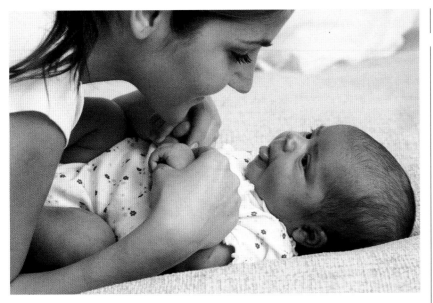

Tête-à-tête Making eye contact with your baby, and laughing and talking to them at close quarters stimulates their listening and language skills.

DEVELOPMENT ACTIVITY: BLACK-AND-WHITE PATTERNS

As they begin to interact with the world around them, your very young baby finds boldly contrasting images and distinctive geometric shapes and patterns visually stimulating. To encourage this stimulation, create a black-and-white design for your baby on card stock, using felt-tip pens to make patterns and shapes (stripes and angles are particularly appealing to babies), or purchase a baby book with similar designs. These patterns develop your baby's focusing abilities and encourage spatial awareness and visual perception. Play this game for a minute or two every day, but don't overdo it. Excessive visual stimulation will distract your baby from the "familiarization process" of getting to know and becoming integrated into their new world.

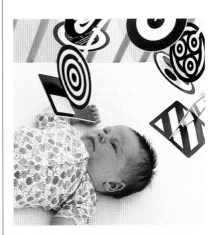

Visual stimulation Bold, moving patterns will hold your baby's attention and also help develop their ability to focus.

Your three-week-old baby doesn't understand the concept of play yet, of course, but at this age "play" simply means engaging and spending quality time with your baby. It affords them the opportunity to learn much more than you might think, and it will encourage a healthy bond between you, as well as promote their emotional health and well-being.

While it is important not to overstimulate them, a few 5- to 10-minute sessions each day, whenever they are calm and alert, will be great fun for both of you, and will help them develop on all levels. Try to gear your play to their mood—if active and alert, try some gentle clapping, tickling games, or carry baby outside and show them around the yard; if in a quieter mood, talking and singing may be more appropriate. The point of play is to learn by having fun, so keep it light and cheerful, and forget about what baby might be learning. That will become clear before you know it!

Vary the games you play together to develop different parts of your baby's body and brain. Babies instinctively "practice" skills. They may try out their new tricks after the games are finished; for example, if you've been encouraging them to poke out their tongue, they may attempt this when they see your face.

Crying

All babies cry to communicate and it can be difficult to figure out what they are trying to say at first. You'll soon learn to differentiate between cries, and find it easier to figure out the very best ways of providing comfort.

On average, even the most contented babies cry for between one and three hours a day, and some seem to cry constantly. Try to relax about crying and think rationally. Most babies cry for the same reasons, and working out what's wrong is the first step to finding a solution. If you are anxious, your baby may pick up on it, which will only compound the situation.

Why is my baby crying?

A crying baby is not necessarily unhappy, just good at conveying their needs. So when you've walked around for the fiftieth time trying to settle them, think positively: you are raising a good communicator! It's time to figure out what's causing the cry.

Use a trial-and-error approach to soothing your baby. What works one day may not work the next, or you may find a trick that works every time. If there is one thing at which all parents excel, it's adapting. Over time, you will begin to recognize your baby's cries—you'll know that they are hungry or lonely, or that it's time for a nap. You'll recognize when the baby needs a cuddle or even a little time on their own. They may not enjoy diaper changes or getting dressed, but you'll create techniques to make these more fun, or become adept at getting them done quickly.

Hunger Babies cry when they are hungry or thirsty and will not stop until sated. During growth spurts,

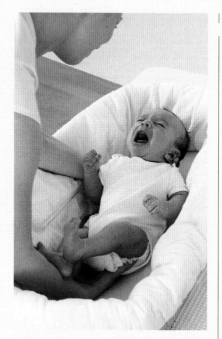

Crying for attention Young babies do not cry without reason; they usually have a genuine need that requires your attention.

when your breasts are struggling to keep up with demand, your baby may be hungrier than usual and cry more. Let them suckle at your breast—for comfort and to build up milk supply.

Feeling too hot or cold Young babies cannot regulate their body temperature. Check that your baby is not wearing too many or too few clothes. Dressing your baby in and putting them to sleep under thin layers can make it easier to cool or warm them quickly. If your baby is

ASK A PEDIATRICIAN

How can I tell if the crying is caused by colic or reflux? About a quarter of young babies suffer from colic. The cause is unclear, but it is linked to excess gas and is characterized by uncontrollable crying (often around the same time of day or night), and drawing up of their knees in clear discomfort. Most babies outgrow it by three months. (For help with easing colic, see p.75).

Reflux occurs when the acid content of the stomach rises into the esophagus, causing burning and discomfort. This can make a baby very irritable. With reflux, crying often occurs during or just after being fed, unlike colic where crying tends to be worse in the evening. Reflux can also cause babies to regurgitate frequently, sometimes in large amounts. If you suspect that your baby has reflux, talk to your pediatrician.

small or slim, they may need more clothing to maintain their body temperature. Chubby babies are often happier with fewer layers.

Wet or uncomfortable A wet or soiled diaper can cause discomfort. Some babies are particularly sensitive and need a barrier cream applied to their skin to protect it. If your baby's skin is red, bumpy, or raw, the baby may have diaper rash (see p.73 and p.373). Leave the diaper off for short periods of time to encourage healing.

Loneliness Babies are sociable and love to be held close. Your baby is stimulated and entertained by your presence and will feel more secure knowing you are there. Don't hesitate to pick your baby up when they cry—there is a genuine need to satisfy.

Understimulation Babies get bored! If the baby has been lying in the cot or car seat for hours, they may need interaction. Gentle play, talking to them, moving them to a different location, or simply a mobile over their crib can help keep them happy.

Overstimulation A little stimulation encourages development, but babies also need quiet periods, during which to consolidate skills and information. They also need to relax in order to sleep well. If your baby is fractious after periods of activity, it may be time to help them wind down and sleep. Baby massage (see p.119) or a long feed can encourage this.

Tiredness Tired babies become irritable. Being overstimulated, or not being given the opportunity to unwind in order to fall asleep, can distress your baby. If your baby seems to be crying for no reason, rubbing their eyes and yawning, rock them until they settle, wrap them up, and lay them down to sleep. Don't try to put them down when they're upset, or you may compound the problem.

Wanting comfort Sometimes babies simply want to be held in a parent's arms, have a cuddle, a gentle massage, or the comfort of suckling—on a breast or a pacifier. While you do not want to encourage "snacking," sometimes nothing else will work.

Feeling unwell An unwell baby may cry as a result of discomfort. Check your baby's temperature (see p.363), which can indicate an infection. It's almost impossible for parents to diagnose illness in a young baby, so if you notice any signs, see a doctor.

TOP TIPS FOR SOOTHING YOUR IRRITABLE BABY

• Babies respond to being held and rocked. If they are eased off to sleep by rocking, bring the stroller inside and settle yourself in a position where you can comfortably rock it with a free hand or foot.
• If your baby needs constant comfort, carry them against your chest in a carrier so they can hear your heartbeat.
• Rhythmical sounds, such as low music, or even the sound of the vacuum cleaner, soothe many babies.

• Many babies like to feel swaddled (see p.53). Try wrapping your baby snugly in a crib sheet before settling them down.
• Some babies need to suck to get to sleep, or to calm down, which is why they feed almost constantly when they are upset. If they're not hungry, they may find comfort from a pacifier.
• Calm them down by giving a light massage (see p.119).
• If crying begins after feeding, after switching from breast milk to formula,

or after switching formula, talk to your pediatrician. The formula you are using may not be suitable.
• Take a deep breath, and relax yourself. If necessary, put baby down safely for a few moments and leave the room to give yourself some space to calm down. Crying babies can be exhausting, and you may be at your wits' end. It won't do them harm to be left in a safe place for a few minutes while you take a quick break.

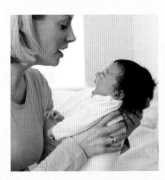

Face-to-face talk Look into your baby's eyes and talk to distract them from crying.

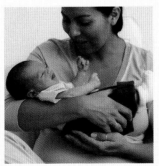

Rocking Simply rocking your baby gently back and forth can soothe and comfort them.

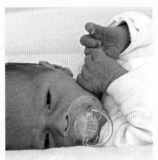

Pacifier Babies like to suck for comfort and a pacifier can help soothe a restless or upset baby.

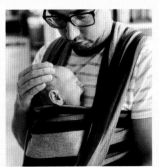

Baby carrier Your baby may love being held in a carrier, but make sure their neck is well-supported.

Copycat

Your baby mimics your facial expressions, opening their eyes and mouth as you do, and copying the tone of your voice when they coo.

When a newborn's parent sticks out their tongue and moves it from side to side, their baby responds in kind. Researchers conclude that imitation is the key learning tool in your baby's "kit" of instincts. Babies watch and imitate other people, then practice the new skills to hone them.

What's more, if you regularly make the same faces when you play, your baby will consider them "familiar" and respond more quickly. Imitation is a sign that your baby is processing information in a sophisticated way:

not only do they need to figure out what you are doing, they also have to control different parts of their body to copy you. This process can start hours after birth, and continues throughout the first months of her life. Your baby will also cry with an inflection that matches your accent, which they have picked up in the womb. Researchers have found that babies cry in a way that mimics mom's "native" language (for example, French newborns cry with a rising "accent," aiming to form an early bond.

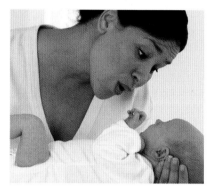

Making faces Using exaggerated facial gestures frequently when you talk will make it easier for your baby to copy expressions.

Baby sounds

Your baby is already learning to talk. "Oohs" and "aahs" will soon develop into babble that is the basis of early speech. Listen carefully!

Crying is your baby's primary method of communicating, but they'll begin to utter little sounds when they are alert, and may respond with sounds when you speak to them or stimulate them, in response to being startled, or when they recognize something like your face or your partner's voice.

The first sounds will be vowel sounds, usually "ooooh" and "aaaaah," and little cooing noises. Apart from attempts to talk to you, you can expect to hear plenty of hiccups and sneezes as well!

Encourage your baby to "talk"—move close so they can see your face, and talk to them. When your baby responds with sounds of their own, "reply" by mimicking those sounds. Your baby is starting to understand basic communication and will respond to this interaction. Talk constantly; tell them what you are doing, for example, when you are changing a diaper. They'll become familiar with the words you use, so when it's time for speech, they'll have a good vocabulary to draw from.

YOUR PEDIATRICIAN

You probably selected a pediatrician while you were pregnant, and you may have even interviewed several doctors to see who's a good fit. If you haven't done this yet, or you're reconsidering your choice now that your baby has been born, ask your ob/gyn for recommendations, then schedule a checkup for your baby.

"Baby wearing"

All babies love being held. Carrying them against your chest will not only calm and reassure them, it will also encourage bonding.

Your baby was tightly confined in the womb for many long months, and due to this experience became dependent upon touch to feel secure. After the birth, touch is equally important—and reassuring—for babies. Research has found that touch is calming and helps babies adapt to their new surroundings. It encourages bonding and promotes healthy growth, development, and even immunity. In fact, newborns need constant soothing touch to become healthy, happy children.

Studies in orphanages have found that babies who are not soothed or nurtured by touch fail to thrive, are slow growers, and develop social problems later in life.

While there can be nothing more rewarding and relaxing than holding your new baby for hours on end, there are things that you will need to get done to keep the household running. Using a carrier to carry your baby is a good way of keeping them in close proximity to you while you do the housework.

Your baby is likely to sleep for longer periods when they are held close to you, or rocked gently to sleep listening to your familiar heartbeat. Your breathing patterns will stimulate theirs, and they will be reassured by being able to feel you right there, next to them.

ASK A BREASTFEEDING EXPERT

Can I express yet? Unless you need to express your breast milk right away, it is recommended that you wait until both you and your baby feel happy and confident with breastfeeding before you start expressing. This is because sometimes babies can experience "nipple confusion" (see p.85) as the muscles and movement that your baby uses to latch on and suck a nipple are different to when latching onto your breast. However, there may be a variety of reasons you wish to express milk, including if your baby is premature or in the NICU, you are returning to work or school, if your breasts feel uncomfortably full, or when your baby is unable to latch on or to suck well.

SOOTHING YOUR BABY THROUGH TOUCH

Your baby will respond very positively to your touch, and will be soothed and reassured by it, so use touch often, especially when they need to be comforted and calmed. Hold them close while bottle-feeding or breastfeeding them, ideally with their bare skin against yours (see p.45). Be tactile—stroke their little face, gently rub their back, pat their hands, and feel and explore their body with your hands. Rock or hold them close when they're crying—letting a newborn baby cry sends the message that you are not always there for them, and makes them feel insecure. Infancy is no time for "sleep training." Cuddle with your baby after their bath—they'll be relaxed and ready to settle down when you put them to bed, resulting in a deep, restful sleep.

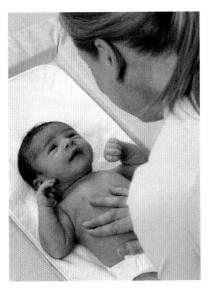

Gentle strokes Softly caressing your baby's body and talking to them as you change a diaper can help them feel less vulnerable.

Feeling lonely?

If your partner has gone back to work and any other help has headed home, you may find yourself alone with your baby for the first time.

Not only can it be difficult to learn how to take care of your baby on your own, but also you may find that long hours without adult conversation can be a little boring. Find out about parent and baby groups in your area, where you can meet other new parents, and engage in a new activity. If you took childbirth classes, try arranging get-togethers, taking turns to host. If your baby's grandparents are nearby, you could arrange regular visits, to give you something to look forward to. Talk to your partner about your feelings, too; they may be able to check in by phone more regularly, or arrange to come home earlier sometimes. Ultimately, though, take this time to adjust and put your feet up while you bond with your baby. Why not watch a favorite movie or binge-watch a show if you get the chance!

ASK A PEDIATRICIAN

Can I give my baby water to drink?
Breastfed babies receive a perfect balance of fluid from breast milk and don't require anything else, even if a little dehydrated during illness. Bottle-fed babies should get the fluid they need from formula, but if it's very hot outside, or they have a bug, a little water can be offered. Use previously boiled, cooled water or bottled water in a sterilized bottle.

Breastfeeding in public

Many new moms may feel apprehensive about breastfeeding in public, but breastfeeding in public isn't just accepted—it's protected.

At first, you may feel self-conscious about breastfeeding in public. But it doesn't have to be a difficult experience, and your confidence will grow the more you go out with your baby. You have the right to breastfeed in public and should never be made to feel uncomfortable about nursing.

Preparation is key—practice different breastfeeding positions at home so you can find one that feels most comfortable and helps your baby to latch effectively. Look online for local breastfeeding-friendly places to go. You may also wish to go on your first few outings with your partner, a family member, or a friend for moral support and company.

Breastfeeding is a convenient way to feed your baby, and there are many ways of doing it discreetly. Try wearing a loose top that can be easily lifted or use a shawl or large, light blanket to cover your breast and baby. Look online to find feeding-friendly clothes (see p.107) or try layering tops so you can tuck your baby underneath one and still be fully covered. Choose a bra that you can easily open, ideally with one hand. Try out a few options to find what feels best for you.

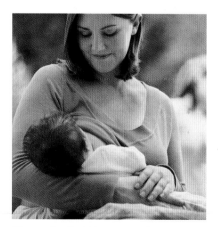

Discreet feeding A loose top will allow your baby easy access to feed and will not reveal too much of your flesh.

Your baby's thermostat

Babies cannot regulate their own body temperature until they are much older, so it's important to check that they are not too hot or cold.

Babies' bodies are unable to regulate temperature effectively. They lose heat from their heads when very hot but, otherwise, rely upon their caregivers to keep them at the right temperature.

It isn't necessary to take your baby's temperature (see p.363) unless they feel very hot and may have an infection. Instead, examine them regularly by putting your hand against their cheek, which should feel warm to the touch, and checking that their feet and hands are cool, but not hot or cold. Dress baby in layers, which can be added or removed as necessary. You'll need to use your instincts to assess the right balance.

Aim for a bedroom temperature of around 60.8–68°F (16–20°C), which is just right for babies. Overheating has been linked with SIDS (see p.31). At night, dress your baby in a onesie and sleep suit, then add a swaddle or baby sleeping sack until they seem cozy.

During the day, your baby should wear roughly the same amount of clothing as you, plus one extra layer. Avoid putting their recliner next to a vent or fire or in direct sunlight. Keep baby away from drafty open windows. Hats are a good idea when it's cool outside, but babies should not wear hats in bed unless very small or premature, so they can cool down when necessary by losing heat from the head. Babies often become very warm in the car, so they don't need a blanket over them unless it is very cold or you have the air conditioning on. Always remember to remove your baby's outdoor clothing when inside.

Most importantly, relax. In most cases, your baby will look and/or feel obviously cold or hot, and you'll soon know at a glance whether to add a sweater or remove socks!

CONTRACEPTION

You should decide on the form of contraception you want to use now, and discuss it with your doctor. While the time it takes for fertility to return is very variable, it's important not to take chances. Exclusive breastfeeding day and night gives 98 percent protection against pregnancy until your baby is 6 months old, if your period has not returned. However, it's possible to find out your are pregnant again within weeks of your baby's birth. Your periods usually return between 4 and 10 weeks after birth if you are bottle feeding or combining breast and bottle.

DEAL WITH DIAPER RASH

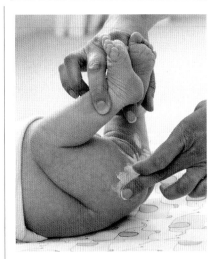

Barrier cream Zinc oxide topical cream can soothe any inflammation as well as protect your baby's skin when their diaper is soiled.

Contact with urine or feces irritates your baby's delicate skin and can result in diaper rash. To prevent this, change your baby's diaper frequently. If their bottom does become sore, let them play and kick about without their diaper on at least twice a day, to allow the air to get to the area. If you use reusable diapers, give them an extra rinse. Apply barrier cream to encourage healing, but if the rash does not clear up in a couple of days, see your pediatrician who will check for thrush and may prescribe an antifungal cream.

Getting your baby to sleep

If you can recognize when your baby needs to sleep, you can catch their wave of tiredness and send them off into a peaceful slumber.

An overtired baby can be difficult to calm, so settle them down to sleep as soon as you notice they are tired, when they will be more likely to fall asleep quickly and sleep deeply. The length of time that your baby goes between naps will be individual to them, so it's important that you recognize when they are ready to sleep. In general, it will come after a period of wakefulness.

Throughout the day and night, your baby will have drowsy periods when they are more ready to fall asleep. If you miss one window, you may have to wait an hour or so for the next. Look out for yawns and eye rubbing—obvious signs of drowsiness. They may cry a little for no obvious reason, or make little grunts of growls that eventually reach a full-blown cry. Some babies frown when they are tired, while others become a little jerky—probably in frustration! Don't try to your baby awake when they're tired—overstimulation takes that much longer to unwind.

ASK A DOCTOR

My baby brings up a little milk after each feeding. Are they sick? It's normal for babies to "spit up" a little milk after being fed—a result of trapped air surfacing, bringing up a little milk with it. It doesn't cause any pain or discomfort. To prevent spitting up, handle your baby gently after a feeding and when burping. If they are bringing up large amounts of milk, they may have reflux (see pp.369–70), so go see your pediatrician.

Taking a break

Although it can be tempting to take total charge of your baby, especially if you are breastfeeding, regular breaks will refresh you.

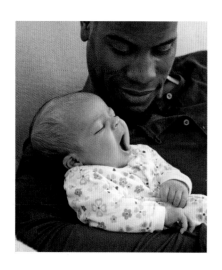

Family time Family members need to get to know your baby and understand their care, too.

You may be one of the many parents for whom it's difficult to relinquish control. However, it's important to take time off to recover fully from the birth. Whether you have a long soak in the tub, meet a friend, exercise, or get some sleep, a break from routine will make all the difference to your physical and emotional health.

Your partner, or other family members, will welcome the chance to hone their skills and spend time bonding with the baby. They will develop confidence in their care, reducing the pressure on you. Set up a regular time for them to take over—perhaps bath time, or on weekend mornings. Even short periods help establish their relationship—and give you a rest.

After around four weeks, if you are breastfeeding you can start to express milk (see p.28) and your partner or other family can take over feeding from time to time. You can then go farther afield during your breaks.

Responsive feeding

Your baby is learning what hunger feels like, and by satisfying that appetite you reassure them and help them feel more secure.

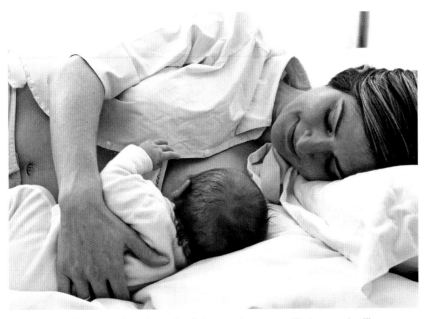

Food and security Let your baby breastfeed whenever they want to. Their tummy is still tiny and can only take small amounts, so they need to nurse on a regular basis.

It is important to continue to feed your baby on demand because they are learning how to respond to their own hunger cues. They will let you know when they are hungry, and when you satisfy that hunger you are not only encouraging trust and security by meeting their basic needs, but you are also teaching them to eat when they are hungry. This can help prevent issues in later life.

By now, your baby may be going three or even four hours between feedings, but don't be surprised if this pattern suddenly shifts. Growth spurts and increased physical activity during the day can make them hungrier, and they may seem to nurse endlessly as they work to build up your milk supply.

DEAL WITH COLIC

To ease symptoms of colic (see p.68) burp your baby after feeds (see p.49). Try a warm bath to calm them down, then rub their abdomen and lower back with warm olive or grape seed oil, in circular motions.

A breastfed baby may react to mom's diet. Reducing the amount of dairy products you eat can make a difference, as can avoiding processed foods that contain milk protein. Avoiding garlic, onions, cabbage, beans, and broccoli can also help. If you do try eliminating these foods, add them back after a few days if you don't notice a difference. Babies and mothers benefit from a wide variety of foods. If you are bottle-feeding, try an anti-colic bottle, which can reduce the amount of air your baby takes in while feeding. You could also try a different formula, but ask your pediatrician first. Colicky babies are soothed by motion, so try a ride in the car or stroller, or gentle rocking in a sling. For babies over 1 month, gripe water (an herbal remedy with baking soda), may help. Colic normally subsides at around 3 or 4 months old—but if you are finding it hard to cope, and nothing seems to be alleviating your baby's symptoms, call your pediatrician.

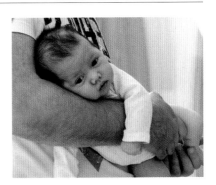

Colicky babies Hold your baby face down along your forearm with your hand firmly between their legs. Try walking around a little, too.

Conflicting advice

There is no harm in listening to well-meaning advice given by friends and family, but don't feel under any obligation to act on it.

Everyone, from your mother-in-law to the butcher, has very clear ideas about how babies should be treated and cared for, and how children should be raised. It can be very disconcerting to find that, in the eyes of some people, you are doing everything, well, wrong.

One of the most important skills you can learn as a new parent is to sift advice—develop a thick skin, listen politely, and then ignore what doesn't fit in with your parenting philosophy. This skill will be useful not just now but throughout your parenting years. When people are offering advice, no matter how experienced, remember that times change, and that everyone has their own ways of doing things. So what may have been standard 20 or 30 years ago may not be appropriate now. Also, every baby requires tailor-made care. Trust your own knowledge, and politely deflect advice and criticism. Try anything that sounds useful, and take in practical tips if you want to, but stick to your instincts and do things your way.

ASK A PEDIATRICIAN

My baby's scalp has large patches of loose, dry skin. Is this eczema? Your baby has cradle cap, a common condition characterized by yellowish, oily, scaly patches on the scalp. To help control the itching and discomfort, lightly massage a baby-friendly emollient (moisturizer) onto their scalp to loosen the scales. Using a soft brush, gently brush over their scalp to loosen the scales, then carefully wash your baby's scalp with baby shampoo.

Little explorer

Your baby is starting to show an interest in all the new things in their world, and nothing is more fascinating to your baby than their own little body.

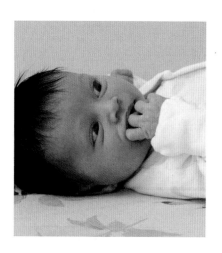

Oral discovery Babies examine and test things out using their tongues and lips.

Around this age, your baby discovers their hands and, possibly, their feet. They'll look at their hands in wonder, and bring them to their mouth. This provides entertainment and develops early hand–eye coordination. Within their of vision, hands are easy to focus on—wonderful "toys" that appear in and out of vision and capture attention for long periods. Your baby won't know the hands belong to them for some months yet, though.

As your baby's neck muscles get stronger, they will turn their head toward noises and try to maneuver into a position to see you. Their eyes may open with interest when a face or a toy is held within sight, and if you move it away, they may try to follow it. This is the beginning of tracking (see p 79). Hang a mobile so the objects are about 12 in (30 cm) from their head. Your baby's eyes will move to examine it.

Switching diapers

Now that you're feeling a little more settled, you might consider different ways of doing things, such as switching to reusable diapers.

Many parents choose disposables in the early days because they are more convenient, and save the presence of an ever-growing pile of dirty diapers threatening your sanity! But as life begins to take on some semblance of a routine, you may find that you can now rearrange your time to wash diapers—or even investigate a diaper service. Babies grow very quickly, so if you have already been using reusables, you may need a new set now.

If you haven't yet used reusables but are thinking about doing so, now could be a good time to make the switch. Once your baby is about 10 lb (4.4 kg), you can purchase diapers that can be adjusted to see them through to potty-training days. So at least you won't waste any money on buying the tiny ones. According to a 2023 review, reusables were more cost-effective and environmentally friendly than disposables. There's also research to suggest that the shape and design of reusables offer better support for your baby's posture, and can help keep their legs apart, in a "frog" position, that benefits the development of their hips.

Of course, disposable diapers have their advantages, too, including being super absorbent and easy to put on and take off. So there's no reason to change if you don't want to. Even if you prefer reusables, disposables are handy from time to time—on vacation, out and about, or even when you're just busy and washing diapers is one task too many.

YOUR POSTPARTUM CHECKUP

There are just a couple of weeks to go until your postpartum checkup by your doctor to make sure you have fully recovered after the birth of your baby (see pp.92–93). In some cases, an appointment will be made for you by your doctor's office, but you should call and check what the procedure is—you may need to make the appointment yourself. It's a good idea to start jotting down any questions or concerns you have now so they don't slip your mind during the checkup.

SMILING YOUNG BABIES

It is possible that you've seen your baby smiling in their sleep, and giving a fleeting grin from time to time. This type of smiling is known as "reflex" smiling, and it can occur from birth until about eight weeks old. It is believed to make infants more attractive so they are cared for. Social smiling, which occurs in response to stimuli (such as your smiling face, or a familiar song) is known as "learned" smiling, and can occur as early as four weeks, although usually at 6–8 weeks. But even contented babies might be 12 weeks before they smile. You'll know it's the real thing when your baby smiles with their entire face, including their eyes.

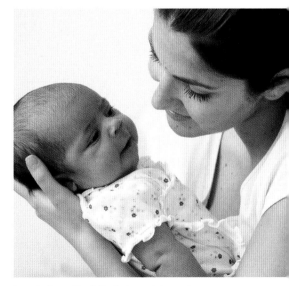

Is my baby smiling? Until about eight weeks, a baby's smile is the result of a built-in reflex rather than a responsive gesture.

1 month

BABIES HAVE MORE THAN 300 BONES; MANY FUSE TOGETHER OVER TIME TO MAKE 206 ADULT BONES.
Although your baby still needs plenty of support, they already trying to hold up their head on their own. They may even lift it briefly when they are resting against your shoulder or on their tummy. Their hands are held in fists for the first few months, but they'll soon start to open and close them.

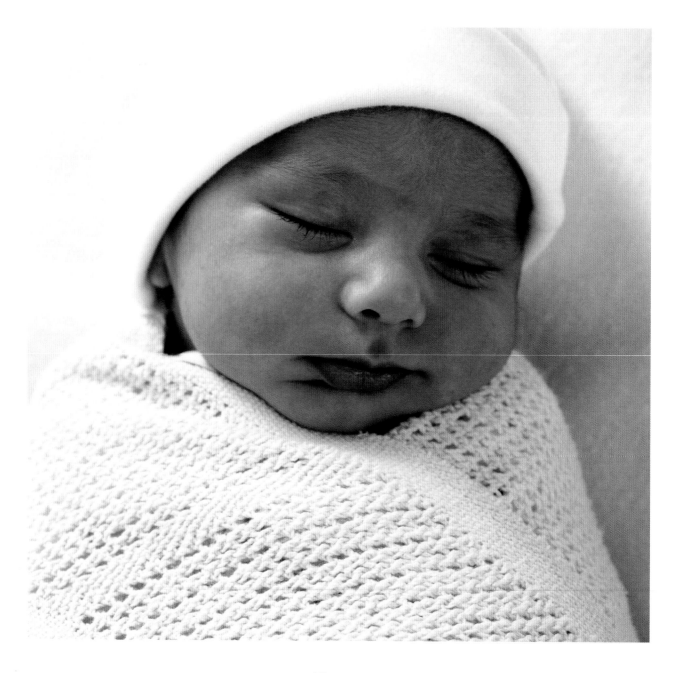

Tracking objects

One of the most exciting developments in your baby's vision is
the fact that they can now begin to "track" an object as it moves.

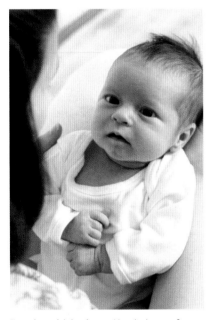

Focusing with both eyes Your baby can focus
but can't see very far, so keep objects of
interest within 12 in (30 cm) of their face.

At first, your baby moves their head
in order to move their eyes, so a
massive movement is required to
keep their eyes pinned on a moving
object. Initially, they move their head
only horizontally to track objects,
largely because it is easier to move a
head from side to side than to lift it up
and drop it down. If you pass a rattle
in front of their eyes, they'll try to
move their head to the side to follow it.

In time your baby will start to move
their eyes independently of their
head and develop "eye-teaming"
skills, in which they use their eyes
together. So don't worry if they look
cross-eyed from time to time—in the
coming weeks, their eyes will be
better coordinated because they will
have more control of the nerves
and muscles to keep them from
crossing.

Your baby will find it easier to track
objects that are highly contrasting—
your face, for example, or black-and-
white geometric shapes and lines, will
catch their attention and encourage
them to focus. Hold the object of focus
in their line of vision and move it
slowly from side to side. Their eyes
will lock on to it. Gentle movements
are easier to follow than fast, jerky
movements.

Over the coming weeks, you'll notice
that your baby will track things longer,
and show much more interest in the
things they track. By three months,
you can begin to encourage their
vertical tracking skills. For now,
though, celebrate their wonderful
new achievement.

FOCUS ON TWINS: TELLING IDENTICAL TWINS APART

Although every parent of identical twins
will tell you that there are subtle
differences between their babies, the
truth is that most parents of identical
twins do struggle to tell them apart from
time to time, especially in the early weeks,
when the different personalities of each
baby are not yet established. It can be
much easier to know which is which
if there is an obvious difference, such as a
birthmark, a fuller head of hair, or a
different timber of cry.

Many parents choose to color code their
children—with red for one and blue for the
other, for example. You can choose to
keep on your baby's hospital band for a
little longer than usual, just to
differentiate between them, and then
color-code their clothes so that you'll
know who is who. Rest assured that,
within a few weeks, their minute
differences will become clear, and these
will become very big differences with
every month that passes.

ASK A DOCTOR

**I seem to be leaking urine when I cough
or laugh. Shouldn't things have tightened
up down there by now?** It can take a while
for ligaments and muscles to tighten up
after pregnancy and childbirth. Like all
muscles, your pelvic floor, which supports
your bladder, needs to be exercised
regularly to become "fit." If you didn't
practice these exercises (known as Kegel
exercises, see p.65) during pregnancy, it
can take longer to tone them after the
birth, but it's never too late to start.

Taking time out

It's easy to forget that you and your partner had a relationship before parenthood. Take up any offers of babysitting and find time to be together.

No matter how much you enjoy being a new parent, there are times when you long for an adult conversation and to get out of the house. Yet, parenting is tricky, and requires plenty of planning, negotiating, and agreement to keep everything afloat.

Your relationship requires the same input and effort that it always did to keep it strong, so it is important that you and your partner spend time alone together. While there is no reason why you can't schedule "dates" at home, it's refreshing to go out and focus on each other, without the interruptions and distractions that life with a new baby brings.

A grandparent or close, trusted friend can take over for an hour or two. Choose a time when your baby is usually happy and fed, or likely to be asleep. Use this time to enjoy your partner's company; try not to talk only about the baby. Talk about other things, and relate as adults in a relationship, not just tired parents. Your relationship will enjoy a new lease on life, as will you!

ASK A PEDIATRICIAN

When will my baby sleep through the night? Most babies don't sleep through until around six months (and sometimes later).Your baby's tummy is tiny and digests feedings quickly, so needs regular refueling, even at night. Also, they need the reassurance of being close to you. Comparatively, breastfed babies sleep lightly and wake more often. Don't panic. Rest when they do, keep nighttime feedings quiet, and remember—this stage won't last forever.

Enjoying sounds

Your baby is now starting to make sense of the world's sounds and will respond to loud and soft noises and, best of all, music!

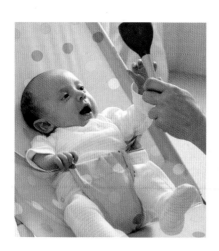

Your baby will listen carefully when a sound catches their attention. They'll turn their head to find out what's causing sounds. Loud noises may startle, and a lullaby may soothe. Watch your baby's response when you whistle or drum your fingers on the table. Play lively music and watch as they kick their legs or listen with interest. Play a softer melody and your baby will likely quiet and visibly relax. Some studies show that music can affect a baby's nervous system, easing anxiety.

Use music in playtime to stimulate and add to the sense of fun. Play different types of music according to your mood and point out the sounds that make up your baby's environment. Your baby will begin to associate sounds with the activities they denote, so they'll hear the water running and eventually realize this means bath time.

Great shakes Your baby will be interested in hearing a variety of different sounds.

Night and day

Many babies don't have their body clocks set to your schedule, spending long hours awake at night, and sleeping through the day.

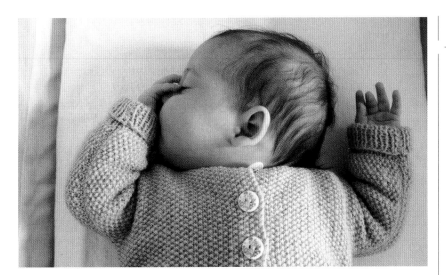

Daytime sleep To help your baby differentiate between daytime sleep and nighttime sleep, keep the room light during the day, and don't block out household sounds.

Although it makes sense to sleep when your baby does in the early weeks, they do now need to be edged more toward a practical sleeping plan so that you both get the rest you need. Babies need plenty of sleep during the day, but there should now be periods of activity between naps. At night, aim for the opposite.

In the daytime, put your baby to sleep in a stroller or bassinet in a light room other than the bedroom. The light entering the room will work on the baby's pineal gland in the brain, which governs sleep and wakefulness, and they'll be much less likely to sleep for very long periods than if the room were dark. Also, they'll be more likely to wake at an appropriate time if there is a little background noise going on.

Make the day stimulating enough to promote sleepiness at night. If your baby is napping and feeding all day, they are unlikely to be physically tired enough for prolonged nighttime sleep. Wake them up from long naps with plenty of cheery talk, play, and songs, and fill the waking day with stimulating activity.

At night, handle your baby very quietly and efficiently, and resist the temptation to talk. Put your baby back into the crib after changing and feeding, making it clear that playtime is not at night. Your baby might fuss, but will soon get the message.

DEVELOPMENT ACTIVITY: MOBILE ENTERTAINMENT

A mobile over your baby's bed, floor mat, or even changing table, if you have one, will be visually stimulating and encourage them to "track" objects (see p.79), which also strengthens their spatial perception. Choose bright colors, which will catch their attention, and, if possible, a model that can be wound up to move in a gentle, baby-friendly circular motion. Music is a bonus, too, since it can soothe, or stimulate, depending on what's best.

Your baby's bassinet or floor mat is a safe place to relax and play, and you can get to other household activities while they watch and listen to this new toy.

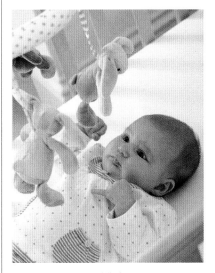

Around they go A mobile hung over your baby's crib gives them something to focus their attention on.

Feeling up and down

Having a new baby changes life dramatically, and it can be difficult to manage to begin with, which can leave you feeling a little low.

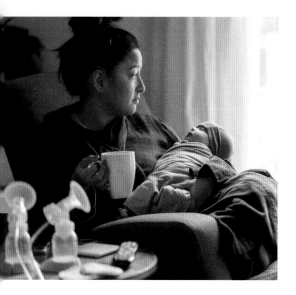

No matter how happily you anticipated your life with a new baby, the reality can be exhausting and a little stifling. You may miss regular contact with friends and colleagues and feel lonely. You may be shocked by the fact that you can't manage to get anything done during the day other than caring for your baby.

Don't feel guilty about these emotions—they don't mean you don't love your baby or enjoy being with them. This is a period of adjustment to

Downtime Taking care of a new baby can be very tiring and it's perfectly normal to have mixed feelings in the early days.

a new way of life, guided completely by another person. Most of us like to feel in control of our lives to some extent, and life with a baby is about as far away from that as it gets. It can help to arrange get-togethers. Pop your baby in a carrier and to go the office to show them off. Get out into the fresh air and change your routine from time to time. Rest assured, soon, life will take on a more regular pattern and you can plan more.

Take some time for yourself. Ask your partner to take over for an hour and give you a welcome respite from baby care while you read a book, or even just feel the sun on your face.

You and your body

Pregnancy and birth can change your body. Although that can feel surprising or strange, the new you is something to celebrate.

After childbirth, you might glow, even if you feel tired; or you might feel a bit flat and body conscious. Your tummy is likely to be less swollen now, and for most, it's good to feel that your body is your own again, free from the rigors of growing a new life! If you're not quite at that stage yet, don't worry. You have adjusted to the physical rigors of pregnancy, and it will take time to restore a sense of

normality in your body. If your breasts are bigger now you're breastfeeding, enjoy your voluptuousness. If you have stretch marks, remind yourself that they'll fade over time. Eat healthily and enjoy some physical activity when you can, and do this to remain healthy and give you energy, rather than feeling you need to fit back into your jeans.

ASK A DOCTOR

I'm breastfeeding and my periods have returned! Is this normal? Although most do not see the return of their periods until around six months, they could start as early as four weeks or as late as a year after the birth. For this reason, do not presume that breastfeeding offers you a reliable form of contraception.

Expressing milk

Expressing your milk allows you to buy yourself a little freedom and your partner to get involved with feeding your baby.

Some women start expressing around now with a view to continuing to breastfeed when they return to work, or because they want more flexibility and someone else to give their baby a feed every so often. You can express milk using a pump (see p.28) or by hand (see box, right). The best time to express is when you are relaxed. You'll soon figure out when in the day you have the most milk—many women find they have very full breasts first thing in the morning. Give your baby a feed from one breast, and either simultaneously express from the other or take a warm bath, pop your sleeping baby in a bassinet next to you, and express what's left.

When you express, your breasts will produce more milk. However, it can take a few days for your milk supply to catch up, so express small amounts and let your baby suckle at your breast often. You might notice that your breast milk looks watery in comparison to formula or cow's milk—but it's the perfect consistency for your baby.

If breast milk is immediately frozen, it will last up to four months. Store it in plastic feeding bottles with secure tops, or you can buy sterile bags made for this purpose. Write the date on the bottle or bag so that you know when you need to use it by. Freezing breast milk destroys some of the disease-fighting antibodies it contains, but its nutritional value is not affected. Defrost frozen milk in the fridge overnight, or place the bottle or bag in a bowl of warm water. Don't use the microwave or the stove to heat milk, since this kills some of its nutrients.

EXPRESS MILK BY HAND

Some women find it easier to express by hand than they do being attached to a pump. Make yourself comfortable, preferably with your baby nearby. A warm bath first may relax you. Cup your breast with one hand and use the other to press the breast so the milk in the milk channels travels downward toward the areola. Now use thumb and forefingers to squeeze the breast tissue to press out the milk, but try not to touch the areola. Keep pressing and releasing—you'll find a comfortable rhythm. It can take a few minutes for your milk to flow. If you are struggling, imagine your baby suckling or even reach over to touch them to encourage let-down. Rotate your hands to reposition them from time to time, which encourages flow by stimulating the sinuses (see p.26).

Have a clean bowl or sterilized bottle ready to collect the milk. Express each breast until the flow slows down—for perhaps five minutes or so. You can go back and forth between them until your breasts feel empty. If you are putting your freshly-expressed milk into the freezer, remember to add a label with the date.

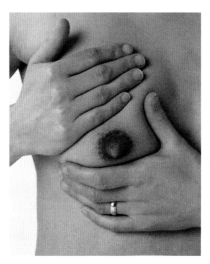

Manual release Press the breast to start milk flow. Then, avoiding the areola, gently squeeze and release the breast between thumb and forefingers, using both hands.

Freshly expressed breast milk can be stored in the fridge for up to five days at 39°F (4°C) or lower or in the freezer for four months at no higher than 0.4°F (-18°C).

Baby talk

Constantly talking to your baby can help them develop
language and communication skills.

You may be surprised to find that you are, quite unexpectedly, narrating your day-to-day activities to baby, speaking slowly, using a high-pitched, singsong voice—and that baby is responding. This is a natural, instinctive method of communication that parents use, known as "parentese," and it occurs in every language in the world. Studies have found that babies pay more attention to and prefer this type of speech. It encourages communication between parent and child and helps babies learn the rudiments of language. Using baby talk doesn't just interest your baby and hold their attention; it helps them pick up words more quickly than without it, and contributes to their mental development.

You may feel uncomfortable speaking in a slow, high-pitched voice with a simplistic vocabulary (or even babble) and lots of repetition, but your baby will find it soothing and will actually begin to understand you—and the nuances of language. Talking to your baby has an incredible effect on their development, so don't hesitate to chatter away as you take care of them. Explain what you are doing as you go along. They won't understand the meaning of words at first, but over the coming months they'll learn that these sounds are labels for your actions or objects around her.

Studies suggest that talking to babies helps them identify where words begin and end, and provides them with the clues needed for them to develop language skills. You'll find that most adults—and even children—adopt parentese when speaking to babies, and this is an instinctive way of speaking that will reap long-term rewards.

Sharing the load

Co-parenting has never been more usual for families than it is today, so if
you plan to share childcare, it's important to start as you intend to continue.

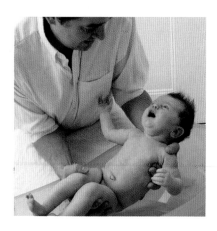

It's good to share baby care with your partner—your baby gets to bond with both of you and ensures neither of you feels less confident than the other. Your baby will enjoy cuddles from you both, and will become familiar with the ways each of you has developed to care for and soothe them.

Taking turns When you and your partner take an equal share in baby care, you divide the load and both learn new skills.

Talk to each other about how to divide the workload of caring for your baby and running the home. Try not to undermine each other's methods— if your baby is happy, it's fine.

If you're bottle-feeding, it's preferable that only the two of you feed your baby in the early days since this is prime bonding time. If you're breastfeeding, once you've settled into it, you can express some milk so your partner can feed the baby, too.

Bottle-feeding know-how

Whether you're using formula or you plan to start, or you've been expressing milk, here's how to ensure bottle-feeding goes smoothly.

If you are breastfeeding, most experts advise against giving babies a bottle before about five or six weeks to avoid "nipple confusion." Sucking from a bottle requires less effort and babies can get used to drinking milk more quickly. However, if you can establish breastfeeding successfully over the first six weeks, your baby will develop the skills needed and find it less daunting to switch between breast and bottle.

Remember that your milk supply is based on your baby's demands. If they are getting milk from a bottle, they won't be "demanding" it from you, and your supply will lessen. If you are planning to return to work, you should introduce the occasional bottle around now. Some babies will reject a bottle if you wait too long. Once you have expressed milk (see p.28 for more on pumps, and p.83 for information on manual expressing and storing breast milk), give your baby a bottle once a week or so to make the transition to bottle-feeding easier. Heat the milk so that a drop on your wrist feels just warm, and discard unfinished milk. Throwing away expressed milk may seem like a waste, but there's a risk of bacteria growing, which can lead to stomach bugs.

Sometimes even babies who have been bottle-fed from birth can experience problems. If your baby struggles when being fed, check the nipple flow. If it takes longer than 20 minutes to finish a bottle, they may need a faster nipple. If baby chokes or splutters, the flow may be too fast.

INTRODUCE A BREASTFED BABY TO A BOTTLE

Choose a time when your baby is calm and not very hungry. Some babies take to bottles easily, while others are more resistant. If your baby is reluctant, try expressed milk rather than formula, and smear a little of your usual nipple cream around the nipple. Choose a slow-flow nipple shaped like a real nipple to mimic the breastfeeding experience, and open your shirt so your baby feels your skin and warmth. It may take a few attempts for them to accept it.

If you are having no luck, try asking your partner to take over. Sometimes babies smell their mom's milk and know that they are being offered something different—and possibly not as pleasant. If you aren't around, they may accept "different" because it is a whole new experience. If your baby becomes distressed, leave it for another day and breastfeed as usual. The last thing you want is for the bottle to have unhappy associations.

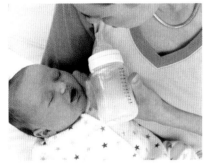

Giving the bottle Gently stroke your baby's cheek to elicit the rooting reflex and insert the nipple carefully into their mouth.

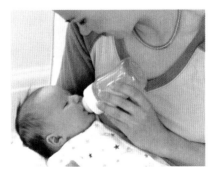

During the feeding Talk to your baby and let them pause mid-feeding if they want. Change sides to give your arm a rest.

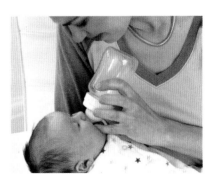

Removing the bottle Gently slide your little finger into the corner of your baby's mouth to stop them from sucking the nipple.

Thinking about safety

Now that your baby has a little more control of movements, use these tips to keep them safe.

Ensure your baby is supported, positioned, and held at all times, so they don't suddenly jerk out of your grasp or roll off the bed. Remove electrical cords and dangling cords of curtains and blinds away from your baby's bed, play, changing, or feeding areas. Never leave medicines, small objects, household plants, or plastic bags within your baby's reach. Always remember to fasten the harness on your baby's bouncy chair and car seat, even when they are sleeping and immobile. Avoid leaving your baby alone, even for short periods, unless they are on a flat, safe surface (ideally the floor) or strapped into their seat or stroller. Keep your baby's bedding tucked safely under their arms, so they don't draw it up and over their face. Similarly, put them to sleep at the bottom of their crib so they don't wiggle down under the covers.

COMFORT ITEMS

Your baby has the mental capacity to remember familiar objects, so now is a great time to introduce a comfort item. A soft toy or cuddly blanket are ideal—buy two, in case one gets lost. If you bring out the comfort item whenever you soothe your baby, they will associate it with comfort. This encourages self-soothing by giving them a tool to encourage happy, positive, relaxing feelings.

Making new sounds

Your clever baby may have increased their vocabulary already, moving on to double-syllable sounds with the occasional consonant.

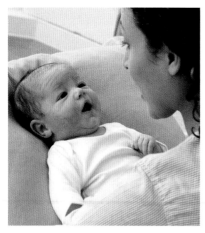

Make baby talk Encourage your baby's communication skills by "chatting" to them.

Cooing and gurgling, and even giggling, may be becoming second nature to your baby, and they'll be excited about communicating with you and other members of the family. Their babbling is their first attempt at speech, and you'll notice huge leaps in their baby vocabulary over the coming months as they practice the sounds they've been learning to make.

Your baby is learning the basics of conversation and the art of listening and responding. According to linguists, babies can tell the difference between similar syllables, such as "ma" and "na," at about four weeks. Repeat the sounds they make back at them. They'll love to know that you understand what they're trying to say, or the emotion they're attempting to communicate. They are most responsive when they are with familiar people, and when they are spoken to in parentese (see p.84).

Vowel sounds, such as "ah," "uh," "ooh," and "oh," are the first sounds babies make. These graduate to double vowel sounds, such as "ah-uh" and "ooh-ah," before a consonant such as "g" or "m" appears. "Ahh-gooo" may become your baby's favorite means of expressing pleasure.

Listening and learning

Your baby's hearing faculty is quite sensitive. This makes them a great listener and means that sound is a good source of information for them.

Even before your baby was born they could hear your voice and the voice of your partner. Now that the baby hears them every day outside the womb, and understands the link between those voices and their continued well-being, they find them highly comforting. Given that your baby likes to hear your voice so much, make the most of it—talk to them (see p.84) and sing songs. Hearing your voice around helps your baby feel safe and secure.

Repetitive sounds

Particularly when they are accompanied by repetitive actions, such as the "pop" in "Pop Goes the Weasel," repetitive sounds help babies learn expectation and predictability, and cause and effect. Some experts believe that repetitive sounds can help to improve babies' memories.

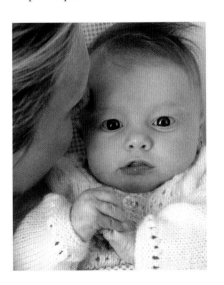

New sounds

Unexpected sounds can make your baby startle—they might fling their arms in the air, raise their knees, or even cry. Reacting negatively to sounds affirms that your baby's hearing is working as it should. Comment on the noises your baby hears to teach that noises are normal and have meaning. Babies who live with noisy siblings may even learn to tune noise out!

Spotting a problem

Your baby should be noticeably calmed or become distracted by your voice—although the pause in their activity may be only brief and you will have to watch for it carefully. In addition, if you clap your hands behind the baby's head, they should startle. If you think your baby consistently doesn't seem to respond to your voice or loud noises, consult your pediatrician, who can arrange a hearing test to ensure everything is developing normally.

Often, though, babies simply learn to ignore the noises around them, especially if they feel secure; also, young babies can sleep through a large amount of noise. Full-term babies rarely experience hearing problems, unless there are other members of the family who have them.

Listening to family Your baby is your most devoted audience; they love to hear your voice.

DEVELOPMENT ACTIVITY: PLAYING MUSIC

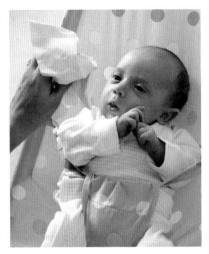

Exploring sounds Introducing your baby to new sounds, such as the sound of crinkling paper, is good for sensory development.

Some studies suggest that babies who are exposed to many musical styles develop a good ear for sound and musical appreciation when older. Music, particularly classical music, may encourage neurological pathways to develop in the newborn's brain, improving thought processes and stimulating "alpha" brainwaves, which are associated with feelings of calm.

Bring different styles of music into your baby's life. Perhaps play lively, upbeat music in the morning, sing nursery rhymes at playtime, and play soothing classical music when you want to create a sense of calm for a sleep.

Downtime for baby

Raising a relaxed child partly depends on how relaxed you are, so
it's important to include a little bit of wakeful downtime every day.

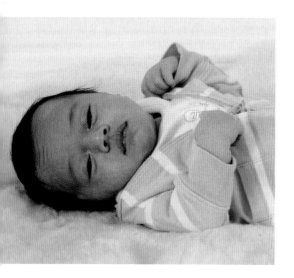

Quiet time Give your baby quiet time on their
back to explore the world on their own.

It is healthy for babies to spend some time each day looking around, taking in their world without you directing them. Otherwise you will have an irritable, overstimulated infant. It takes time to find the balance between playtime and downtime, but as you learn to read your baby's signals this will become easier.

Downtime is important, but make sure your baby has short bursts of tummy time every day, too. Be mindful of the amount of time your

baby spends lying on their back, particularly if they are awake and active. When your baby is born, their skull is soft. Too much time lying flat can result in some babies developing flat head syndrome causing the head to look asymmetrical (plagiocephaly) or to widen causing the forehead to bulge out (brachycephaly). Usually, neither problem is a cause for concern and both are quite common, affecting about 1 in every 5 babies at some point. Over time, the head shape usually improves by itself requiring no medical intervention.

Your social network

Meeting friends lifts your spirits, gives you a change of routine,
and introduces your baby to the idea of social company.

Whether you meet up with friends, visit a parent-and-baby group, or join an online parents' support group, sharing experiences, swapping tips, and enjoying adult conversation can be invaluable. Having other parents to talk to can reassure you that your concerns are likely to be common.

Spend time with positive people who respect your philosophies. If you come away feeling as if you are not living up to collective expectations, it

may be the wrong group for you. This should be an uplifting experience that increases your confidence.

Be mindful of what you post online; "sharenting" is the action of parents using social media to share news, images, or videos of their children. This practice raises issues around consent and leaving a long-lasting digital footprint, which may have implications long term.

ASK A PEDIATRICIAN

My baby hates tummy time. Is there any way to encourage them? Babies need about 30 minutes of tummy time each day in order to develop important muscles, but it doesn't have to be all at once. Plan three 10-minute sessions. If your baby fusses, distract with a song or a toy to eke it out! Choose a stimulating play mat, and get down on your tummy, stroke their back, and talk to them.

It's bedtime

Now that your baby is almost six weeks old, they'll probably respond well to their bedtime routine and feel better about being left alone.

It will probably be some time before your baby sleeps through the night, and they will continue to wake up frequently to be fed or comforted as the weeks go by. No matter how tired or frustrated you may feel by these night wakings, try to stay calm and respond to their needs as quickly and quietly as you can. A baby who knows that their parents will come when they need them is more secure, and will be more likely to develop self-soothing skills early on.

Good sleep patterns are dependent upon a gentle bedtime routine, which helps your baby unwind and anticipate the series of events that will ultimately lead to longer periods of restful sleep. Rowdiness with a parent who returns from work won't relax them, so keep things calm and quiet, giving a bath, a lovely feed, and a lullaby before settling them down to sleep. Babies love repetition, so sing the same song every night to help them understand what's coming next and anticipate it with pleasure.

Stay with your baby if they need you and reassure them of your presence. Don't tiptoe around the house while they drift off—let your baby hear the familiar sounds of your voice and normal household activities. They'll know you're there, and will get used to sleeping in noisier environments, so won't be startled awake by tiny sounds.

All babies need daytime naps, and babies who have regular naps find it easier to sleep well at night since they are well-rested and used to being put down to sleep. If you get your baby down at the first sign of sleepiness (see p.81), you'll miss that second wind of energy.

Finally, don't sleep train your baby yet or leave them to cry. At this stage, they needs a warm, loving routine that makes them confident enough to fall asleep and settle back to sleep when they wake, knowing you're there if they needs you.

YOUR BABY'S HAIR

When your baby is born, their hair may be thick or thin, dark or light, standing on end, or neatly coiffed as if they've just stepped out of a salon. What a baby's hair will be like at birth is as unpredictable as anything else. Even if both parents have blond hair, the baby may be born with dark hair and vice versa. Very often, if your baby is born with hair at all, it will fall out over the course of the first few months of life, to be replaced by something more in keeping with the rest of the family!

Your baby may develop a bald patch on the back of their head, where their head rests when they're lying down; this is perfectly normal, and once their "real" hair comes in, the patch will disappear.

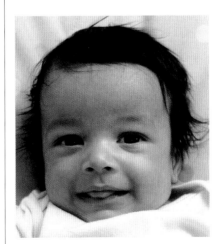 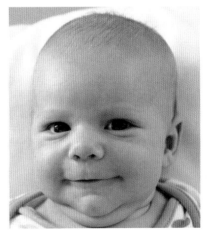

Thick hair Any hair your baby had at birth may fall out in the first six months and then grow back in a different color or texture (left). **Fine hair** Babies born with no hair, or very fine hair, may stay like that well into the first year (right).

Extra feeds

By this time most babies start to sleep longer at night than they do during the day.

Around now, many babies have a growth spurt, making them hungry and demanding, so be prepared for extra feeds during this time. If you're lucky, your baby might smile properly for the very first time right about now. However, many babies don't manage to smile until around two months of age.

Between now and 3 months, your baby will start to respond to certain sounds—first by turning their head and changing their facial expressions, and then by actually cooing and gurgling. They're really beginning to communicate.

First smiles Up until now, a baby's smiles are likely to be a reflex action or as a result of gas. However, they will move on to giving gorgeous, purposeful smiles.

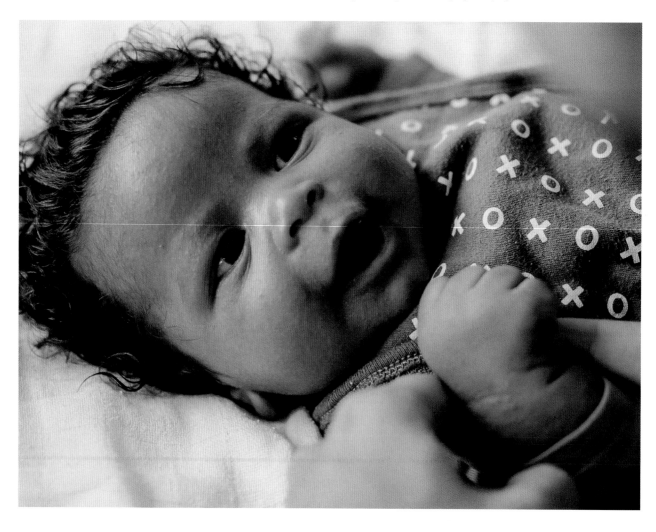

Time for a growth spurt

You can expect a rapid and intense period of growth any time now—sometimes it can seem as if your baby has become bigger overnight!

Restlessness during sleeping, extended periods of sleeping, and, most obviously, an increased demand for food are all signs that your baby might be having a growth spurt, especially when they appear in combination. Many breastfeeding mothers mistake increased restlessness and feeding demands for signs that they are not producing enough milk—however, if these signs occur around the six-week mark, it is far more likely that a growth spurt is the cause.

During a growth spurt, it can be really difficult to establish a fixed routine of feeding your baby, and any routine you thought you'd established can seem to disappear since your baby constantly seems hungry. Your milk supply will respond to your baby's demands, so it's important that you feed them whenever they ask for food so that your body steps up the quantity of milk it produces to satisfy them. It's also important to encourage your baby to empty each breast fully, so that they get plenty of fatty, filling hindmilk. Usually, their feeding pattern will settle down again pretty quickly as the growth spurt passes, often within only a few days.

If you are bottle-feeding your baby, it may be time to increase the amount you give, but only by 1 fl oz (25 ml) at a time. Consult your pediatrician if you are unsure.

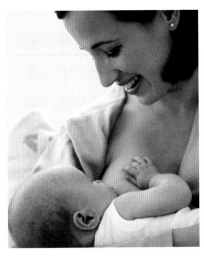

Hungry baby Feed your baby as often as they want; the amount of milk you produce depends on how much they nurse.

NEWBORN SIZE UP

If your baby was more than 8 lbs (3.6 kg) at birth, they may not have worn newborn sizes; however, the average baby normally outgrows the smallest-size baby clothing between five and eight weeks—sometimes sooner. If things are starting to look a little tight (particularly at the feet), keep your baby comfortable by moving them up a size. Clothes designed for 0–3-month-old babies should get them through the month, but be prepared to be flexible. Take your baby along when you go shopping and hold the clothes up against them; allow for shrinkages in the wash and an upcoming growth spurt. When in doubt, go a size larger. They'll be into 3–6-month outfits in no time at all!

ASK A BREASTFEEDING EXPERT

My baby seems hungry all the time. Can I give a bottle of formula as well as breastfeeding? Although your milk supply should now be established, it will increase over the coming months to meet your baby's needs. Around this time, your baby will be undergoing a growth spurt, and want to feed more often to fuel that growth. Nursing will increase your supply to match your baby's new demands, so it is important to put them to your breast as often as they want. It's not a good idea to give extra bottles of formula at this stage because your breasts will not be stimulated to make enough milk for your baby. So if you want to continue breastfeeding successfully, try to avoid this. It usually only takes a few days for your breasts to catch up, so bear with it and feed your baby frequently.

Your postpartum checkup

When your baby is around six weeks old, you will visit your own doctor for a checkup. This routine examination is to check that you are doing well, and that you're coping with your new life as a parent. This is a chance to discuss any concerns you have.

The postpartum checkup, also known as the six-week check, is usually done by your ob/gyn in their office. By the six week mark, your body should have recovered from the birth. Your uterus should be back to its normal size, the lochia flow has likely stopped, and any stitches should be healed.

Checking your physical health

It is likely that, as with your prenatal appointments, the first checkups your doctor will perform will be to take your blood pressure and, possibly, to test a urine sample. Six weeks after birth, your blood pressure should have returned to normal levels (below 140/90), even if you suffered from either high or low blood pressure during your pregnancy. Your urine may be checked, especially if you had high blood pressure during pregnancy, have high blood pressure now, have any urinary symptoms, or if you had gestational diabetes.

If you are breastfeeding, your doctor will ask you about your breast health—whether you have any soreness or cracked nipples, and so on—and will perform a physical examination if you want one. They will also be ready to answer any concerns that you may have about breastfeeding.

Increasingly, doctors are conscious you should adopt good dietary and exercise habits after giving birth to speed your recovery and to help you achieve appropriate weight loss. For this reason, your doctor may weigh you and advise you, if necessary, about an appropriate diet and activity that will help you reach your pre-baby weight. It is advisable to wait until you have this checkup before embarking upon any significant exercise program, because your body will take at least six weeks to recover properly from childbirth.

Your doctor may ask if you would like them to check any stitches and healing in your perineum if you had a tear or episiotomy. They will ask if your vaginal bleeding or discharge has settled down and if you've had a period yet. You will also be asked whether or not you have had intercourse, and if so whether you experienced any pain. This is also a good time to talk about contraception, and whether you have any concerns. If you haven't had a pap smear test in the previous three years, the doctor will encourage you to have one done once the baby is more than three months old.

Checking your emotional health

Your doctor will want to know how you are feeling emotionally following the birth. They will ask if you have experienced any low times, how well you are sleeping, and how you are coping with the demands of being a new parent, including asking about your support network. None of these questions is intended to find flaws,

ASK A DOCTOR

My baby's belly button sticks out. Could there be a problem? Belly buttons come in all shapes and sizes, so how your baby's umbilical stump will detach and what their belly button will look like is entirely unpredictable. However, if it protrudes significantly, especially when your baby strains or cries, they may have an umbilical hernia. This harmless condition occurs when there is weakness in the muscles around the umbilicus, where the cord was attached. Most umbilical hernias clear up on their own in the baby's first year without medical intervention. Occasionally, however, babies need a simple surgery. It's a good idea to mention a protruding belly button to your pediatrician, so if there is a hernia the condition can be diagnosed and monitored.

When will my hemorrhoids go away? Hemorrhoids are common in pregnancy, and can also occur as a result of pushing during labor. In many cases, they disappear within a couple of months of the birth, and you can encourage this by eating a diet rich in whole grains, fruit, and vegetables, drinking plenty of water, and exercising regularly (including Kegel exercises, see p.65). Raising your feet when using the toilet can help when moving your bowels. If it's painful, not improving, or you have bleeding, see your doctor.

and it's important that you answer honestly, voicing any worries or concerns you have (about any aspect, physical or emotional) about your own or the baby's well-being. Your doctor will be careful to look for signs of postpartum depression so that, if you do seem susceptible, you can receive the support you need as quickly as possible.

Questions about birth control

Birth control options depend on whether you are breast- or bottle-feeding. Bottle-feeding moms can use any form of birth control, but breastfeeding moms are limited to those that don't contain estrogen, since it can affect milk supply. Ask your doctor about the forms of contraception suitable for you. Condoms are a good option, as is an IUD.

It is likely that your six-week checkup will go smoothly and not bring to light any serious concerns. However, if your doctor has any worries about any aspect of the checkup, they will suggest appropriate follow-up appointments to make sure that any potential problems are caught and tackled, or dismissed, at the earliest opportunity.

AFTER A CESAREAN

Your doctor will check that your incision is healing, and that you don't have any discomfort. By six weeks, most women can do many of their essential everyday activities, such as bathing, housework, baby care, and some gentle lifting. However, some women continue to find it difficult to lift heavy things and to have sex until much later. Don't do anything that feels uncomfortable. You can drive again as soon as your doctor confirms that it's safe. And you've probably been able to carry around your newborn for a few weeks now with little or no discomfort.

CHECKS FOR YOUR BABY

Your baby also receives a checkup at 6 to 8 weeks of age at the pediatrician's office. The examination is similar to the one they had at birth. You'll need to undress them, so dress them in clothes that are easy to put on and take off, and take a spare diaper.

• **Bones, joints, and muscles** The doctor will lay your baby on their back and gently manipulate each leg to check that the hip joints have the full range of movement. The doctor will straighten your baby's legs to make sure they are the same length, and check that the spine is straight and other joints are functioning properly. The doctor will check that your baby's fontanels have a healthy appearance (that they aren't bulging or sunken; see p.97), and may check how the neck muscles and head control are developing, either by observing your baby as you hold them on your shoulder or by observing some tummy time.

• **Heart** Your doctor will check your baby's heart sounds and pulses to help rule out congenital heart problems.

• **Reflexes** Your pediatrician may use some simple tests to check how your baby's reflexes are developing.

• **Eyes** Looking into your baby's eyes with an ophthalmoscope will reveal any congenital problems, such as cataracts. The doctor will also check that your baby can track objects (see p.79).

• **Other** Your doctor will feel your baby's abdomen to check for hernias. If you have a boy, the doctor will check that the testes have descended properly into the scrotum sacs.

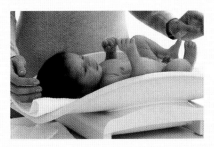

Weight check Weighing your baby and plotting the reading on their growth chart will help make sure that they're gaining weight at an appropriate rate for their age.

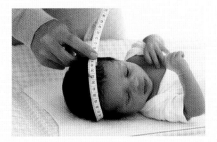

Checking baby's head Your baby's head circumference provides an indicator that growth is normal and that there are no problems beneath their skull.

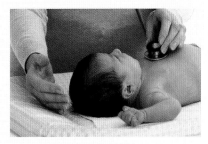

Heart check Listening to your baby's heart with a stethoscope enables a doctor to check whether there are any abnormal heart sounds or murmurs.

Little smiler

Your baby's first smile is one of the most precious moments of parenthood, since it shows things are on schedule and they're happy.

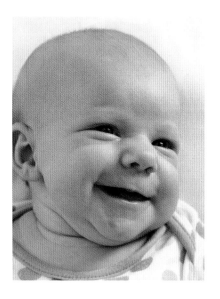

Babies don't smile until they are ready to—even the most contented babies may not break out their first smile until about seven weeks old, sometimes later. However, evidence does suggest that talking to your baby, smiling at them, and making lots of eye contact helps the process along. Baby boys may be slower to smile than girls, but are equally open to encouragement. Once your baby does break that first smile, they'll be so happy with your reaction that they'll do it again and again.

First smile The more you smile at your baby, the more they'll try to copy you and smile back.

Your baby's first smiles will take place in response to familiar auditory stimulation, such as the sound of your voice. By two months, as their vision improves, they'll begin to smile in response to things they see—usually favorite people: you and your partner.

Once your baby has learned to smile, they have reached the first milestone in their ability to communicate in a manner other than crying. This first smile seems a wonderful reward for all your work! Soon they'll be smiling at other familiar faces, such as siblings and grandparents. The bigger the fuss you make of their smiles, the more they'll repeat them.

Grasp reflex

Your baby has little control over their movements yet, but they'll try to grasp if you give them something to reach for.

Your baby will automatically grasp anything that is placed in their palm, because their newborn grasp reflex is still in place. However, they're also becoming more aware of what's around, so if they see something that attracts them, they may try to stretch out or wave their arms and grasp it.

Instead of just watching that toy, your baby may lift an arm toward it in an uncoordinated motion. It will be a long time before they can actually open their hand and then close it around the object in a conscious movement, but they may well grasp something by accident rather than by design, even if many of their movements are undertaken with a clenched fist. Now's a good time to make sure there's nothing within reach that they could pull down upon them. Your baby may also reach for dangling hair, jewelry, or scarves, so watch out!

Your baby's kicks and arm motions are still a little jerky, but they will slowly become more graceful and intentional as their muscles and nervous system continue to develop. They may also start to kick and wave their arms in excitement or enjoyment.

Improving vision

By now, your baby's eyesight will have improved dramatically compared to how it was at birth.

At birth, your baby could focus on objects that were about 12 in (30 cm) away—roughly the distance between your breast and face. They are now able to focus at distances up to 24 in (60 cm). This increase is due to brain development, as the brain becomes more effective at interpreting data and processing it into clear pictures. You may also find that they start to focus on parts of their body, particularly the hands (see p.106).

Your baby has developed some special cells called binocular cells that help improve their ability to distinguish depth. However, they still can't move her eyes in perfect unison, and their ability to perceive depth properly is still a month or so away.

Color and shape
It takes a while for the brain to distinguish colors, especially shades of a single color. By the time your baby is six weeks old, their brain will begin to decipher red, green, and yellow, with blue coming a little later. They prefer distinctive shapes to straight lines, and research suggests that a special part of a baby's brain is attuned to recognizing faces, which is why they will focus on a face, and learn to smile in response to it.

Movement
Your baby should be able to follow movement with their eyes, if only briefly (see Tracking objects, p.79).

(see p.106).

ASK A PEDIATRICIAN

My baby boy has an undescended testicle—will he have to have an operation? Normally, the testes (testicles) develop inside your baby's abdomen, then drop into the scrotum during the second half of pregnancy. By the time your baby is born, his testicles should have descended into his scrotum. Sometimes they remain in the groin, and this is known as "undescended testes." If they are not released into the scrotum, they will not be able to produce sperm later in life—and are at an increased risk of developing cancer. Try not to worry. In some cases, testes move down on their own, usually by 12 months. If your baby's testes don't, he may need an operation known as an orchidopexy, which would be carried out just before his first birthday. Your doctor will monitor the situation, and talk you through the procedure.

Sometimes when I'm washing or changing my baby I notice he has an erection. Is this normal? Yes, this is normal. The penis is very sensitive and all baby boys have erections from time to time, some more than others. They have even been observed to have erections in the womb.

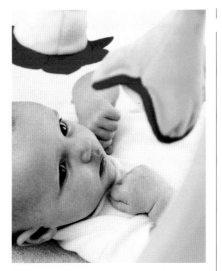

Seeing in color At six weeks, your baby's brain starts to decipher the colors red, green, and yellow, and, a little later on, also blue.

EYE EXAMINATION

A follow-up physical examination is available for babies up to the age of eight weeks old to identify any problems not picked up at birth. As part of this examination, your baby's eyes will be checked. While the examination is not painful, your baby may find parts of it uncomfortable. Using a special light, the pediatrician will look into your baby's eyes to check how their eyes look and move, and for any signs of eye problems.

Resuming intimacy

Sex might not be high on your list of priorities right now, but making time to be intimate together keeps you connected as a couple.

Between six and eight weeks after the birth, your body should have almost completely recovered. Any stitches or tearing should have healed, bleeding (lochia) should have stopped, and your vagina should have returned to its pre-pregnancy size. If you had a cesarean birth, your incision site should be on the mend.

However, after birth, most women experience a significant drop in estrogen levels, which can lead to vaginal dryness. For most new parents, however, lack of desire has more to do with fatigue and adjusting to new parental roles than with hormones.

If you're worried that intercourse might be painful, talk to your partner and let them know what you are comfortable with. If you don't feel ready for full intercourse, consider foreplay instead. Be sensitive to each other's needs and patient with one another. If you want to have intercourse, take it gently at first and try using lubricant to ease penetration.

Finally, be aware that sex can trigger the let-down reflex, which may cause milk to leak from your breasts during lovemaking. Also, you'll need to use some form of contraception if you don't want to get pregnant again, even if you are fully breastfeeding and have not had a period.

Peak period for crying

If your baby seems to be wailing nonstop today, take heart: studies show that crying is at its most fervent around this time.

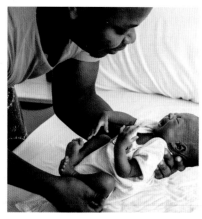

Frequent crying At around six weeks, crying is often as bad as it will ever be and should become less of a problem by three months.

Usually babies cry because they want attention, a feeding, or a diaper change, but there are also other likely causes.

Some doctors believe colic (see p.68) peaks at six weeks, causing persistent bouts of crying, often during the evening, which can be distressing for all. If this is the case for your baby, there's little you can do except to wait and reassure yourself that it is usually significantly reduced between 10 and 12 weeks old.

A growth spurt (see p.91) makes your baby more hungry and more liable to fuss. Some theories suggest that this is because crying triggers the body to manufacture more milk to meet the baby's increased demands.

Learning new skills, such as smiling, and becoming increasingly alert, can be tiring for young babies and crying provides a release for this.

Carry your baby in a sling or rock them gently in your arms to reassure them. Take comfort that this phase will pass. Enlist the help of friends and family if you're struggling to get things done or need a break for an hour or so. If you are finding it difficult to cope, your pediatrician can support you.

Starting to get active

If you were given the all clear at your six-week health check, now might be a good time to start easing your body back into physical activity.

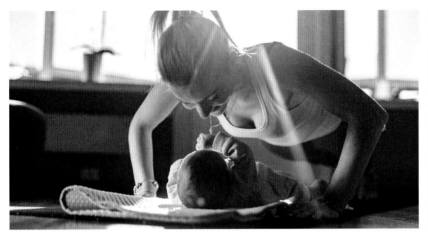

Making time for movement Some postpartum yoga classes incorporate baby yoga, too. Yoga can help you regain strength in your back, stomach, and pelvic floor muscles, in particular.

Every female body responds to pregnancy in its own way—so be realistic. If you were very toned before becoming pregnant, and if you had an active pregnancy, you are likely to regain your fitness more quickly—but it isn't a foregone conclusion. Whatever your underlying fitness level, make your goals achievable and don't expect too much too soon—the truth is that you may never get back the same body you had before, but you can certainly be as healthy, if not healthier.

Take it easy
Pregnancy and childbirth put your body through a major trauma. Ease yourself gently into exercising, taking things at a slow pace to start with. Your joints and ligaments will still be loose for around three to five months, so stick to low-impact exercise and avoid anything too vigorous or jerky, which could potentially cause injury.

Spend some time both before and after exercising doing a few gentle stretches to warm up and cool down. If, at any point during exercise, something hurts, stop immediately.

How much, how often?
Initially, aim for about 5–10 minutes of toning exercises every day, and 20 minutes of gentle aerobic activity three times a week, if you can. You can increase both as you become more fit and your body feels stronger. Never push yourself beyond what feels comfortable or achievable.

You'll have to figure out ways of making time for exercise with a baby:

THE FONTANELS

There are two soft spots on a baby's head, one at the back and the other on top of the head. The fontanels allow a baby's head to pass through the birth canal. The posterior, triangular fontanel, located at the back of the head, will close when a baby is about four months old, while the one on the top of the head (the diamond-shaped, anterior fontanel) takes between nine and 18 months to close.

It is normal to see your baby's head pulsating in time with their circulation. When your baby cries, the fontanels may bulge a little, and then return to normal. If they bulge more than usual or become sunken, contact your pediatrician. Sunken fontanels may be a sign of dehydration while bulging fontanels might indicate a serious illness, head trauma, fluid buildup, or internal bleeding. Seek medical advice if your baby shows signs of distress.

perhaps sharing baby care with a friend so you can take turns to exercise. You could even take your baby with you to a stroller-pushing exercise class held in a local park.

Include your pelvic tilts and Kegel (pelvic floor) exercises (see p.65) to help prevent postpartum incontinence. And try yoga. Postpartum yoga classes adapt the yoga postures to account for the fact that you have recently had a baby.

Active baby

Your baby is beginning to practice their new muscle control—wiggling a lot more, kicking, and twisting their body from side to side.

This is the perfect time to introduce a baby gym. Your baby's control over their body has improved, so they will enjoy batting at hanging toys, and reaching out toward things. They may even manage to grab them, although they won't be able to intentionally close their fist around them yet. If you put something in their hand, they'll hold on—and chances are, they won't let go!

Their arms and legs will wave furiously when they are excited—or even angry—and diaper changing will become much more trying. You may find that they respond to music by slowing down their movements or speeding them up, accordingly.

Your baby's new interest in using their body may keep them awake at night as they work on honing their skills and inadvertently kick awake. Some parents introduce a baby sleeping sack at this time, so baby stays warm throughout the night. If Your baby has a low-hanging mobile, move it up a notch, since they may decide to bat it down.

ASK A PEDIATRICIAN

Is it okay to let my baby have a pacifier? A pacifier won't harm your baby's health or development provided you use it responsibly. If it helps soothe them, there's no reason why not. But do be careful if you're breastfeeding that you don't give your crying baby a pacifier when what they really need is feeding, as this could affect your milk supply. Try not to use a pacifier all the time, just when you're trying to settle or comfort your baby.

Studying shapes and colors

Your baby is showing much more interest in complex designs and shapes, and is now able to distinguish more colors.

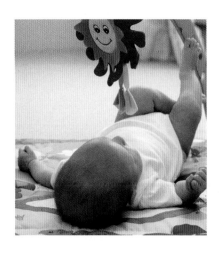

Your baby can now focus both eyes on an object, and will show a preference for more complicated designs, colors, and shapes. They'll still love faces—yours, family members', and other babies'—the most, but they'll be very intrigued by high contrast, colorful objects, which will be able to keep them mesmerized for many minutes at a time.

Colorful toys Your baby will try to reach out for anything that is moving, so surround them with interesting, vibrant objects to stimulate and entertain them.

Encouraging your baby to look at objects of interest will help strengthen pathways in their brain and develop vision—but make it fun and don't overstimulate. Your baby will be awake longer, and have more opportunities to explore the environment.

While your baby could once focus only on black-and-white and bright colors, they can now recognize interesting patterns and a wide range of colors, which is one reason why baby toys are manufactured in a rainbow of colors.

Your baby's vaccinations

An important part of preventative health care is immunizing your baby against illnesses that may seriously harm them later in life. Your baby will be given an immunization timetable, which is important to follow.

While a baby's immune system develops lifelong immunity against illnesses by acquiring them, many are dangerous, with a high risk of complications or death, so over the coming months, your baby will be immunized against serious illnesses. By immunizing your baby, you also help largely to eradicate diseases from the population.

Immunization begins at birth and prepares your baby's body to fight diseases it may catch in the future. For example, the polio vaccine stimulates the immune system to produce antibodies against the polio virus, which later recognize the disease if and when it enters your baby's body, and are ready to fight it.

In most cases, vaccines provide lifelong immunity, although some need a booster every 10 years or so. It is possible to show symptoms of mild forms of some diseases by immunization, but the risk of complications is much lower than if your baby acquired the full-blown disease. It's natural to be concerned that combining several vaccines could overload your baby's system, but there is no need to worry. Your baby's immune system becomes more mature by the day, and is already capable of protecting them from a wide range of organisms causing infections that they come into contact with all the time. Their system can very easily deal with the existing combined injections.

There is a small risk of side-effects, such as a mild fever and some weak symptoms of disease. It is unusual for a baby to experience an allergic response, but natural to experience some tenderness, swelling, and redness at the site of the injection. They may be irritable and fussy, and sleep more than usual. A dose of pain medication and a quiet feeding should soothe them. Rest assured: vaccines have a well-researched, high safety record.

Keeping track

Your baby's immunizations will be noted down on their medical chart, but you may want to keep your own record of the date of each immunization and any symptoms or side effects. Some parents like to note the brand name of the vaccine for future reference, in case they move to another part of the world at some point, or the schedule of immunizations changes for any reason.

Making your baby comfortable

Feed your baby before their vaccination to calm them. Stay calm and talk to them and reassure them in a soft voice, or distract them with a pacifier. It will be over in a few seconds, and they may not even notice it's happened. If they cry, hold them and talk to them gently. They'll be back to their usual, happy self in no time.

IMMUNIZATION SCHEDULE

Birth:
- Hepatitis B (first dose)

1–2 months:
- Hepatitis B (second dose)

2 months:
- Rotavirus (RV; first dose)
- Diphtheria, Pertussis, & Tetanus (DTAP; first dose)
- Haemophilus influenzae type b (Hib; first dose)
- Pneumococcal disease (PCV13/PCV15; first dose)
- Polio (IPV; first dose)

4 months:
- RV (second dose)
- DTAP (second dose)
- Hib (second dose)
- PCV13/PCV15 (second dose)
- IPV (second dose)

6 months:
- Hepatitis B (third dose)
- RV (third dose)
- DTAP (third dose)
- Hib (third dose)
- PCV13/PCV15 (third dose)
- IPV (third dose)

Between 12 and 15 months:
- Measles, Mumps, & Rubella (MMR)
- Chickenpox
- Hepatitis A (first dose; second dose to be given at least 6 months later)

- Vaccines for COVID-19 and flu are recommended beginning at 6 months.

More regular feedings

Your growing baby should have settled into a pattern and be able to take in more milk at each sitting, and go longer between feedings.

YOUR BABY MONTH BY MONTH

ASK A PEDIATRICIAN

My baby seems to be uncomfortable after a feed, and is suffering from diarrhea. What should I do? If you are breastfeeding your baby's poop will often be soft, runny, and yellow in color. Whereas if you are using formula milk, your baby's poop will tend to be firmer and a pale brown, green, or yellow color. It is quite normal for your baby to have occasional runny poops while their digestive system adapts. You will be able to tell if your baby has diarrhea if their poop has a stronger odor than usual, is more watery, causing leaking diapers, or if your baby is pooping more frequently than normal. If your baby's diarrhea persists and they have other symptoms such as vomiting, arrange to see your pediatrician.

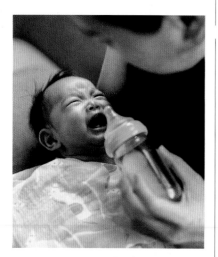

Upset tummy Speak with your pediatrician if baby appears distressed after a feed.

Milk is still your baby's only source of nutrition and liquid, so it's important not to "schedule" them into a routine that leaves them hungry or thirsty. Breast milk is digested more quickly than formula so, a breastfed baby may feed more often than a bottle-fed one, but the gap between feeds will increase over time. Bottle-fed babies often sleep longer through the night than breastfed babies, but that's no reason to make the switch to a bottle.

You'll ideally want to empty both breasts at every feed, so your baby gets the right balance of liquid and nutrition (see p.27); however, you may find that your baby is satisfied after just one breast. Make a note of the times you feed your baby and the breast from which they last fed to remind you which breast to give first at the next feed, and also see if there is a pattern to the feedings. If the baby is not gaining weight as expected, they may be snacking a little too often, rather than taking in a full, long feed.

If you are bottle-feeding, keep a note of feeding times and the amount. At this age, most babies are having six to eight bottles of 4–6 fl oz (120–180 ml) in 24 hours.

If you wish, tweak your baby's schedule in small ways: you may feed on demand during the day, then wake your baby before you go to bed to fill them up so that they sleep longer at night, for example.

LACTOSE INTOLERANCE

Some babies find it hard to digest the natural sugar (lactose) found in both breast milk and formula milk. Babies who are lactose-intolerant suffer digestive discomfort, such as diarrhea, vomiting, and colic, which can cause distress and result in constant crying.

Lactose intolerance is very rare and occurs when there is a lack of the enzyme lactase, which helps the body digest the sugar in both breast milk and formula milk. Lactose intolerance is more common in premature babies as the level of lactase builds up toward the end of the last trimester of pregnancy.

Sometimes, babies can develop lactose intolerance for a short period of time after suffering from a stomach bug or prolonged use of antibiotics.

A baby suffering from a cow's milk allergy may present with similar symptoms. While it is one of the most common baby allergies, it is still relatively rare with less than 2% of babies diagnosed in the US. If you are worried your baby has a cow's milk allergy or is lactose intolerant, you should seek medical advice.

Fun bath times

If your baby has so far been reluctant to take a bath, a few toys and gentle splashing games may persuade them to start enjoying one now.

Bath time can be much more fun now that you can add a few bath toys to the tub for your baby to play with. They may be excited by the fact that they can cause waves by kicking their legs.

Gently splash the water and use a small cup or bath toy to pour warm water over your baby—they'll love the experience, and be interested in the movement of the water.

Sing, laugh, and speak in a gentle, upbeat voice to encourage them to see bath time as something positive. They're more likely to smile and enjoy the bath if they see your smiling face. Singing a relaxing song, or finding one they can begin to associate with bath time, can help keep them calm and happy.

Now that they're a little more mobile, it's a good idea to use a nonslip mat for the bottom of your tub. Make sure you have a good grip on your baby, since they'll be very slippery, particularly if they're trying to maneuver into a different position. If they're still in the sink or a baby bath and displacing most of the water before the end of the bath, it may be time to move on to the tub!

If your baby still resists a bath, consider bathing with them. Gather everything by the tub so you can step into a robe and get baby dried off first. You may need your partner to hold the baby while you get into and out of the water. Remember that babies can't tolerate hot water in the same way we can, so resign yourself to a slightly cooler bath—no more than 99°F (37°C).

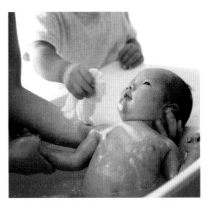

Fun time Bath time is a great opportunity to have fun and to bond with your baby.

Sleeping well at night

Grabbing a nap when your baby sleeps may be your only option in the early weeks, but you will, over time, want a good night's rest.

Being woken in the night can be frustrating, no matter how much you enjoy feeding your baby. If your baby is right next to your bed (or sleeping with you), you can feed them quickly while still half-asleep yourself. If their diaper isn't too wet, you can probably leave a change until later, too. It may sound difficult to believe, but you'll soon go on "auto pilot" at night and feed them without really waking up!

If you do wake up and can't get back to sleep, do some of the relaxation exercises you practiced during pregnancy, and try not to focus on how many hours of sleep you are not getting. Avoid alcohol or caffeine in the evenings. Try a glass of warm milk, a banana, or a bowl of oatmeal before bed; these foods contain the amino acid tryptophan, which will encourage restful sleep. If you are breastfeeding, it may enter your milk supply to help your baby sleep well, too!

Finally, about an hour before bed, have a warm bath (not hot, which can be overstimulating), and take some time to unwind. Doing chores is not an ideal pre-sleep routine!

2 months

AN INVOLUNTARY RESPONSE, THE "GRASP" REFLEX THAT BABIES ARE BORN WITH PERSISTS FOR THE FIRST FEW MONTHS. As your baby's muscles become stronger, they may be able to push up a little when on their tummy. They'll "discover" their hands around now and find them endlessly fascinating. They'll want to reach out and grab things, but may not succeed for several weeks.

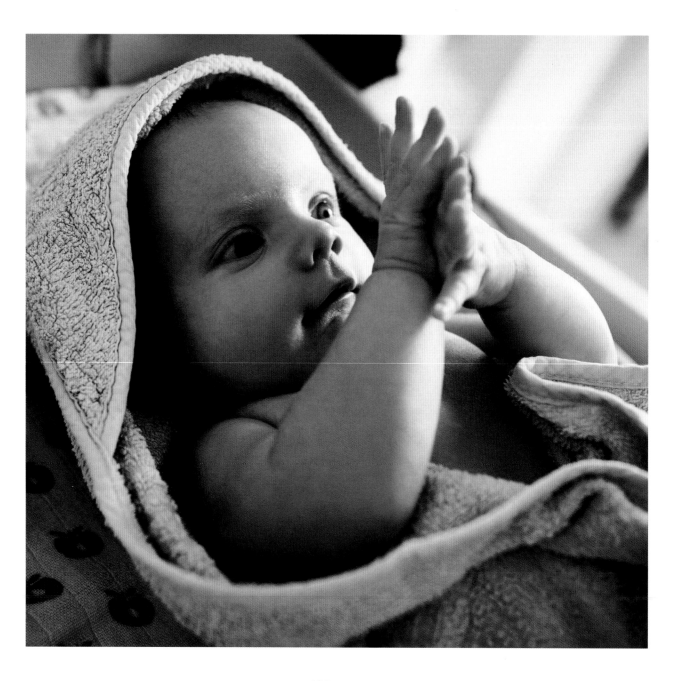

Your baby's immune system

Now that your baby has reached the two-month mark, they may need a little more help from you to protect them from illness.

At two months old, your baby's "reserve" of antibodies (primarily from their time in the womb) begins to run dry, and they are more susceptible to illnesses. This is the point at which babies begin their immunization program (see p.99).

If you are breastfeeding now, you will continue to protect your baby with the five most important types of antibodies. Breast milk also contains a type of white blood cells, called lymphocytes, that help your baby fight illness. This is "passive immunity," because it is passed to your baby rather than developed by them. Your baby will be protected against many, if not all, of the diseases to which you are immune. Breastfed babies have been shown to get sick less often, and experience less severe symptoms when they do become ill. Your baby's own immune system starts to kick into action in the first few weeks of life, but does not mature until later in childhood, which is why children can get so many colds!

Hygiene

Keeping your environment clean will help protect your baby against illness. This doesn't mean dousing the household in antibacterial solutions, but simply keeping anything they could put into their mouth (such as bottles, teething rings, equipment for making up bottles, and pacifiers) scrupulously clean. This will prevent a buildup of bacteria that could cause

stomach upsets, and also prevent the transmission of viruses from other members of the family.

Vet your guests

Although it can seem absurd to turn away visitors who are suffering from a cold or another illness, it is a good idea in the early weeks of your baby's life while your baby is less able to fight off the infection. Bacterial infections can also be very dangerous in little ones. Ask guests (and family members) to wash their hands regularly, dispose of any used tissues, and avoid holding your baby until they are healthy.

Sick babies tend not to feed well, and even a little weight loss can affect a baby's overall strength and development. Any baby with a fever should be seen by a pediatrician as a precaution (see p.369).

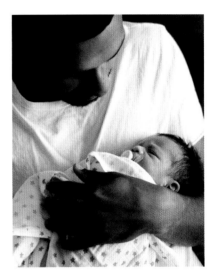

A close eye If your baby seems sick, monitor them and call your pediatrician if they worsen.

ASK A PEDIATRICIAN

How can I tell if my baby has an ear infection? It's difficult to know without seeing a doctor. Ear infections are common after a cold, but there aren't many specific symptoms. The ear won't be red, and although some babies will rub or bat their ear, many also do this when tired. Crying, irritability, high temperature, vomiting, and even diarrhea can all be due to ear infection (see p.378). There may be a discharge from the ear, which suggests that the

infection has perforated the eardrum. At this stage your baby may appear better, but it's still important to see the doctor. Antibiotics aren't routinely given since many ear infections are viral, but the sicker the child, the more likely they are to get antibiotics, and this is often the case with babies. Ask your doctor what medicine is appropriate to relieve your baby's discomfort.

Dressing up

Spending a fortune on baby clothes isn't practical, but shopping for a special occasion will be fun and provide some priceless photos!

A special occasion may give you just the excuse you need to buy something beautiful for your little one.

Before you head straight for the frills and tiny suits, consider the nature of the occasion. If your baby will be passed around to lots of people, or expected to get through a whole day outside their usual environment, try to be practical. Go for something that won't make their skin itch or make them feel uncomfortable, and ensure that it can be fastened and unfastened for quick changes. Tiny buttons, tight collars or waistbands, or anything that constricts your baby's movement or causes them to overheat probably aren't ideal.

Avoid anything too expensive—one leaky diaper or heavy spit-up and off it comes! (Washable is essential.) It may also be a good idea to go for separates so a quick part-change can save the day. Bring along a couple of spare tops and/or bottoms, just to be on the safe side.

DRESSING TWINS

If you have to dress twins for a nice occasion, two outfits will obviously hit your bank balance harder than one, so look for secondhand outfits. Most special outfits only get worn once or twice before babies outgrow them, and nice clothes are often given as gifts and never worn, so you may be able to find something new or almost new, for very little outlay.

Developing memory

Your baby is developing their "recognition memory," which means that they can remember and identify familiar people and objects.

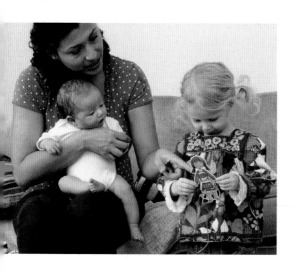

From birth, or shortly afterward, your baby was able to recognize your voice and smell, and soon showed a preference for familiar faces. Now, they will be able to make some general associations. For example, if their older sibling always makes the same silly face, your baby may try to imitate it when they see them. They may gaze at a rattle, waiting for it to make its familiar sound. They will associate you with milk and comfort.

Tuned in Your baby identifies objects and people and remembers more than you think.

Your baby is now building associations based on the repeated link between an action and a feeling; for example, you hold out your arms toward them and they anticipate a feeling of being safe. Over the next few months, these and other associations build rapidly.

This type of memory is a natural, protective instinct that encourages babies to form strong attachments with their primary caregivers. Remembering and preferring familiar faces and objects is a method of keeping themselves safe from danger.

Healthy eating

Being a new parent is demanding work. One of the most important things you can do for yourself is to eat healthy and be well-nourished.

All new moms need plenty of healthy, nutritious food. Dieting now, especially if you're breastfeeding, can leave you short on nutrients, making you prone to illness, fatigue, and mood swings. And if you're preoccupied with your weight, it will affect your enjoyment of motherhood.

Try to base your diet around fruits and vegetables, whole grains (such as whole-wheat bread or pasta, and brown rice), proteins (such as lean meats, dairy, eggs, fish, nuts, seeds, and legumes), and healthy fats (olive and sunflower oil, avocados, and oily fish). Eating this type of healthy diet will provide the essential nutrients you need for optimum health. These, in turn enter your breast milk, so you'll enhance your baby's diet, too.

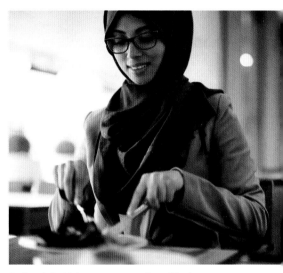

Eating right It's important to eat lots of fresh fruits and vegetables that are nutrient rich.

BOOSTING YOUR ENERGY LEVELS

A good way of maintaining energy as you deal with the demands of early parenthood is to eat little and often. Cheese with apple slices or crackers, or some dried apricots can keep you going between meals and keep your metabolism active. Try the following to help you feel healthier and energized.
• Get a little gentle exercise every day. Walking, swimming, aerobics, and/or yoga (with your baby, of course) can help build muscle, which encourages your metabolism to work efficiently.
• Stay hydrated. Thirst is often mistaken for hunger, and breastfeeding (if that's relevant for you) is thirsty work. You'll need about 2.8 quarts (2.7 liters) of water every day to make up for lost fluid.
• Take all offers of meals made by friends, and get into the habit of batch cooking when you do get a moment in the kitchen.

With a small baby, having some standby meals is always a good idea. If you've got a freezer full of nutritious soups, casseroles, or even delicious fruit-and-oat muffins, you are more likely to eat well, and you'll be less likely to rely on highly fatty or salty prepared meals. It's just as easy to make a quick salad as it is to make a prepared meal, and you will reap the rewards.
• Keep plenty of healthy snacks. Cut some carrots, celery, or cucumber and pop them in some water with a squirt of lemon juice to keep them fresh. Buy salsa, low-fat dips, or hummus. If you long for something sweet, make a fresh fruit smoothie, eat a couple small squares of dark chocolate, or try a bowl of whole-grain cereal with fruit compote and yogurt.

ASK A NUTRITIONIST

How many more calories should I eat each day while breastfeeding?
Breastfeeding moms use up about 500 extra calories each day, but you don't necessarily have to replace them. If your diet is much the same as it was pre-pregnancy, you will naturally lose about 1 lb (450 g) per week without making any changes, as your fat stores will be called upon. If you are exercising a little, you are likely to lose even more. It's best not to think about calories: if you focus on eating a healthy diet, your body will find balance, and that means you will feel and look healthy, too—and your baby will be getting the nutrients they need.

Sleeping like a baby

Your baby may now be going longer between feedings, and sleeping more soundly at night. You'll probably get more sleep as well.

It is more likely that your baby will sleep well if they are comfortable, so it is important to alternate their sleepwear and bedding as outside temperatures change. A hot or cold baby wakes up frequently, even if tired. Keep the bedroom cool, even in winter, using layers of thin sheets or blankets that can be easily taken off or put on. If it's hot outside, it's fine to put your baby to bed in just a diaper and a

onesie, plus maybe a pair of socks. To keep air circulating around the room try using a fan, facing it away from your baby's bed. A gentle breeze will keep them comfortably cool.

If your baby is starting to kick off their covers at night, tuck the ends firmly under the base of the mattress, or around their legs. If your baby is waking themselves up in the night with little jerks and startled

movements, consider swaddling.

A baby sleep sack might come in handy to keep your baby warm no matter how active they are. Choose a quilted cotton sleep sack that fastens at the shoulders for quick nighttime changes. Sleep sacks are available in "togs," much like duvets, so choose a weight that suits the temperature in your baby's room.

Fascinating hands

Your baby's favorite "toys" at the moment are their own hands, which entertain them as they move in and out of their line of vision.

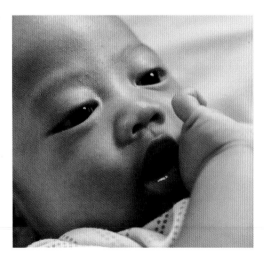

Increased dexterity Your baby now has better control of their hand movements.

Now that your baby is starting to open and close their own hands, they may begin to stare at them in fascination, bringing their hands or fingers toward their mouth, or even aiming them in your direction touching your face or body. They may attempt to bat at objects dangling above their bed or baby gym, or at a toy if you hold one out to attract their attention.

Your baby is a tactile little person and will enjoy feeling new textures. They may unconsciously stroke their own face, clothes, comfort blanket, or anything they come into contact with. Your baby may look up in

amazement when you offer something new with an exciting texture, such as a soft toy with fur or a textured teething ring. Everything is new and interesting, and your baby will enjoy exploring using their mouth and hands.

Try offering a rattle to hold for a moment (they are likely to drop it) or attach a wrist rattle to your baby's arm to attract their attention. Give your baby the space to explore and find out what they can do by themselves.

Stylish nursing wear

If you have breastfed since birth, you're probably ready to ditch the baggy T-shirts and functional nursing bras and update your look.

There's not much point in buying anything new at first, especially while you're using nipple creams, leaking breast milk, and trying to get used to the mechanics of the breastfeeding process. While there's no reason to change or buy new bras unnecessarily, be aware that your breasts do change size during these early months. For this reason, it's worth your time to go for a professional re-measure every so often to be sure you are wearing the correct size. If you do need new bras, there's now a much wider range of colorful, feminine maternity lingerie to choose from, so this might be a good opportunity to treat yourself.

It's a similar situation with clothes for breastfeeding. At first, the most important consideration is comfort, but once you start to feel more like your normal self again, you may want to shop for "normal" clothes in your favorite stores. You can still follow fashion when you're breastfeeding— just go for wrap tops, or low scoop-neck and loose-bottomed T-shirts that can be lifted up and tucked over your feeding baby. Choose cotton and other natural fabrics that won't cause you to get hot while your baby is pressed against you feeding. Look for clothes that will be easy to wash and dry. Take the time to try on any purchases—your shape may have changed. Some stores offer a personal styling service, so take advantage of expert advice.

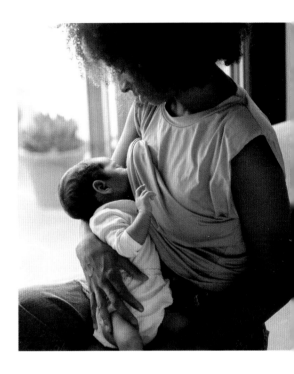

Nursing top There are tops available that are both practical and stylish.

DEVELOPMENT ACTIVITY: FUN WITH SOUNDS

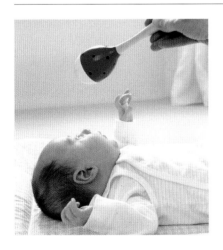

Rattles are wonderful toys for young babies, and as your baby becomes more interested in the world around them, they'll be mesmerized by the sight and sound of their favorite toy in action.

Whether you choose a rattle that attaches to their wrist or a handheld model that can be put in their hand, you will be providing your baby with a perfect first toy. They'll learn hand–eye coordination and develop their muscle control as they figure out how to operate it. Choose a brightly colored rattle that makes a sound easily. The idea is that they will be able to make the toy work themselves—even if it is not through conscious effort. Most toys will end up in your baby's mouth, so choose something soft and easy to clean. The handle should also be easy for their little hand to hold. Be careful, too: their movements are still very jerky and they can easily bop themselves on the head in excitement.

Rattle stimulation Offer your baby a rattle that is light enough for them to grasp. They will no doubt want to mouth and taste the rattle, too!

Getting used to a crib

Help your baby familiarize themselves with this new space, by putting them in their bassinet first before moving them into the crib.

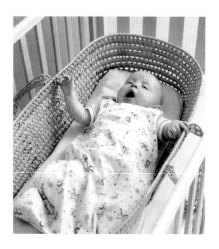

Your baby might be touching the sides of the bassinet by now—and even waking up when they do so. If this is the case, you'll want to move her into a crib. A big crib can be daunting for a baby who is used to a smaller and cozier environment, so it's a good idea to get them used to it gradually before you put them down to sleep in it for the first time.

If you've already bought a crib, it can be a safe place for your baby to play while you do other things in their room. A mobile and a few toys scattered around, or a baby mirror fastened to the side, will capture their interest. They'll become accustomed to the space, so when it is time for them to sleep there, it will be familiar.

Before you make the transition, put their bassinet inside the crib (or nearby) for a few nights. If, when you do first move your baby, they seem distressed at the beginning, try putting them in the crib for daytime naps only. This way, they'll be able to see what's around them and grow more confident. When they're settling nicely in the day, you can consider moving them at nighttime, too.

Moving to a crib Placing your baby's bassinet in the crib for a few nights makes the transition easier for your baby to deal with.

YOUR BABY'S CRIB

If you haven't bought a crib yet, now's a good time to do so. It needs to be strong and sturdy, with no jagged edges or sharp points. Keep in mind:

• If you are buying a new crib, check that it conforms to the new federal requirement. Any crib sold after June 28, 2011, must have stronger slats and mattress supports, anti-loosening devices to prevent cribs from coming apart, and more stringent safety testing. Drop-side cribs, immobilizers, and repair kits can no longer be sold.

• It's better to buy a new crib than a used one, but if you get a used crib, don't use one more than 10 years old or that has been modified or broken. Buy a new mattress, even if your crib is used. It should fit the crib snugly.

• A teething rail is a protective covering—usually made of clear, nontoxic plastic—that lines the side rails of the crib. This protects your baby's gums (and the crib) once they're teething and start to chew.

• When assembling, check that all screws and bolts are secure, so there is no danger of it collapsing. Also, badly installed screws could scratch your baby or even work themselves loose and pose a choking risk.

• Cribs more than 30 years old may have been finished with poisonous lead-containing paint. In this case, the paint must be stripped and the crib repainted to make it safe. Also, the slats may be too far apart, or the side rails not secure

ASK A PEDIATRICIAN

What do I need to consider when positioning my baby's crib? You should keep your baby's crib in your bedroom for the first six months to reduce the risk of sudden infant death syndrome (SIDS, see p.31). Also, position the crib so that it's out of direct sunlight and well away from windows, blind cords or strings, heating vents, lamps, bookshelves, and hanging wall decorations or pictures.

Is a used mattress OK? Always buy a new mattress, even if your baby's crib is secondhand. It should fit the crib snugly, so your baby can't slip between the crib and mattress. Check that it conforms to current safety standards and does not contain fire-retardant polybrominated diphenyl ethers (PBDEs).

Your baby's sleep cycle

Just when you think you've got your baby to sleep, they stir and wake up. What's happening as your little one settles down to rest?

Babies, like adults, experience two different types of sleep: deep sleep or "NREM" (non-rapid eye movement) and light sleep or "REM" (rapid eye movement) sleep. In deep NREM sleep, the body and mind are quiet, breathing is shallow, and limbs are relaxed and loose. In light REM sleep, the eyes move under the eyelids and the brain is more active, which is when dreams occur.

Sleep and brain activity

Over an eight-hour night, adults typically spend 75 percent of the time in deep NREM sleep and 25 percent in light REM sleep, which occurs in cycles throughout the night. In the first few months of life, babies sleep for about 18 hours a day, half of which appears to be spent in light REM sleep. One theory is that lots of REM sleep during the steep learning and growth curve of early life, helps the brain develop new and complex interconnections. Blood flow to the brain nearly doubles during REM sleep, so your baby may appear restless, with fluttering eyelids and twitching arms or legs. Your baby is unlikely to adopt any kind of regular sleep pattern with identifiable NREM/REM cycles until about 4 months old. At this point, they'll probably spend about 35 percent of their sleeping time in light REM sleep and 65 percent in deep NREM sleep.

What to do when

If possible, put your baby down just before they drift into light sleep, so they get used to settling themselves. Once they drift off, avoid moving them from one place to another, since they're likely to wake.

If they seem about to wake up, resist the patting them on the back or talking. Leave quietly, and they'll be more likely to drift back to sleep. As your baby grows older and enjoys longer REM

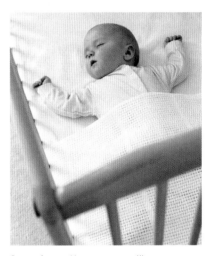

Sweet dreams Your presence will reassure your baby, helping them feel safe and secure.

sleep cycles, they should sleep more soundly during these periods and be less likely to wake.

ASK A PEDIATRICIAN

Does my baby dream? There is evidence to suggest that babies not only dream from the moment they are born, but have been doing so for several months in the womb. Dreams take place during REM sleep, when your baby isn't sleeping quite so deeply and their brain is active, and because they have so many more hours of this type of sleep than we do, they'll be dreaming frequently. Their dreams will usually be based around their experiences of the day, which consolidates learning, emotions, and development. They may have upsetting dreams from time to time, but will be calmed by your soothing voice.

When can I sleep train my baby? Your baby will sleep as much as they need to, whenever they need to, and won't be ready to sleep through the night without a feeding for some weeks. Sleep-training techniques aren't generally started until babies are several months old, and involve encouraging them to sleep longer at night with minimal attention from their parents. This doesn't mean letting them cry, but helping them feel safe enough to fall asleep, knowing that their parents are close by. But it's not too early to adopt a calming bedtime routine, such as a bath, feeding, and a story or lullaby, so that your baby begins to associate this soothing sequence of events with sleep.

Post-baby health issues

If you can't seem to shake off the baby blues and still feel low or upset, it's possible that you're experiencing postpartum depression.

The baby blues affect moms about three days after the birth as a result of hormonal changes wreaking havoc on their emotions (see "Ask a doctor," p.49). The baby blues should usually ease within a couple of weeks, so if you continue to feel low or exhausted, you may be experiencing postpartum depression (PPD).

What is PPD?

Feeling distressed as the weeks go by, having a sense that other moms are managing when you are not, or becoming low during your baby's first year means it's likely you're suffering from postpartum depression. PPD can last for a few weeks or for months—but the sooner you get professional

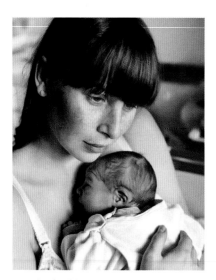

Long-lasting blues If you are still feeling upset, teary, or depressed, don't hesitate to ask your health professionals for advice.

help, the more quickly you are likely to recover.

Typical signs of PPD include:
• Feeling exhausted even when you've just woken up;
• Crying often; feeling empty and sad;
• Guilt and shame that you're not happy or don't love your baby enough;
• Being overanxious in general or fearful for your baby;
• Feeling scared to be alone or go out.

One or two moms in every ten will suffer from postpartum depression. The important thing is to recognize that you aren't well and to get help as soon as possible. Your pediatrician and ob/gyn will recognize your situation and know how to get you help, often suggesting local services to support you. Your doctor may recommend medication, such as antidepressants, and may refer you for counseling.

Postpartum psychosis

A very few women (about 1–3 in 1,000) develop a condition called postpartum psychosis, symptoms of which include severe depression, delusions (believing everyone is conspiring against them or they or others are possessed), hallucinations, and an inability to think clearly. It is essential if you feel this way to visit your doctor. Medication, such as antidepressants or antipsychotics, and therapy mean postpartum psychosis can usually be treated in a few weeks.

POST-BABY HORMONAL CHANGES

The pregnancy hormone relaxin softens collagen and elastin in the tissues. It remains in your body for up to five months after birth. If you are breastfeeding, prolactin, the hormone that produces milk, has a similar effect. As a result, your gums may soften and be prone to bleeding, which can lead to tooth decay. See your dentist to have your teeth cleaned and the state of your oral health assessed.

After pregnancy, hair follicles enter a "resting phase," causing excess hair loss (molting). This occurs any time between two and nine months after the birth. Once your hormones return to pre-pregnancy levels, molting stops and your hair will regrow.

Breastfeeding affects your bones. Moms lose 3–5 percent of their bone mass while breastfeeding, although this is recovered within six months of your periods resuming, or weaning your baby from the breast. This won't have any bad effects; in fact, breastfeeding prevents osteoporosis (thinning of the bones) in later life, but breastfeeding moms do need plenty of calcium in their diet—roughly 1,250 mg per day.

Your wider family

Cherish your relationships with your extended family. They'll provide a support system for you and your baby for many years to come.

Over the past couple of months, you may have seen more of your relatives than ever before, as they admire the new addition to the family. No matter how independent you have been until now, relying little on extended family, and perhaps only meeting on special occasions, all that is about to change. You may already have found that your bond with your own parents is strengthened. Now you may realize how important other family members will be in your baby's life. Though not every parent has close family ties, there are many ways to find a support network (see p.170).

Encourage relationships with family and friends and create frequent opportunities for visits. Relations can become strained when you have conflicting views on caring for your baby, and you may be the recipient of plenty of unsolicited advice. Gently encourage loved ones to respect your ideas and approach, even if they don't agree. Allowing them to establish a loving relationship with your baby is the most important thing.

If you are a single parent, your family and friends will be more valuable than ever for support and guidance, as well as love. It's hard raising a child on your own. You may feel you lack opportunities to talk about your baby's development or even your worries. It can be a pleasure to share your baby's milestones with loved ones.

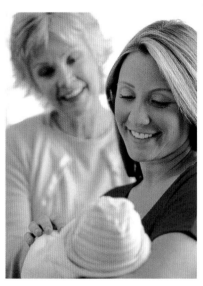

Staying close A strong bond with your extended family will enrich your baby's life.

Distracted baby

Your baby is fascinated by everything that's going on around them, and attracting their attention while feeding and changing may be difficult.

It's easy for your baby's attention to be drawn elsewhere now, which can be challenging when you're trying to nurse. Try feeding your baby in a quiet room that offers fewer distractions. Turn off the TV when you are feeding and talk to your baby quietly so that their focus remains on you. Gently turn your baby's head back to you if they become distracted. Try to establish feeding times when they are genuinely hungry and want a long feed. If your baby is snacking or feeding for comfort, you may find yourself putting them back to your breast or a bottle again and again.

When changing their diapers or clothes they may resist you or wiggle and roll around in order to see what's going on around them. Try to engage your baby by making diaper-changing a more interesting experience: hang a colorful mobile over the changing mat, tickle or talk to them, and work fast so you don't have to deal with their wiggling for long!

Seeing in color

Your baby can now discern a variety of colors and is also starting to develop depth perception, marking the progression to seeing in 3D.

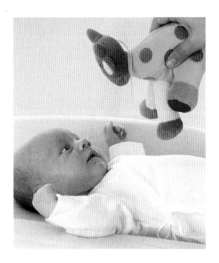

Depth perception will not be fully developed for another four months (usually at least six months), but as your baby's brain and coordination develop, they will be able to discern an object's position, size, shape, and relative distance more effectively. This will eventually allow successful reaching out and grasping to take hold of things. Before this can happen, though, their eyes have to be able to work together. You'll notice your baby's depth perception slowly improving—their eyes will move together but won't always be coordinated in the early weeks, but gradually that will get better and better. It takes a while for babies to see their world as a complete picture.

Depth perception will eventually help keep your baby safe by preventing them from crawling off the edge of the porch, for example, but bear in mind that being able to discern the distance is not all that's needed to stay safe—curiosity will often get the better of them.

Toy time Fun toys that are different shapes and colors will hold your baby's attention.

Hygiene and allergies

Good hygiene prevents illness but don't go overboard with the antibacterial wipes: some contact with germs is important for your baby.

Overuse of antibacterial cleaning products has now been linked with a higher incidence of allergies—probably because a baby's immune system will not be given the opportunity to develop properly without having things to fight. Allergies are a sign of a dysfunctional immune system, and anything that hampers its development in baby- and childhood could make your baby more susceptible. The general rule should be to keep things clean, rather than sterile.

This will ensure that your baby's environment is safe from harmful germs, yet suitable to allow their immune system to develop properly.

Hot water and ordinary bars of soap are perfectly adequate for cleaning your baby's toys (although these should still be sterilized once in a while). If plastic, the toys may be able to go in the dishwasher. Stick with natural cleaners wherever possible around the house. Filling your baby's environment with a host of chemical cleaners can also trigger an allergic response, as well as overload their sensitive system. Normal cleaning products, soap, and water will be enough to keep your house clean and fresh the natural way.

Don't worry about a little dust settling;studies have found that early exposure to dust mites can prevent allergies to them, and it will take the pressure to clean off you. The same goes for pet dander (see also "Pets and your baby," p.122).

Relationship roles

Your lives have changed dramatically and you may feel unsettled and excited by the altered dynamics of your relationship.

No matter how much you adore your baby, if you worked before the birth you may feel baffled by how much your life has changed, and resentful that your partner is able to go out to work while you take on day-to-day baby care. Your career may be on hold and, although it may make financial sense for you to stay at home until your baby is older, you may worry about taking time off from your career and the effect on your progress in the future.

What's more, because you're at home, it probably makes sense for you to take on more of the domestic chores. This can cause an imbalance in the way you perceive your relationship—and the equality within it. In addition, if you're not working, you may not enjoy the same financial independence, which can be difficult to adjust to.

Work out a fair division of labor, bearing in mind that some workplaces now permit new parents to share childcare in the first year. Proactively approach home-life imbalances, by talking respectfully and openly, before they become problems.

ASK A DOCTOR

I had a cesarean and although the incision has healed, I'm still feeling low and tired. How long will it be before I'm back to normal? Every woman recovers from a cesarean birth differently, and although the visible scars may heal within six weeks, some women will take up to six months to regain their full energy. It's also quite common for numb areas on your skin to persist many months after the surgery. Try to take each day as it comes, as with any new mom, and rest if you feel tired. If you experience any pain in the pelvic area, or you feel low and tired, talk to your doctor: there may be a reason (such as anemia or postpartum depression) which can be treated.

I've noticed some very slight spotting of blood following intercourse. Should I be worried? Sometimes, just the manipulation of the cervix, which is still healing, or orgasm (which makes the uterus contract) can cause light spotting. It could also be related to hormonal fluctuations, or if you are using contraception, notably birth control pills. Occasionally, small skin tags form at the site of tears or incisions, which can bleed when rubbed against. Certain infections, such as chlamydia, can also cause spotting after sex. If you have any bleeding after sex, make an appointment to see your doctor.

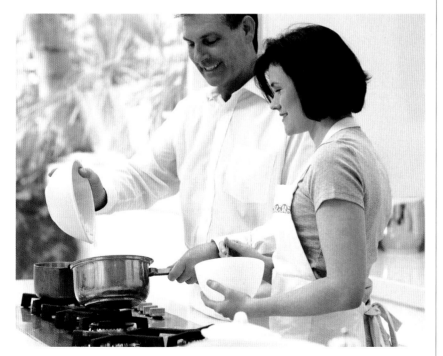

Feeling valued It's important that you both feel that you are sharing the responsibilities of family life as fairly as you can, even though your home life will have changed to adapt to parenthood.

Planning child care

Going back to work may feel a lifetime away, but it's important that, sooner rather than later, you think about who will take care of your baby when you return to work. Deciding on the right child-care strategy is not something you want to feel rushed into..

The best way to begin your search is to draw up a shortlist by word of mouth—ask friends to recommend day-care centers, nanny agencies, and babysitters in your area. You can then check them with your local or state child-care regulatory office. Your baby's well-being is paramount above all other factors. Also, child care may be your single biggest expense once you go back to work, so it's vital to get it right.

Nannies

Hiring a nanny means you'll have someone to care for your baby in your own home. Use a reputable agency and interview each nanny on your shortlist. Have a list of questions ready, covering such topics as how they handle discipline and what kinds of games they would play with your baby. If you need them to be able to drive, ask about that, too. Start by drawing up a full job description, describing every aspect of your baby's day-to-day care—and what you'd like to see happening in the future. Talk these through with each interviewee to make sure that their working practices, beliefs, ideas, and ethics match your own.

Make sure that you interview nannies with your baby, and watch how they interact. You'll want someone who is interested, playful, and affectionate with your baby. Check references and ensure that they have emergency first-aid training.

Make sure they're licensed or accredited, do a thorough background check to ensure they can safely work with children, and talk through issues such as nutrition, exercise, stimulation, and TV watching. Ask for an example of a daily routine, and assess how flexible they might be. If they have to leave on time every evening, you might find that won't work for you. It's also worth asking where they see themself in five years' time. If you are hoping for continuity over the coming years, it would be good to know now if they are planning to move away!

You should draw up a formal contract of employment and meet your legal obligations as an employer, such as paying taxes and social security contributions.

Family childcare

A caregiver takes care of your baby in their home, probably along with several other children. Once again,

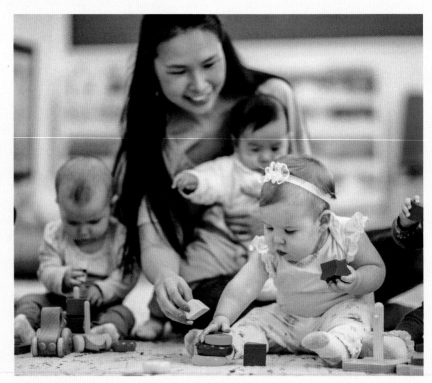

Choosing a babysitter Your prospective babysitter should have plenty of experience with taking care of young babies and juggling their needs with those of older children.

always take time to visit prospective caregivers in their own environment, and bring along your baby to see how they fit in. You'll need to go through all of the issues that you would discuss with a nanny, and ensure that your family child caregiver has plenty of experience with babies and very young children. Is the house clean and welcoming, with lots of suitable toys and books, and space to play outside? Is there a smoker in the house? Or a lot of TVs? Is your caregiver flexible? You don't want to end up with extra charges when you are running a little late. Consider the number of children in their care, and ask how they balance the needs of differently aged children. A young baby needs a great deal of individual care, and you need to be certain that your baby will get the necessary attention. If both you and your baby feel comfortable in the caregiver's home, chances are your baby will be happy there.

Daycare center

Daycare centers provide child care from three months old (although some take babies from as young as six weeks). Visit every daycare center on your list to get a feel for whether or not it has a loving atmosphere and an ethos compatible with your own. Ask about staff turnover, since long-serving staff suggests a happy, supportive environment. (For more tips on choosing a daycare center, see box, right.) The best daycare centers have long waiting lists, so it's never too early to start looking.

Other alternatives

If a nanny, family childcare provider or daycare center doesn't seem right for you, brainstorm to see if you can find a creative solution. You may be

able to plan your schedules so both you and your partner can take on some of the childcare, and get extra help on the days you can't. You may decide to work at home, and try to juggle work and your baby—perhaps with the support of an au pair or a babysitter. An au pair is required to have extra training to have continuous sole charge of children under the age of two, but can help around the house or supervise older children. Ideally, use a recognized, approved au pair agency.

Sometimes grandparents are happy to step in and take care of children, but this is an arrangement that should be treated with respect, and carefully discussed in advance. Payment may not be necessary, but you should be flexible and also feel confident that your approach to childcare is honored. It can work beautifully when you establish good communication. Equally, however, it can lead to resentment on both sides, so tread cautiously.

Finally, you may want to consider working part-time, or changing your hours so childcare is less frequently required; for example, if you can work from seven until three every day, and your partner takes over the early-morning care, you may be able to get away with just five hours of care a few days a week. Talk through the different scenarios with your partner, and make sure you are both in agreement. If you are a single parent, make sure you have some backup support so your baby will be cared for when you are running late, or the baby or your caregiver is sick. Being solely responsible for a baby can be overwhelming at times, so take any offers to help you out when you just can't be there.

CHOOSING DAYCARE

When selecting a daycare center, above all else, trust your instincts. If you see happy babies and warm, caring staff, you are probably on the right track. If it feels good, it may be right! Focus on centers with:

• A high staff-to-child ratio. There are laws about the number of little ones that can be cared for by each responsible adult; you are looking for better-than-average ratios.

• An arrangement in which younger and older children are separated, so babies get the right care without the distractions of older children.

• A strong, fair discipline policy that matches your own beliefs.

• Permanent staff members with good first-aid experience, and experience dealing with childhood illnesses and providing medical attention. If your baby has health concerns, check that caregivers can manage them effectively.

• Well-trained, experienced staff who constantly update their knowledge, and understand child nutrition and development, and common issues of childhood.

• Warm, loving staff with affection for and interest in the children.

• A designated staff member for every child, to ensure that individual needs are met.

• A sound policy and clear evidence of safety and security.

• A good selection of clean, neat toys, and age-appropriate books.

• Plenty of opportunities for your baby to be stimulated.

• A quiet place for babies to sleep and a clean place for them to be fed.

• A policy of updating parents on their babies' progress daily.

• A good open-door policy, so you can visit at any time.

Target practice

Your baby's hand–eye coordination is developing fast. They are working hard to get their arms and legs to go where they want.

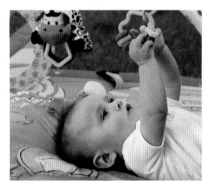

Coordination Your baby will enjoy practicing skills, such as reaching and grasping.

By now, your baby will have realized that when they hit an object it moves, thereby making a link between cause and effect. Each time your baby reaches out for a toy important information is being fed back to their brain about muscle and body movement. They will now hit and grab with greater meaning.

Lay your baby on their tummy and put a toy a little away from them to encourage them to move toward it. Help your baby grasp the toy by placing it in the palm of their hand: grasp reflex will cause their fingers to tighten around the toy.

Place your baby under a baby gym and position them so they can easily reach one or more of the hanging toys. If your baby is successful some of the time at reaching and grasping the hanging toys, they will enjoy the experience much more. In the coming months, your baby will be able to target objects more accurately and pull them toward them.

Tummy time

It is safest to put your baby to sleep on their back, but they also need dedicated time to lie on their front to develop upper body strength.

Your baby should now be able to lie on their front and attempt to lift their head to look up or to the side. They may try to lift their head by using their forearms to push upward. It will be another month or two before your baby pushes up with confidence.

This important milestone in their development is the start of the motor skills that will lead to rolling over and, eventually, crawling. Your baby should have dedicated time to lie on their front when they are alert, as studies show that because babies sleep on their back, tummy time gives them practice in looking and pushing up. Always stay nearby while your baby is on their front. Their neck muscles are still relatively weak and unable to hold up their head for long, so they may become anxious or distressed if left on their front for too long and will need you to rescue them.

Put toys around your baby to encourage them to reach out and even move (see "Target practice", above). Lay your baby on your chest while you're on the floor. It will make them happier to see your smiling face when they lift up their heads.

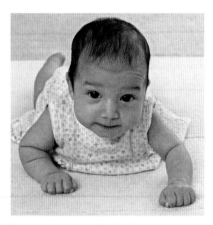

Developing muscles Your baby can probably lift up their head to see what's around them.

Out and about

Your baby can see quite well now and their sight is improving all the time, so give them lots of opportunity to explore the world around them.

If you haven't used a stroller yet, you can now consider one that allows your baby to sit upright with support. Some strollers are designed to face outward, while other models face inward so your baby can see you.

Some experts say that inward-facing strollers are best, since they allow your baby to continue bonding with you, learn from your talking and facial expressions, and be comforted by your visible presence. A stroller that faces outward, on the other hand, encourages your baby to look at what's passing them by. If they're daunted by your absence, talk to them as you walk, and reach over and stroke their face to remind them you are there. Occasionally, crouch down in front of the stroller and have a reassuring little chat. They are learning information about speech, content, tone and rhythm as you talk, even though they can't understand the meaning of the words.

Stay safe

Always fasten your baby's harness carefully, and check that they are comfortably upright, not slouched forward. Adjusting their bottom so that it is a little farther forward should help them to sink back in comfort. You may also want to invest in a headrest or neck support, to make them feel more secure. A good stroller will fully recline so you can gently ease them down, ideally without waking them if they're asleep. Don't forget to put the brake on whenever you stop, even if there is no obvious incline. Accidents can and do happen. Avoid hanging heavy bags on the handle of the stroller; it can easily fall over. It's best to invest in a stroller that allows you to store items under the seat, which gives it a good, firm base. Keep in mind that upright collapsible strollers with only one seat position are not appropriate until six months.

For parents of more than one child, there are many double (and triple) strollers, some more practical than others. Some parents like the "one-in-front-of-the-other" (tandem) set-up (since it allows them to negotiate tighter spaces), although these can be hard to maneuver and require brute force to turn them. "Twin" strollers tend to be popular because your babies can see, hear, and communicate with one another easily. This form of "entertainment" may be invaluable if an outing takes longer than expected. The drawback to this type of stroller is its width and use in narrow entrances and aisles.

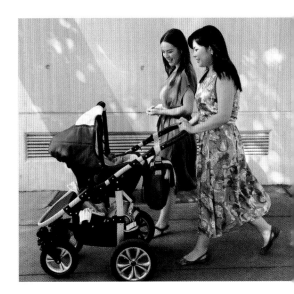

Out and about Being in, or out, of their strollers gives babies opportunity to experience the new world around them.

DEVELOPMENT ACTIVITY: BOARD AND FABRIC BOOKS

Brightly colored books with faces of babies and/or animals are perfect for your baby's stage of development, and they will love to gaze at the pictures.

Sturdy board or fabric books are good, since they can often be easily cleaned and can double up as toys for your baby when they want to entertain themself. Books that have a variety of different textures on their pages will appeal to your baby. Encourage them to reach out and touch the pages. Make up your own stories as you go, or repeat the name for the object on the page to help them learn.

Reading your baby's cues

Sucking fingers? Yawning? Reading baby cues is an important first step in communication. It lets your baby know that you understand and will respond.

As you repeatedly offer your baby what they want as soon as you see the signal, they learn that you will meet their needs without having to resort to crying. The baby will build up a larger repertoire of cues and gestures to get messages across, and in the coming months will begin to anticipate your response. In this way, your baby's communication and trust are starting to develop.

Looking for clues

You can probably already recognize the different pitch and tone of a cry that means "I'm tired" compared to the one that tells you "I'm hungry." Now it is time to look out for more specific vocal and nonvocal signs. You should watch for cues such as leg-kicking, a reddened face, and fist-waving because these signs or actions may mean your baby is overstimulated, frustrated, or in need of a diaper change. Look for mannerisms that suggest tiredness— perhaps rubbing eyes, yawning, or sucking on fingers. As you gain more understanding of your baby's signals, you'll predict ever more quickly what it is they need.

To play or not to play?

Your baby can also give you signals about whether or not they're in the right frame of mind to play, or whether they need time to unwind quietly on their own. These are known as "withdrawal" and "approach"

cues. If your baby becomes still, looks at your face, reaches out to you, moves their arms and legs smoothly, turns their eyes (wide and bright) or head toward you, coos, smiles, babbles, and raises their head, these are classic "approach" signals. Your baby is letting you know they are in the mood for interaction!

If your baby turns away their head, arches their back, squirms or kicks, pulls away, turns their eyes away from you, wrinkles their forehead, hiccups, or frowns, these are "withdrawal" cues. They are a sign that your baby needs a break or a rest from what is going on. They may want to stop playing, feeding, or even being held. It may be time for a change in activity or even a nap.

ASK A PEDIATRICIAN

My baby doesn't pass a stool every day. Are they constipated? Babies' stools can vary greatly, but a change from what is normal for your baby may suggest a problem. Babies can move their bowels anywhere from three times a day to once every other day. Breastfed babies tend not to get constipated since breast milk contains the right ingredients to keep the stool soft. Lots of babies strain when having a bowel movement. This is normal. Signs of constipation, however, can include hard, pellet-like stools, straining without producing stool, or painful bowel movements, sometimes with a tiny amount of fresh blood on the diaper due to a small tear in the anus. If bleeding occurs, consult your pediatrician.

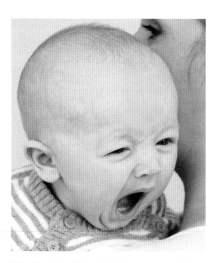

What do I mean? Sucking on fingers could signal tiredness, hunger, or watchfulness.

Winding down Your baby's yawn means that playtime is over and they are ready for a nap.

Baby massage

Massage can relax and soothe your baby, help ease the discomfort of gas and colic, and even promote restful sleep.

There are plenty of baby massage classes if you want to learn the right techniques (your doctor may be able to recommend one locally), but you can also use gentle strokes you practice every day as you rub your baby's back to soothe them, or play with their hands or feet. The main goal of baby massage is for you to have fun together, and for your baby to enjoy your loving touch.

Try to choose a time when your baby is relaxed—so not just after a feeding or when they are hungry—and make sure that the room is warm and your baby is lying comfortably on a soft surface. Try stroking their arms and legs firmly to begin, then massage their abdomen lightly in a clockwise direction. Talk to your baby as you massage and watch their cues: if they seem unhappy at any point, stop the massage. Try a mixture of gliding, fluttering, and rotating strokes to see which they like best.

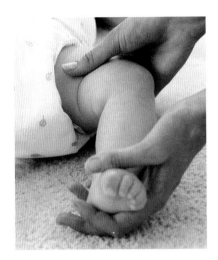

Legs and feet Start by gently squeezing the thigh, and then rub the ankle and foot.

Your social baby

Your baby is smiling more and may be gurgling and cooing to "talk" to you. Your social baby is emerging.

You and your partner have the greatest influence on your baby's social development. As you talk with your baby, wait for them to respond and then react. In doing so, you are teaching them how to engage in two-way communication.

Your baby's smiles are now becoming more frequent and you will find that they smile not just in response to your smile, but even perhaps in response to your voice. They will also begin to smile at other willing adults who might grin at them. These are all signs that your baby is now widening their social network. Spend plenty of time throughout the day having face-to-face time. Look into their eyes, mirror back their expressions, speak and then wait for your baby's reaction.

Around this age, babies become aware of who is familiar and who is a stranger, and may even begin to express preferences for certain people. You can help your baby feel relaxed around trusted others by ensuring grandparents and friends get lots of cuddling time and opportunities to smile at and coo over the baby. Babies are also fascinated by other babies and often become mesmerized by another baby's face, perhaps even smiling at it. It will be a while yet (up to two years away) before your baby makes real friendships, but early interaction is good for long-term positive sociability.

Smile!

A baby's mouth has more nerve endings per square millimeter than any other area of the body.

Because your baby's mouth is supersensitive, they explore the world by mouthing anything they can get hold of. Your baby also learns by watching. They have "mirror neurons" in their brain, specialized nerve cells that enable them to imitate the facial expressions and movements of others.

Even though your baby may smile and excitedly wave their arms when they see you, they may not be so friendly with strangers. That's because they're beginning to develop the ability to remember people and objects. When they are unfamiliar, they may get a little anxious and need reassurance.

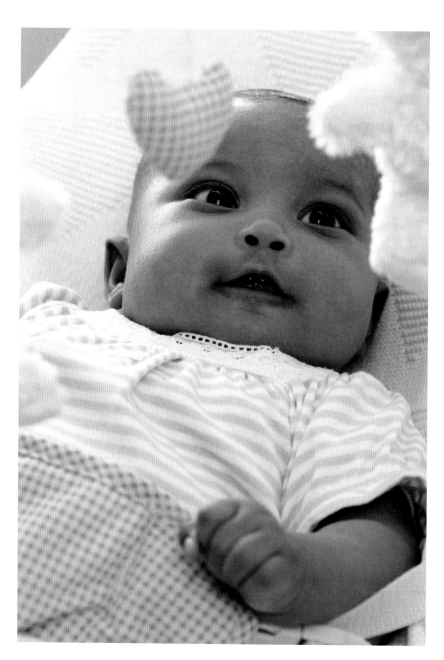

Do as I do Your baby will copy your facial expressions, from smiles to frowns to tongue-poking! Have some fun making faces at each other.

Listen + watch = learn

Everything your baby sees and hears helps them learn how to adapt to their new environment, so what's fun for them is also good brain fodder.

Your baby was born with plenty of brain cells already connected so they could perform essential tasks such as sucking and swallowing right away. Also, all the baby's senses have been soaking up information from birth onward. Every experience forges connections between brain cells, which means learning. Your baby will also copy your facial expressions and make a sound after you've spoken.

Imitating your baby's facial expressions teaches your baby to express their feelings without words, learning that others can do what they can do—psychologists believe this plays a crucial role in developing a sense of self, others, and belonging.

At 11 weeks of age, your baby is gleaning more and more information, creating a detailed picture of their environment. From watching siblings dance to music to looking at a light, then turning away from it, the baby has myriad nerve impulses firing through the brain to make connections between music and movement and light and dark.

Bright colors stand out best at this stage, and your choices for stimulation don't have to be expensive or elaborate. Put the baby next to a mirror (as long as they can't break it), or on a warm day, seat them in the shade beside a brightly colored pinwheel that spins in the breeze.

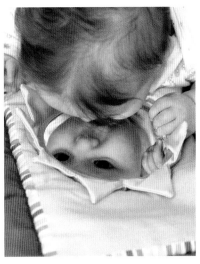

Mirror play Your baby will be fascinated by their own reflection in a mirror.

Time out as a family

A family outing can be a welcome change of scene and gives your baby the experience of different environments.

Now that your baby is increasingly interested in all sights and sounds, an outing can be refreshing and stimulating. Seek out some family-friendly experiences to share. Try to keep car trips relatively short and look for places that will give new smells, sights, and sounds. A simple picnic in the park, lying with you on a rug under some trees watching the

pattern of leaves and branches moving is enough. Even a walk through the park or along the busy streets in the stroller provides scope for entertainment.

What's more, whenever you do things together as a family, at home or away, you are building up a store of shared memories and stories to tell relatives, especially details of your

baby's cute or amusing reactions to new experiences. You are also beginning a tradition of family activities that will become a positive habit as the years pass.

Take plenty of photographs of these early experiences. As your child grows older, they will love to look through them and see what they did with you when they were a baby.

Pets and your baby

It's not only your own pets that you need to be careful about,
but also friends' and family's animals, too.

It will still be a while before your child is old enough to build a safe relationship with pets. For now, be mindful that even the best-trained animals can become unpredictable, and it is important never to take anything for granted between your baby and your pet.

Animals, and dogs in particular, can become jealous of the new kid on the block. If you have a dog, try to give it special attention when you can, so it doesn't feel neglected. Make sure your dog still gets routine walks and meals at normal times so the baby's presence doesn't disrupt life too much. Don't

let the dog go upstairs if this is where your baby sleeps; install a stair gate if necessary to keep the dog away.

As your baby nears three months old, they have grown used to being able to grab and pull the objects they can reach. When this is a pet's tail or ear, there is risk of a warning shot from the animal—a nip or a scratch, for example. Never leave your baby unattended around your pets, and keep the pets out of the room while your baby is free to play. Under no circumstances should any pet be allowed to sleep in your baby's bed. Cats, in particular, may go looking for

warmth in a crib (or a stroller), which makes them especially dangerous. Always use a cat net to prevent this.

Health-wise, make sure your pets are regularly immunized and kept worm- and flea-free. Pets, especially puppies and kittens, may carry parasites that cause toxocariasis, so always maintain proper hygiene to minimize the risk of infection. Never allow either cats or dogs to lick your baby, especially on the face. If you're visiting friends who have pets, the same precautions apply—keep your baby safe and within sight.

DEVELOPMENT ACTIVITY: DANCING

Do you have a favorite song that you love to dance to? If so, why not make this song the anthem of a regular activity that you or your partner can share with your baby? Put on the favorite song, hold your baby securely, and sway with them to the music. You can make the movements rhythmic and gentle or a little bolder as the music dictates, as long as your baby is safe. They will love the feeling of being moved around in their parents' strong arms, and may even chuckle as you move around with them.

In time, they will learn to associate the music with a positive experience, and hearing it will make them feel good, even if one of you is out at work—or if you both are and you have left your baby in a trusted person's care.

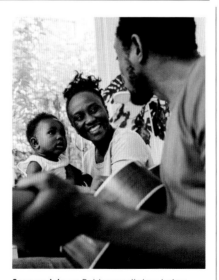

Song and dance Babies usually love being rocked to music—and at this age, they won't be embarrassed by your dancing!

PET SAFETY

• If you own a cat, buy a cat net to cover the baby's crib and always use it.

• No matter how trustworthy you think your dog or cat is, don't leave them unattended with your baby: the slightest movement or baby swipe could cause the animal to lash out.

• Wash your hands after handling pet food or pet bowls to reduce the risk of spreading pet-food-related diseases, such as salmonella infection. Also, wash your pet's food and water bowls in a separate sink or bucket.

• Reptiles are associated with a high incidence of salmonella infection that can be caught by handling them. Some experts recommend that they should not be kept as pets if children are under five years old.

Exploring by mouth

Your baby's mouth and lips are full of nerve endings and taste buds to provide information on flavor, texture, and consistency.

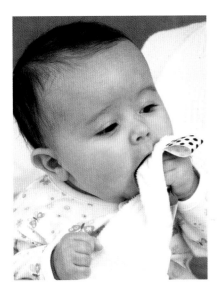

Your baby will by now be putting their fingers into their mouth and trying to grasp objects and bring them up to their mouth. They will enjoy exploring each item, discovering its taste, its feel, and the resistance to pressure as they bites down.

Mouthing helps your baby practice moving their tongue, lips, and jaw so that, over the coming months, they gain finer motor control of each. This will aid speech development, chewing, and swallowing.

Exploring their world Your baby will mouth objects to get a sense of their feel and taste.

Your baby will be indiscriminate about what goes into their mouth, so just make sure there's nothing within reach you wouldn't want them to chew on. There are plenty of toys available that are specially designed for babies to chew, including cloth books with rubbery edges. Teething rings are good, too, especially when they double as noisy rattles. They're narrow, too, so they're easy for tiny hands to hold.

You might find that your baby enjoys sucking on the corner of a soft toy or burp cloth—babies often do this for comfort, as a sort of alternative pacifier.

Caring for your baby's skin

Babies often suffer from dry skin, bumps, and rashes, so it's important to treat their skin gently and ensure that they're comfortable.

Babies' skin is thinner, more sensitive, and less oily than adults', making it particularly prone to drying out, especially during winter when the air indoors is dry and overheated.

If your baby's skin is dry, try not to bathe them too often (once every 3–4 days is fine, with a sponge bath at other times) and avoid using soap or bubble bath. Plain warm water with a drop of hypoallergenic or organic

baby bath is enough. Keep bath times brief and afterward, pat your baby dry and apply a little hypoallergenic moisturizer or emollient cream.

Landry detergent residues can cause irritation, so use a baby-friendly detergent and fabric softeners, and put baby clothes through an extra rinse cycle. Avoid clothes made from scratchy fibers and synthetics.

Tiny pimples on your baby's face are known as neonatal acne. Leave them alone—they are common and will disappear on their own. If your baby has a bright red rash around the neck, armpits, or diaper area, they may have heat rash, especially if the weather is hot. Remove clothing to allow air to circulate and cool their skin. Sometimes a red rash is a sign of thrush (see pp.373–374).

Keeping track

Your baby's weight gain is probably fairly steady now, but it's still reassuring to get them weighed at the pediatrician's office during regular checkups.

Although every baby is different, most gain an average of between 4–7 oz (120–200 g) each week until they are about six months old. By this age, they have usually doubled their birth weight, and weight gain then gradually slows.

Breastfed babies tend to grow more rapidly than formula-fed babies for the first three months, but then they grow more slowly and, by the time they are 12 months old, breastfed babies are on average just over 1 lb (0.5 kg) lighter than formula-fed babies.

You'll have plenty of appointments at the pediatrician's office during the early months to find out your baby's weight and have it plotted on their growth chart. If your baby is following roughly the same percentile line, their rate of growth is perfectly healthy. Growth spurts or bouts of illness may lead them to jump up or down to the next percentile occasionally, but what you are looking for is a fairly regular pattern of growth overall.

If your baby's weight gain does dip, or increase significantly over an extended period, talk to your pediatrician—they can assess whether or not there might be a problem, and refer you to a specialist if there is cause for concern.

Toward sitting

Your baby's neck muscles are probably strong enough to support the weight of their head for a few seconds now.

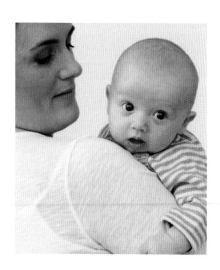

In order to sit upright, your baby needs to be able to support their neck and back, and figure out how to use their legs to steady themself and their arms to stop from toppling forward—that will probably take until they are about seven months old, but they can certainly start to practice.

Even if your baby can perform confident push-ups, they will need to develop greater neck stability. Tummy time (see p.116) is great for this, as is carrying them on your shoulder.

You can help your baby develop core stability by propping them up in a reclined sitting position. Make sure they are well cushioned to the back and sides and stay with them at all times. Be ready to pop them back on their back or tummy when they tire.

Once your baby is strong enough to hold their head securely for prolonged periods, getting the balance right is a matter of practice—and lots of cushions to fall into.

Stronger neck muscles Carrying your baby so they can look over your shoulder encourages them to lift their head.

Traveling with a young baby

Your baby's stronger now and also very adaptable, so if you've been thinking about going out of town, this could be a good time. With a little advance planning, there's no reason why you shouldn't all enjoy a relaxing, hassle-free vacation.

Now that your baby is two months old, they should be quite a good traveler. They're less fragile than they were and probably won't mind too much where they sleep. Also, they're still too young to have a set routine yet, so a little disruption shouldn't disturb them too much.

Planning ahead

If you intend to stay in a hotel and your baby sleeps in a crib, you'll either need to take your own travel crib, or reserve a crib for your room. If you are renting a car at your destination, it's important to reserve an infant seat when you make the reservation. If you're traveling internationally, you'll also need a passport for your baby. If you plan to travel to a country where vaccinations are needed, check with your pediatrician to learn whether your baby is old enough to have them. Some, such as yellow fever, are not safe for babies under six months.

MALARIA

The WHO advises against taking infants to areas with malaria. If you decide to go, seek expert medical advice on how best to protect your baby and yourself, especially if you are breastfeeding. Seek immediate medical help if your baby develops a fever during or after a trip to a malaria region, even if you have taken all the precautions.

Traveling by car

In some respects, car trips are the most straightforward—if you have plenty of trunk capacity—because you can load up everything you need. Fit window sun shades to protect your baby's eyes and skin, but remove their outdoor clothing. Make sure that the car seat is secure in the back seat and that the seat belts are properly threaded. If you have a long trip ahead of you, try to avoid traveling at rush hour, and consider driving at night, when your baby can go a bit longer between feedings.

Traveling by plane

Check your airline's baggage policies. Diapers, creams, clothing, formula, feeding equipment, and other necessities add a lot of weight, so book extra allowances in advance. Weigh your luggage before you leave.

You are allowed to take enough baby milk and sterilized water (in a baby bottle) in your carry-on luggage to last you the journey. In some cases, this may be more than 3 fl oz (100 ml). You may be asked to verify the liquid (or baby food) by tasting it.

You can often take your baby in the stroller all the way to the plane door, at which point you'll need to collapse it so it can be taken to the hold. Or you can use a baby carrier.

Packing Being prepared for every eventuality is the key to successful traveling with a baby.

ASK A PEDIATRICIAN

When is it safe for my baby to fly? It's safe from two days old, but you're unlikely to fly so early. If you plan to travel internationally, your baby will need to be two weeks old to get their passport. Mothers who've had a Cesarean will be unable to fly until 10 days after the birth. It's advisable to check with your airline to find out their policy.

Give your baby a feeding during take-off and landing: swallowing will help prevent ear discomfort due to changes in cabin pressure. Most planes have special child seats, and changing tables in the lavatories.

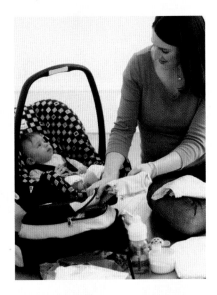

3 months

CHARACTER TRAITS PRESENT FROM BIRTH ARE PART OF WHAT MAKES UP YOUR BABY'S PERSONALITY. Your baby's eyes now work better together and vision is becoming more three dimensional. Their muscles are stronger, and they may be surprised to find they can flip from tummy to back. They like to kick, which strengthens their leg muscles in preparation for crawling and walking.

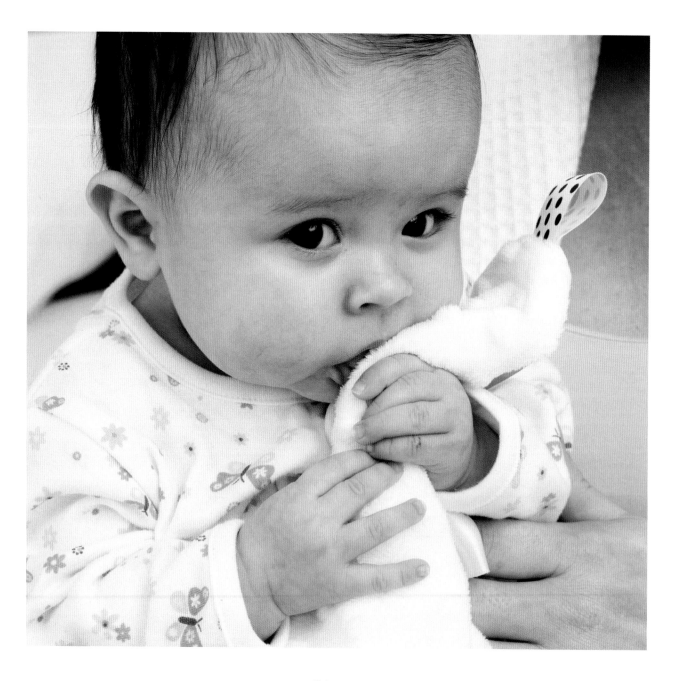

Another growth spurt

Your baby's due for a second growth spurt at around three months, so prepare for another feeding frenzy—and a restless night or two.

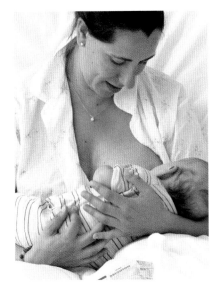

Supply and demand Your baby's frequent demands for milk are nature's way of making your body step up its milk production.

Now that you're more settled, the three-month growth spurt shouldn't come as too much of a surprise. Your baby may demand food as frequently as every two hours for a few days, which can be exhausting for you, but there's no fighting it, so try to go with the flow. If you're breastfeeding, stock up on healthy snacks, drink plenty of water, get a good book to read while nursing, and prepare to be in demand for a while. Your body will increase milk production to meet baby's needs.

Formula feeding

You may need to make up an extra bottle for your baby during the day, or increase the quantity of each bottle by 1 fl oz (30 ml). Be guided by your baby's appetite and be careful not to overfeed. Your baby shouldn't have more than 5 fl oz (150 ml) of milk per 2.2 lbs (1 kg) of weight per day. So, if your baby weighs 13 lb 3 oz (6 kg), they shouldn't have more than 30 fl oz (900 ml) over 24 hours. Keep some emergency cartons of formula in your home, which can provide a good backup, too.

Sleeping

You may find your baby sleeps more during the day and is restless at night, perhaps waking up more than usual. Or they may wake up earlier from naps because they're hungry. This sleep disruption may last a couple of days to a week but it will pass.

FOCUS ON TWINS: DEALING WITH GROWTH SPURTS

To have two babies going through a growth spurt at the same time or one after another can be exhausting. Routines tend to be disrupted, so one baby may wake frequently for feedings (that is, has entered a growth spurt), while the other doesn't. To relieve the burden, express some breast milk so someone else can give the baby who is going through a growth spurt an extra feeding.

Alternatively, when the twin demanding extra wakes to be fed, you wake the other one, too, even if it's for a smaller feeding. Many parents find this simply means the less hungry baby eats little and often, but remains happy. However, once the growth spurt is over, you may find that you have established a routine of frequent feeding in both babies that you then have to break.

Most importantly, sleep when your babies sleep, and enlist the help of friends and family to keep the rest of the household running smoothly.

Twice the work To feed two babies as they each experience a growth spurt will require plenty of patience on your part.

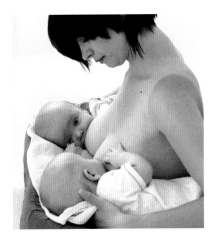

Looking farther afield

Everything your baby sees is new and exciting, and they'll begin to focus intently on objects that are farther away.

Your baby will be fascinated by everything they see, near and far. By three months, their eyes are more coordinated, working well together. They will not look quite so cross-eyed and can track a slow-moving object with much smoother eye motions. Their depth perception is improving, and their world is becoming more three-dimensional. Their distance vision is beginning to develop, and they can now make out the shape of your face when you enter a room. You'll notice your baby watching things that are several yards away.

Provide your baby with plenty of things to look at. Hold the baby turned outward so they have a chance to see what's going on around them, and point things out to them. Call from the other side of the room, and watch their delight when they see your familiar face. Shake noisy toys from a little farther away, encouraging your baby to turn and look.

Up to about 12 weeks, many babies may squint as their vision develops. This is a normal phase of growing, but if your child continues to squint after three months, tell your pediatrician so they can catch any anomalies early and take steps to correct your baby's vision, if necessary.

Doing the flip

Your baby may be about to flip over from tummy to back. Watch out! The acrobatics could soon begin.

Tummy time (see p.116) helps strengthen the muscles used to roll over. It's easiest for babies to flip from front to back, so this usually occurs first. In most cases it will just happen by accident. It's unusual for babies to be able to do this at 12 weeks but it does happen. As soon as they flip over once, they'll be capable of doing it again and again in sequence. So be aware about where they might end up and what's within reach. Leaving your baby on the bed or changing table, even for a second, is definitely not an option now. Keep in mind that some babies never roll. Skipping this milestone is nothing to worry about.

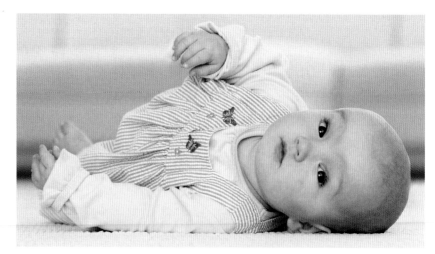

Rolling over By three months, your baby's movements will become smoother. They may lift their head and shoulders high, perhaps to roll over and get closer to you or investigate a toy.

Your baby's personality

Babies, like the rest of us, have their own individual personality. Getting to know your baby's unique traits and characteristics will help them flourish.

In the first few weeks and months, your baby's personality will start to show. They may be easy to please, excitable, or even a little grumpy and difficult to calm. If you have a child already, you may be surprised to find your new baby has a very different temperament.

Your baby's personality is shaped by a combination of inherited traits, present needs, and environment—including your reaction to your baby. You may find it interesting to ask your parents whether you were similar to your own baby at this age: perhaps you were placid or difficult to comfort, just as your baby is. Your reaction to your baby and state of mind can affect how baby responds on a day-to-day basis, too.

If your baby is calm, responsive, and smiling, you may find them easier to parent and to respond to; however, if they are less calm, perhaps distressed because of difficulties such as colic, you may find you have to be particularly alert to their needs and spend more time soothing them and introducing activities such as baby massage (see p.119) which can relax and quiet them.

Some babies are less social and easily overwhelmed and overstimulated by groups of people and noisy, bright environments. If your baby has opportunities to meet new people in a warm and welcoming way, they'll soon overcome any natural fears.

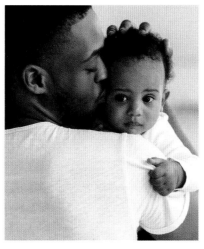

Sensitive soul Babies who are less eager to go to new people need extra reassurance.

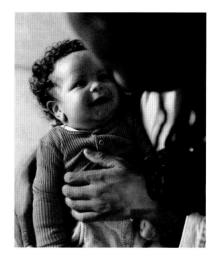

At ease Some babies enjoy more interaction and cope better when visitors come along.

Your baby may be energetic and enjoy physical exercise, or calm and laid-back, and take everything in stride. They may be easily unsettled and need a routine to feel secure. All babies are unique. Getting to know and understand your baby's personality can help you adapt and learn which activities to offer. Try not to label your baby; embrace them for who they are and they'll flourish in your care.

SUN AND SAFETY

Babies need vitamin D from sunlight for strong bones and teeth, but their delicate skin can burn easily, and they can easily overheat. Avoid direct sunlight and keep your baby in shade when sun is strongest (from 10 a.m. to 3 p.m.). Babies under 6 months shouldn't be in direct sunlight. Dress your baby in lightweight, long-sleeved outfits with pants when outside to avoid exposing too much skin. When impossible to avoid direct sunlight, it's OK to apply sunscreen sparingly to the face, hands, or other exposed areas. Use sunscreen (SPF 30–50), that blocks the sun rather than filtering it, and is hypoallergenic. It should also protect against UVA and UVB rays. Put a sun hat on your baby and keep in the shade at all times. Offer plenty of feedings if you're breastfeeding; bottle-fed babies may need a little extra water to stay hydrated.

Working parent

If you need to return to work, you will undoubtedly have some juggling ahead of you. Remember that you don't need to be superhuman.

Depending upon the demands of your career, you may decide to return to work while your baby is still very young. The key to a smooth transition is to find excellent childcare that will give you the confidence in your baby's well-being while they are away from you. Don't rush this process—take your time to find the caregivers who perfectly suit you and your family.

Remember that daily reunions with your baby, when you walk through the door, will nourish the bond between you both. Hold off on chores and instead spend as much quality time as your schedule allows soothing, chatting, and playing quietly together at the end of the day. If you can make it back for bath time, this is a great opportunity to bond. If you are worried about keeping the house tidy, do a quick surface clean after your baby is in bed, or if appropriate, consider paying for a weekly clean to give you more time with the baby when you're home.

Time to connect

Don't worry about taking shortcuts. If you can't manage to put together a meal from scratch every night, investigate some of the quality, ready-prepared meals now available that can be put into the oven when you get home. Or batch cook over the weekend while your baby is napping or being entertained by your partner, friend, or family member, and use your freezer to make workday meals

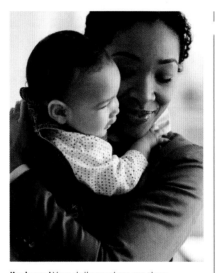

I'm home! Your daily reunions are time to reconnect.

simple—just a case of defrosting and serving. Sauces and stews are great time-savers, too—while heating them up, boil pasta or rice, or hydrate some couscous. Even a hunk of bread dunked in a reheated stew is a quick and tasty option.

Over time, things will settle into a routine, and you'll find the best ways to manage both work and home life. Making time for your baby and your partner while you're at home will reap rewards in years to come—a little dust or clutter now is a short-term problem. With a supportive and healthy home life, you'll be surprised at how capable you feel, ready to tackle anything and everything!

ASK A DOCTOR

I'm still feeling very tired and low—could I be anemic? Many new parents feel tired and generally low, not as a result of anemia due to iron deficiency, but because they are trying to cope with the challenges of parenthood on little sleep. If you are birth mother, it could also be a sign of postpartum depression (see p.110) or an underactive thyroid gland. Anemia can also cause the following symptoms:
• shortness of breath;
• heart palpitations;
• cravings for particular foods or substances, such as crunchy vegetables or ice;
• food tasting different than normal;
• sore tongue;
• headaches.
   If you have any of these symptoms or feel excessively tired, see your doctor.

VACCINATIONS

Now is a good time to schedule your baby's 4 month check-up with their pediatrician. They will be due for a second set of vaccinations. Try not to be anxious when you take the baby for their shots or they'll pick up on this and experience more distress while they're there.

Naps and nighttime sleep

Your baby may now be awake longer during the day, but will still need three naps and a good night's sleep to get enough rest.

By around three months, your baby will be sleeping about 15 hours in every 24-hour period. About 10 of those hours will take place at night (probably punctuated by one or two feedings) and the other five will be broken into three naps during the day.

Some parents complain that their babies don't nap, but if you put in place a good sleep routine, you'll find that your baby will eventually settle down into a good pattern of daytime naps and a long nighttime sleep.

Babies who don't get enough rest during the day can become overstimulated and take much longer to settle down at night. Putting them down regularly during the day—even if they just kick and play in the crib—will get them into the nap habit, and they'll soon learn to accept that this quiet time is for sleep.

ASK A PEDIATRICIAN

My baby never seems tired—particularly around bedtime. How can I settle them down? It's normal for babies to get a second wind when it's time to put them down. This is a sign that they are overly tired and getting energy from adrenaline. Try moving bedtime to half an hour earlier to catch them while they are genuinely tired, and watch for their sleep cues (p.124).

Little kicker

As your baby's legs get stronger and become more coordinated, they'll enjoy kicking so much that they'll even wake up at night to practice.

Kicking and stretching the legs prepares leg muscles for crawling, walking, and rolling over. To promote leg development, offer colorful toys just out of reach, and provide a safe environment to explore. Curiosity will encourage baby to become mobile in a few months' time, but they'll build up the skills and strength to do this by moving toward things of interest.

Tummy time mainly encourages the development of your baby's upper body, neck, and arms, and also provides an opportunity to bend the legs back from the knees, and to push forward with them later on. When they spends time on their back, they'll perfect their bicycle kick and a wide range of leg movements. You can encourage weight-bearing by carefully holding the baby upright. When you do this, the baby will naturally bounce—don't let go!

Now is the time to be extra cautious; your baby will wiggle and use their legs to move. They might even begin "creeping"—slowly and steadily moving from one place to another.

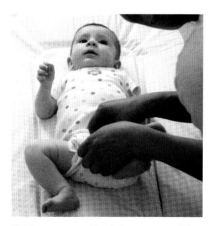

Kicking up a storm Your baby may try to kick away their clothes during diaper change.

131

Observing the world

Babies often gaze intently at objects of interest, as if observing and memorizing every little detail.

Your baby will follow you with their eyes, and will enjoy taking in the sights, sounds, and smells around them. They are beginning to understand and react to their world. Their social skills are starting to flourish, and they will try to communicate in new ways to attract your attention, They may smile, coo, or gurgle.

Although your baby was born with a full set of primary teeth, they were hidden underneath the gums. Their first few teeth may now be making their way upward, making their tiny gums feel uncomfortable, and causing your baby to become unsettled.

Look and learn By watching you and others around them, your baby will be learning how to react to changes they may observe.

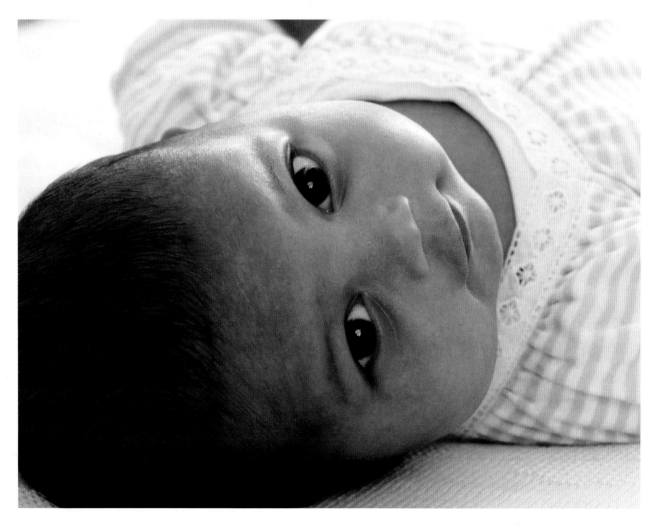

Cooing baby

Your baby's early attempts at speech represent their new way of communicating with you, so make sure you respond to them!

Your baby will love to engage you in conversation, and you may notice them listening intently when you talk. But most of all, your baby will enjoy practicing all the new sounds they have been learning to make. Babbling is an important stage of your baby's overall development and acquisition of language. They will voice the sounds that make up the languages they hear, without creating any words you can recognize. It's a bit like running through the alphabet phonetically! Your baby is gathering together and consolidating all the sounds so they can effectively use them when ready.

As your baby's language develops, they will start crying less and start to make cooing sounds and noises to communicate. Your baby will attempt to imitate sounds and intonation, and will begin to experiment with making "bubbling" sounds caused when their tongue contacts their lips, and also "raspberry" sounds when they squeeze their lips together. This stage is very important for your baby, because it allows them to practice and develop control of the muscles they will later use to talk. Encourage your baby to develop their own memory bank of sounds. Engage in conversation with your baby as often as you can, giving them lots of praise. They might not look as if they are listening, but they are absorbing it all.

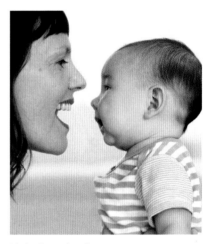

Little chatterbox Encourage your baby to use their voice by giving them opportunities to speak, and showing clear pleasure when they do.

Teething and sleep

Most babies will experience some teething discomfort, waking frequently at night, often wanting the comfort of a feed, even when they're not hungry.

There is no doubt that teething is uncomfortable for most babies, and you may find that your little one wakes frequently at night, gnawing on their fist, batting at their ears, or just fussing. A breastfed baby might want to nurse for comfort and may settle for nothing less, even in the middle of the night.

Although the jury is out on whether teething can cause a baby to suffer bouts of diarrhea, most parents find their babies' stools are looser for short periods during teething, requiring more frequent diaper changes.

If you know your baby is teething, it's important to ensure they're comfortable before going to bed. Give a warm bath and gently massage their face around the jawline and under the chin. This helps to relax the area and ease inflammation. You can rub a drop of teething gel onto the affected area of their gums. (Follow the manufacturer's recommendations as to the amount and don't use more, since this could be dangerous for your baby's health.) Feed them before bed and make sure they get as much as possible, so that hunger doesn't wake them up too early.

Peekaboo!

Gradually, it will dawn on your baby that an object they can't see may still be there—and peekaboo games help them understand this.

The understanding that objects continue to exist even when they cannot be seen, heard, or touched is known as "object permanence," and is a major milestone in a baby's first year. The term was first used by child psychologist Jean Piaget, who believed that most babies grasp this concept between eight and 12 months old. However, all children are different, and some babies have been known to begin to develop this concept as young as four months old. Games of peekaboo now are great fun, because your baby will be pleasantly surprised each time you cover your face with your hands and then "magically" reappear again. They also test your baby's memory: they're learning to anticipate, so they will wait excitedly for your face to appear, and to hear you say "Peekaboo." If you leave your hands over your face longer than usual, they may reach out to prompt you to move them! Learning that things—including you—can still be there when they can't see them is also good for their emotional security. When you vanish for a few moments, they won't feel as concerned as they may have previously.

Learning to sit

Your baby is not ready to sit unsupported but they'll love to be propped or held in a sitting position to get a different view of the world.

Your baby is ready to start gaining the muscle strength and coordination that form the basis for sitting upright. If they can lift their head during tummy time and roll confidently, you can introduce some play ideas to build readiness to sit. For example, prop your baby up securely so they have a stable position then give them noisy, bright rattles to reach for, or encourage them to stretch to grab a cloth draped over their legs. Each time they lean out they're refining their balance. They will topple over, so be ready to hold them, and make sure there are plenty of cushions around to break a fall.

When you prop your baby up do not leave them alone even for a few moments. Until their muscles, coordination and balance are improved they will tire easily and even become frustrated, so watch for signs that they'd rather do some less strenuous play. At this age they may not be ready for this sort of activity at all and that's fine, too. The average age for sitting is six months, with some babies not reaching this milestone until around 10 months.

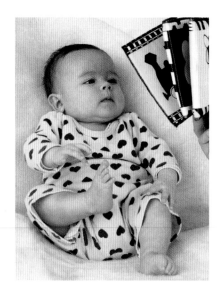

Good vantage point While your baby's sitting propped up, it's a good opportunity to hold up a book so they can see it easily.

Making associations

Even the most acquiescent baby will go through a stage of expressing not just their likes, but also their dislikes—and you'll know about it!

As your baby's memory develops, they will begin to make positive and negative associations. Soon, they will light up when you walk into the room, smile at an older sibling, and gurgle when they see their baby gym. However, their car seat may produce an instant cry of protest; they may actively resist being laid down for tummy time, and your attempts to leave them alone in his bed at night may well end up in tears of frustration—and even anger! They're starting to know their own mind and express their opinion. In fact, browse any baby forum on the Internet and you'll see that 12-week-old babies have a wealth of dislikes, including their cribs, the family dog, bedtime, front-pack carriers, the bath, getting dressed, and even being burped. So get ready for a few disagreements!

Positive associations

In the early days, the best way to deal with dislikes is to try creating positive associations. Maybe your baby has been stuck in the car seat too long in the past, so a few short trips with the nursery rhymes on and a favorite stuffed animal or board book next to them may make a difference.

Change your routine slightly if they're showing a dislike for the bath or bedtime. Perhaps take a bath together. If they dislike being put into the crib, try staying close by, putting a containing arm around them while they lie there. Softly tell them stories,

Distraction often helps—hum, or sing to them; hang a mobile over their changing table; festoon their car seat with new toys; put them in a carrier facing outward; dress them in a different place and play "This little piggy" while you do it.

Gentle guidance

Ultimately, this is a developmental stage that you'll have to work through. Most activities to which babies object are necessary, and you'll have to guide them through—gently, kindly, and patiently. Talk to them, make them laugh, maintain eye contact, and try to control your own frustrations. Until your baby can use words to express themself, try to negotiate, and understand why they must do things they dislike, you'll have to persevere as best you can.

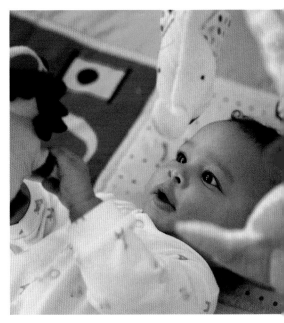

Changing course If your baby dislikes their bouncy chair, they might be better off somewhere else for a change, such as under a baby gym that offers colorful distractions.

ASK A PEDIATRICIAN

My twins don't enjoy the same activities; how can I keep them both occupied and happy? Try to encourage solo play. Set each baby up with an activity they enjoy, putting one baby on each side of you. There will be some turning back-and-forth involved to keep them both occupied, but you'd probably be doing that anyway. It is good that your babies are expressing their individual characters, however hard it is to facilitate two very different sets of needs. If one hates the bath, sponge bathe that baby and put them in their baby seat while you bathe the bath-friendly sibling. If one resists bedtime, settle down the happy twin first and introduce a new element to your bedtime routine for the other. As they get older, they'll begin to look with interest at what the other is doing, and probably want to join in. Be as flexible and creative with your arrangements as you can, and keep in mind that this is just a stage.

Routines to suit you

Your baby's sleeping and feeding patterns are now more predictable, so try adjusting their schedule to work better for you.

By now, your baby may be able to be a little more flexible than they were previously because they can go longer between feedings and, probably, sleep for extended periods of time. Many parents find this a positive development. It means that you are not quite so tied to your baby, and they will be much more amenable to getting into a routine that suits you a little more.

You can now anticipate when they're likely to be hungry, and squeeze in a good feeding before heading out for lunch with friends or a shopping trip. When they're usually alert and happy, you can set them up in the bouncy seat with a couple of board books, or in the baby gym surrounded by toys, in order to do some chores, make phone calls, or sift through your emails. Adjusting your baby's routine slightly from time to time will help them become more flexible and buy you a little freedom. Routines are great for providing young babies with security, because they learn to anticipate what comes next; however, they can become overly binding—the last thing you need is to find yourself in a position where all lunchtime social engagements are put on hold while your baby has a nap. Don't hesitate to create a little time for yourself by involving others, too. If both you and your partner can take turns with the bedtime routine, you'll both develop a knack for settling baby down—and they'll be equally happy in either scenario. Life will soon be getting much easier!

DEVELOPMENT ACTIVITY: PLAYTIME

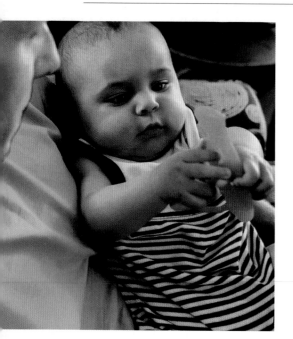

Your baby will enjoy exploring their toys while held securely on your lap. Encourage them to reach for, grasp, and examine toys with different textures, sounds, and shapes. Noisy toys will get their attention, leading them to look, reach, and turn. Scrunch a crinkly toy, or shake a rattle a bit above and to the side of your baby and encourage them to reach and grab. These activities help hand–eye coordination, muscle control, and the ability to grasp by opening their hand and curling their fingers around a toy.

Busy fingers Your baby will love to grasp things, and any new toys will be grabbed and examined carefully.

COLIC

If your baby is still crying frequently and you are convinced they have colic, take heart that most babies outgrow colic around this time, and the distress, discomfort, and bouts of crying should soon stop completely.

In some cases, colic can go on for up to four months, or more. If your baby's colic continues much beyond three months, and nothing helps make them more comfortable, see your doctor to ensure that nothing else is at the root of the problem, such as a reflux disorder.

New challenges

Your baby is ready to play with toys they can grip, shake, and squeeze—they're ready for a new challenge!

The mobile, floor gym, activity quilt, and textured toys are still important to your baby's development, but you can add toys with new textures, sounds, and even buttons. Give them a rattle or squeaky toy and they'll learn that they can make things happen. They will enjoy waving it, and squeezing and shaking it to make a noise, and will in time grasp the concept of cause and effect.

Toys with a variety of bright colors, lights, and sounds will be popular. Babies of this age also find toys with friendly faces comforting as well as fascinating. Your baby will respond well to a toy face, especially if you help them identify it by pointing out

the toy's facial features, then your own, and then gently touch your baby's face as you name each part.

Don't box up old favorites. Babies benefit from being able to master a toy easily, along with learning about more challenging ones. A mixture means there is always a successful activity at hand.

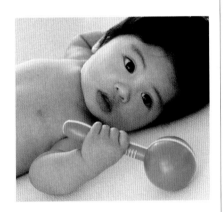

Great shakes A rattle is an ideal toy now because it helps your baby learn that by shaking it, they can cause it to make a noise.

MONTHS 0–3

FUN TOYS FOR NOW

Your baby's favorite plaything will always be you, and the time you spend with them is invaluable for their emotional development. But there are some toys they will enjoy playing with, and that are great for this stage of development.

- **Rattles** are a perennial favorite and they help your baby learn to control their movements.
- **Textured fabric books** are great fun, as are chunky board books with firm lift-up flaps.
- **Blocks** with "surprises" in them will entertain your baby endlessly. Make sure they are chunky enough for baby to grasp—eventually.
- **Stacking pots** make a satisfying noise when banged together; and they'll enjoy learning to stack them.
- **Bath toys** that squeak, leak, and float will make bath time enjoyable.
- **Toys that can be clipped** to your baby's stroller will keep them occupied when you're on the move.
- **A music box** that responds to your baby's touch with nursery rhymes or lively music will delight them.
- **Toys that pop up** when buttons are pushed, such as a jack-in-the-box, will provide endless entertainment and encourage your baby to develop hand–eye coordination.

TOYS AND SAFETY

Always give your baby age-appropriate toys. Toys intended for children over three years old may have small parts that could come off and cause choking. Make sure stitching is firm in soft toys, and that labels are well sewn in.

Do not attach toys to your baby's crib or playpen using string or elastic: a length of 12 inches (30 cm) or more can wrap around a baby's neck and create a strangulation hazard. And remember that your baby can't yet tell a toy from a household implement, so make sure you put anything that should not

go into their mouth well beyond their reach.

If you have older children, store their toys separately, and try to teach your older children to keep their toys away from the baby so they don't choke on something—but never take it for granted that they will always remember the rules.

Most importantly, never leave your baby alone when there is anything within their reach, or with anyone who is not responsible enough to make sure that they do not put into their mouth something that might cause them to choke.

What a giggle!

Your baby has probably blessed you with smiles over past weeks, but any time now their first giggle will melt your heart all over again.

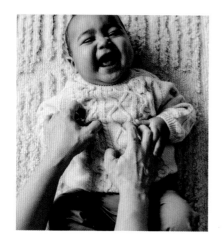

Tickles Many babies giggle when tickled. Make a fun game of tickling your baby to get them to laugh with you.

Finding something that makes your baby laugh becomes addictive. Babies respond best to eye contact, so looking them straight in the eye and smiling is the best way to start. To turn their return smiles into a giggle, you can try tickling their toes, under their armpits, or gently squeezing the fleshy, ticklish parts of their thighs.

They will likely respond with a squeal or a giggle that lets you know they find it funny. Try making a funny face (such as an exaggerated look of surprise) while you tickle their thighs or toes, to add another humorous dimension to the game to help bring on the laughter.

Babies are more likely to be engaged and remember things if an experience stimulates more than one sense. So if you make a funny sound as you tickle your baby, they are even more likely to find it funny.

Forming attachments

Your baby can now identify your face, voice, and smell. When they hear you speak or sing, they will know you are just around the corner.

At around 14 weeks, your baby's sight improves dramatically. As you walk around the room, their eyes follow you more, because they now have greater muscle control. As they become more aware of your coming and going, they may object or begin to cry if they can't see you any more.

Talk to them in reassuring tones as you move around. If you leave the room momentarily, tell them that you will be back in a second—they will soon begin to make connections between what you say and your actions. When you come back, smile to let them know all is well.

As babies begin to understand that they are a separate person from you, having something comforting to hold on to can help them feel secure. It's wise to have two identical comfort objects, so if one gets dirty you can replace it while it's being washed. Your baby may also get attached to its odor, so an occasional wash is useful to ensure the baby doesn't reject it when it smells fresh!

ASK A PEDIATRICIAN

Why does my baby drool? All babies will drool either a little bit, or a lot, from time to time—this is normal and nothing to worry about. Drooling is something they will grow out of over time. Most babies drool more when they are teething, or if they have a cold or a stuffed nose. Saliva contains protective proteins that provide a germ fighting barrier against bacteria, so drooling can be helpful when your baby reaches the stage of automatically putting everything they pick up in their mouth.

Accidental rolls

At three months old, it can happen that your baby will begin to roll, but this is more often by accident rather than by intent.

Once your baby has achieved the flip from tummy to back (see p.128), they'll be working on mastering the art of rolling over—every which way! Most babies can roll over by the time they reach six or seven months old, so it's unusual for them to be doing it now, but not unheard of.

Once they've done it once, that doesn't mean they have mastered rolling: it takes muscle strength, coordination, and planning to make this happen each time they try.

Encouraging rolls

Short periods of tummy time and encouraging your baby to lift their head and push up with their hands are great practice for this milestone. Since it is much easier for a baby to roll from front to back, put your baby on their tummy. If they can support themself well on one arm, hold a favorite, easy-to-grab toy next to, but slightly above, your baby—just out of reach. Try to coax them to tip their head back to look up and reach for the toy. As they reach, move the toy farther behind them and see if you can coax them to lean toward the toy, encouraging them to flip over onto their back. If they do, reward them with cheering, clapping, and lots of reassuring smiles, especially if they seem a bit confused by what just happened, and be sure to give them the toy. Encourage them to turn to both sides.

Rolling safety

Never leave your baby lying on any raised surface. Change them on a changing mat on the floor. Keep one hand on them as you reach for things. Never leave your baby unattended in a room that hasn't been babyproofed.

DEVELOPMENT ACTIVITY
BACK-TO-FRONT ROLLS

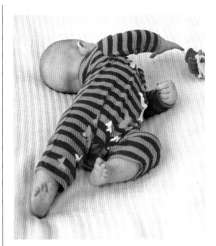

Reaching out Once your baby twists their body and leans over in one direction, they'll soon learn to take the movement all the way over into a back-to-front roll.

The back-to-front roll happens only once the reflex that forces your baby's arm out as they turn their head is overruled by their improving coordination. They also need enough muscle tone to support their head, body, and legs, and the coordination to be able to pull in their arms so they do not prevent the roll. To encourage a back-to-front roll, lay your baby on their back and place a toy next to them, just out of reach. Get them to reach for the toy. If they reach far enough, their center of gravity will shift to bring them over onto their front. Once they've mastered the move, they'll combine it with the front-to-back roll, and will enjoy the freedom rolling across the floor gives them.

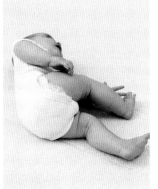 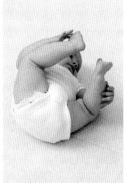

Tummy time to rolling All it takes is one stronger-than-usual push up with one arm and a slight rocking motion from side to side, and your baby will tip over onto their back.

Your baby's financial future

It may seem early to be thinking about saving for your baby's future, but some early planning now really can pay off later on.

Saving now for your baby's future can reduce the financial burden of being a parent when your baby becomes a teen or young adult. A small regular investment now will grow into a decent sum by the time your little one reaches 18 years old.

Grandparents or relatives may want to give you a lump sum to invest on your child's behalf. It can make sense to open up something in your child's name to benefit from special tax savings that may apply. Talk to a financial adviser, or look for financial advice online. You can also check your local bank branch to find out what accounts are available for kids.

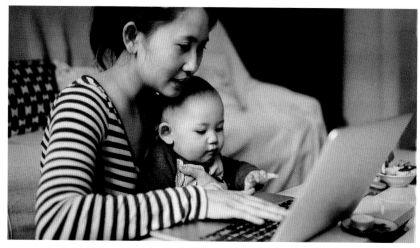

Do your research Whichever type of investment you choose to make for your baby, make sure you put some time into researching where to find the best deals.

Savings accounts

Savings account options vary by bank, but there are a few basic guidelines:
• Your baby will need a Social Security number in order to have an account, so apply for one if you haven't already.
• A parent or guardian will be expected to be a joint account holder until the baby is 18 years old, so be prepared to give your personal information, too.
• Shop around to find a plan that's right for your situation: an account with no minimum balance, a competitive annual interest rate, or another feature that's attractive to you. You'll be able to give your baby a financial head start before they even know what money is!

529 plans

An attractive way to start saving for your baby's college fund is through a 529 plan, which is a tax-advantage savings plan to help you save for post-secondary education. Most 529 plans are sponsored by states, and they offer special tax incentives to state residents who enroll in their plans. You don't need to live in that state to enroll in its program, though.

Savings bonds

Many babies receive US savings bonds as welcome presents from relatives. They're sold at half the face value and earn a fixed interest rate for 30 years, maturing at 20 years—just in time to help with college expenses.

SMALL CHANGE SAVINGS

One lovely way to save a little for your baby—with the added dimension of handwritten notes to discover later—is to make or buy a "sealed" piggy bank (sometimes called a terramundi) that you can pop loose change into over the weeks, months, or even years—slowly, slowly building up a little stash of cash to spend on something fun in the future. From time to time, write a little note about something funny your baby did or a milestone they reached, and push it through the opening. Invite visiting family members to do the same. In years to come—perhaps a 13th, 16th, or 18th birthday—your "baby" can crack open the bank, pocket the spoils, and read all the memories of their younger years.

Structuring sleep and feedings

Your baby's tummy can now hold enough milk to allow them to sleep for longer periods, and so your baby will be settling into a more regular routine.

In the morning, wake your baby when you get up so they're more likely to sleep when you want to relax for the evening. At this stage most babies need six to eight feeds in a 24-hour period, including breakfast, mid-morning, lunch, mid-afternoon, and dinner. If your baby wakes in the night to feed, try instead waking them for a feeding just before you go to bed. Keep them calm, with stimulation at a minimum. In the daytime, introducing playtime after a feeding will help your baby distinguish between night and day.

On average, babies sleep for about 10 hours at night now and 5 hours during the day, but each baby is different. If it suits your baby, try a midmorning nap, an afternoon nap, and, if necessary, a short power nap in the evening. If you want them to go to bed at about 7 p.m., try two longer daytime naps instead.

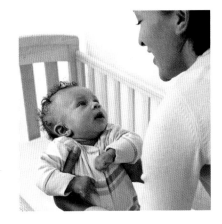

Good morning Waking your baby will help them adapt to your routine.

Physical play

Now that your baby is stronger, physical games such as knee rides and tickles encourage confidence and physical awareness.

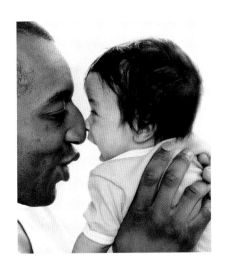

Whether it's tummy time, tickles, or bouncy play, your baby will benefit from having the opportunity to move and take part in activities that make them aware of their body.

With your baby on their front, roll a ball in front of them. They may move their legs and body to reach it. Sit on the floor with them and prop them securely in a baby nest, or hold them safely between your legs, then

Fun faces Hold your baby close to your face as you make faces, make funny noises, and rub noses—you may even elicit a giggle or two!

build towers of soft blocks. They will try to reach out to bat them, and will enjoy watching the bricks scatter across the floor. Your baby will love to be rocked from side to side if they are supported well. If they protest, stop, or try rocking more gently. If they can hold their head up, raise them into the air, and "bump" noses as you bring them down. Try water play: in a bath or baby pool, sit with your baby firmly in your arms. Let them splash, and use a toy watering can to sprinkle water over their arms. Never leave them unsupervised near water.

Being active

So your baby may not be up and toddling yet—but when it happens,
you'll need to be fit and healthy, with lots of stamina!

It can be difficult to motivate yourself to be active, especially if you're feeling tired. However, regular physical activity will help decrease feelings of stress, and promote relaxation and better sleep, which in turn will leave you feeling more energized. Among the benefits of exercise for new parents are: healthier and stronger bones, muscles, and joints; lower body fat and better weight control; better balance, coordination, and agility; improved self-esteem, and a more positive mental outlook.

If you're a new parent, physical activity will help reduce your likelihood of suffering from postnatal depression, anxiety, and low mood. For breastfeeding parents, invest in a quality sports bra that offers good support to ensure you have a comfortable workout.

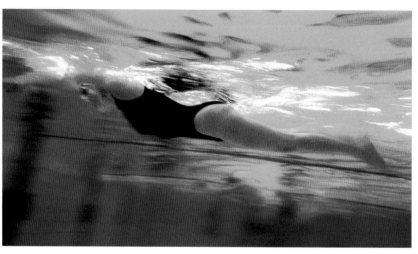

Resuming an athletic activity A few quick laps at your local swimming pool, a stroller-jog in the park, or a game of tennis with a friend are all great ways of getting some exercise.

What kind of activity?

About 14 weeks after giving birth, your body will have regained enough strength for moderate aerobic exercise. Cycling, swimming, dance, pilates, and yoga are all good options. Aim for becoming slightly out of breath but still able to hold a conversation. If it hurts, stop.

Fitting in the baby

Some gyms and local sports centers offer daycare facilities, and some will take a baby at three months old. The prospect of leaving your baby in someone else's care can be daunting, but classes often last only up to an hour. The feel-good factor of doing something for yourself can be a just reward for an hour's separation.

If you are not comfortable leaving your baby in a nursery, try to find a window for physical activity once your partner is home, giving them some bonding time with the baby, too.

If you can't get to a gym, you could enroll in a program of online dance or aerobic classes, or join a park stroller walk, organized by local groups, where you are likely to meet other like-minded parents. Also, there are community centers that run outdoor activities that allow you to take your baby along.

FEEL-GOOD FACTOR FOR YOU

It is very easy in the first weeks of having a new baby to become completely tied up with the business of parenthood and forget that you need taking care of, too. This week, agree on a time for your partner to take care of the baby so you can go to the salon; or have a pedicure, facial, or massage; a lunch or a trip to the movies with friends; or just an hour out in a local café with a good book. It's even better if it's something that requires an appointment, so you don't get tempted to cancel. Whatever you choose, it should feel like a treat, and you should come out of it feeling great.

Feeding and teething

Babies often experience the symptoms of teething before their first tooth is perceptible under the gums, which can cause them discomfort.

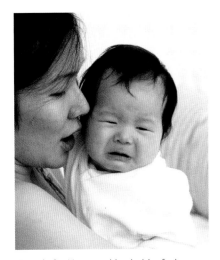

Upset baby Many teething babies feel irritable and restless and, sometimes, pain as the tooth cuts through the gums.

Many babies lose their appetite when teething because their gums are so uncomfortable and painful. If your baby has flushed cheeks, red gums, is drooling excessively, or chewing on toys or fingers more than usual, or if their sleep is disturbed, they may have a tooth coming through. Some associate a low-grade fever with teething, but doctors are reluctant to make this link. If your baby does have a fever, or seems sick, do not assume this is due to teething. Instead, ask your doctor to check for an infection.

Each tooth pushes up through the gums to become visible in your baby's mouth. You may be able to feel a hard, protruding bump in the mouth if you rub their gums with a clean finger, and the area may look inflamed.

Some breastfed babies respond to teething by wanting "comfort" feedings, and this may be the best way to settle your baby down. Other babies find being nursed uncomfortable, cry, and come on and off the breast, only to want it again soon afterward as they are still hungry. This is frustrating for you both, but keep offering your breast as usual until your baby settles.

Bottle-fed babies may also fuss while teething. A little teething gel before a feeding can ease the pain long enough to get some milk into them. If you have any worries, see your pediatrician.

ASK A BREASTFEEDING EXPERT

My baby has a tooth and bites me when I breastfeed! How can I discourage this?
Babies bite when they are experimenting with their new teeth. If baby bites, release them from the breast while saying "ouch," then reattach. They'll begin to understand the meaning of the word. If your natural reaction is to shout in pain, this may shock them and be enough to stop them doing it again! They're more likely to bite if they're not hungry, so take them off your breast when they've had enough. Does baby have a cold or congested nasal passages? If so, they may be clamping down with gums and teeth to hold your nipple in place as they breathe through their mouth. For a remedy to this, call your pediatrician.

TEETHING RINGS

Invest in some non-PVC teething rings that can be cooled in the fridge, never the freezer. These are invaluable if your baby's gums are inflamed or sore. Although it may be a few weeks, or even months, until the first tooth emerges, getting them used to gnawing on a teething ring now can help prevent symptoms before they start, and your baby will know what to do when those first teeth start appearing..

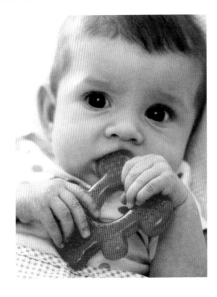

Cool relief Keep a few teething rings in the fridge so there is always a cold one on hand to help ease your baby's discomfort.

Help from family

If your parents or other trusted family members are willing, you may want to consider enlisting their help so you can take a whole night off.

RECORDING YOUR BABY'S VOICE

It may seem impossible to believe that you could ever forget the sound of your baby's earliest sounds, but each stage of a baby's development is so absorbing, it can be easy to lose track of those momentous, heart-warming attempts at communication. Make time to record them as they chatter to their heart's content. Perhaps you can continue to do so regularly, each time making a note of the date. Record the gurgles, coos, and other sounds using your smartphone and email the recordings to family and friends, or just download them to an external hard drive to keep your recordings safe for that trip down memory lane in the future.

LONG-DISTANCE GRANDPARENTING

Relationships with grandparents can be rewarding for your baby—and on into adulthood. Getting things right in the early days can ensure that relationships flourish. If your baby's grandparents live far away, they may feel they need an invitation to visit—always articulate the offer, even if the practicalities make accepting it tricky. Don't assume they simply know the offer is open. Keep them involved by chatting with them using video calls with your baby on your lap, or send them weekly emails with lots of photos. Don't forget to report all those amazing firsts to keep them in the loop.

Now that your baby's routine is more established, you've got expressing down pat (if breastfeeding), and taking care of their needs has become easier, you might want to think about indulging in some time with your own friends or your partner, or time out to enjoy your own passions or need for unfettered me-time. If grandparents, other trusted family members, or close friends are able to babysit for the night, you can plan a trip to the theater, dinner out, or even a night away—a real break that gives you time to focus only on each other or on yourself.

While some parents don't feel comfortable about leaving their baby early on, others find that the benefits to their relationship or self-care outweigh their anxieties. Letting your nearest and dearest help out allows your baby to begin to develop a loving and significant relationship with them—and those significant others will almost certainly relish the opportunity to spend bonding time with your baby. However, leaving your baby for the first time is a very personal choice, and in the end it comes down to what feels right for you.

If you agree that the time is right to get away, decide whether your baby will be staying at your home or the home of the person or people entrusted to look after them. At this age, your baby will probably sleep wherever they are. Then talk through every aspect of their care: when to

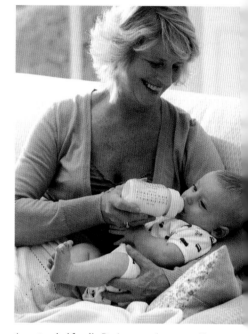

An extended family Doting grandparents will enrich your baby's life, especially if the bond with them is developed early on.

feed them; change their diaper; put them down to sleep; and what to do if they wake up. Make sure that your family or friend knows how best to offer comfort if your baby becomes upset. It's important that you feel you have covered every eventuality. Once you have left clear instructions and contact numbers, there's no reason to worry. Ask your baby's caregivers to call you immediately if they have any concerns.

Encouraging social skills

Your baby will gurgle, chatter, and coo in your company, and be pleased to meet new people if introduced to them carefully.

Babies naturally favor their primary caregiver, so you can make things easier for your partner and other family members by encouraging your baby's social skills. At 15 weeks, your baby is ready for this—social skills are developing apace.

Make sure you set a good example by interacting positively with the people around you. After a busy day with just you for company, your baby will be eager to see and play with someone new. Give your partner a moment to get through the door, but don't keep your baby to yourself. A shared hug makes a nice handover as your baby transfers interest to their other parent. Spend time together as a family as much as possible, so your baby witnesses how you relate positively to each other. Your baby will learn and take cues from you. Make sure you share childcare duties between you and your partner. As long as you stick roughly to the same routine, it won't matter if your techniques differ slightly. As long as your baby spends time with both of you, they won't mind if one of you changes their diaper or sings their bedtime song differently.

A parent-and-baby group gives your baby contact with other adults. All babies are unique in their willingness to go to others. If your baby is reluctant, introduce new people gently, shortening visits or interactions, if necessary, until your baby builds up confidence.

Reading as a habit

Developments in your baby's vision and comprehension mean that they are now able to enjoy books and stories much more than before.

Reading aloud to your baby teaches them about communication; encourages their listening skills, memory, and vocabulary; and introduces concepts such as "story sense" (which is essential for reading skills later on). Books provide an exciting view on the world, in an entertaining and comforting way.

Sit down with your baby at least once a day to explore books. Encourage them to look and listen as you point at and talk about the pictures, and lift flaps so they can see what's underneath. Fill your voice with emotion and expression to capture their attention, and help them experience positive social interaction with you during reading, which promotes healthy emotional development.

Babies love repetition, so your baby may want the same book over and over. You'll be encouraging memory skills by repeating the same stories.

Most things go straight into the mouth at this stage, so choose books that can withstand a good chew. Sturdy, colorful books with rhymes, pictures of babies and animals, and interactive elements (such as lift-up flaps and textures) will engage your baby and involve them in the story.

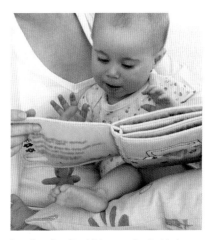

Reading time Establish a reading habit that your baby can enjoy alone when they're older.

Reaching and grasping

Now that your baby knows their hands belong to them, they will start to practice their reaching and grasping skills in earnest.

Your baby has been batting at and trying to grasp objects for a few weeks now. They have figured out that their hand is their own, and the goal now is to direct the hand toward an object without looking at it first.

Once your baby can confidently direct their hand toward an object, they will be able to reach out and grasp small, easy-to-grip, brightly colored toys. These will probably go straight to their mouth, although they may spend time looking at them, dropping them (usually by accident), and reaching for them again.

At this point in your baby's development, reaching and grasping occur at the same time. Your baby can't yet correct any mistakes while reaching. If they can't get ahold of an object that they see the first time, they'll try again, reaching and grasping together. They'll close their hand when they see they've reached that interesting toy. With every attempt, they will improve their hand-eye coordination.

To encourage your baby to reach out, surround them with light, sturdy toys that fit easily in one hand. Choose a variety of shapes, but make sure each one is easy to grip and has a shape, edge, or texture that would fit into your baby's palm. Offer your baby both still and moving objects— there are plenty of toys that vibrate, or can be rolled to draw attention. Praise their efforts to reach and grab. Move toys a little closer if they're

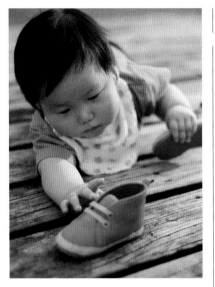

Practice makes perfect With practice, your baby's attempts to reach out and touch or even grab things will become more accurate.

just that bit too far for eventual success, to avoid your baby becoming disheartened. Try not to intervene and do things for them, though. Your baby needs to practice and learn from own their mistakes.

Once your baby can grab things, keep hazards well out of reach. For example, remove your handbag (which may contain small items they could choke on); hot drinks or food; pets; strings or cords; hard or unhygienic items (which will end up in your baby's mouth); electrical cords; houseplants; and medication.

DEVELOPMENT ACTIVITY: CLAPPING GAMES

Although your baby will not be able to clap their hands until about 7–9 months, or later, clapping games, in which you move their hands gently to make a clap, give the experience of bringing their hands together in front of their body. Sing songs while you clap hands together. Let their hands fall, then clap your own hands, singing as you do so. Encourage them to grasp your hands, one in each of theirs, then bring your hands together again— baby is clapping your hands now! The song "If you're happy and you know it, clap your hands" is perfect for this activity. They'll associate it with the actions, and will be ready to join in as their own ability to clap develops in the coming months.

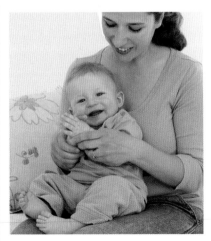

Clap and sing Babies love the drama of clapping their hands and will enjoy singing songs and playing games, too.

What baby sees now

Your baby's vision is improving all the time. They're still drawn to bright colors, but can distinguish more subtle color contrasts now, too.

Your baby's eyesight has notably sharpened and now they will be able to notice objects across the room, although they will still prefer to look at objects close-up.

Your baby's eyes should move together smoothly and follow objects and people around the room. If you notice crossed eyes or any other vision problems, mention them to your pediatrician.

Your baby may now be able to distinguish between more subtle color contrasts, such as red and reddish orange, although subtle differences between pastel shades may still prove elusive. You may also notice that your baby's eyes are starting to change color. Lighter-colored eyes may go through several changes before settling on their final shade at about six months.

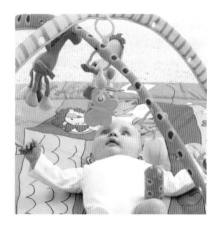

Maturing vision At around this time, your baby will be able to see color and perceive depth more accurately than previously.

Changing friendships

Having a baby shifts your life and focus dramatically, and you may find that some friendships alter as your needs change.

It may be that many of your friends and family share your enthusiasm for your baby. Others, however, may find your new focus bewildering.

It is natural for friendships to wane and surge throughout our lives. You may well make a new set of friends among your baby crowd, and probably have more in common with them at this point. Equally, however, old friendships are not dispensable, and you may need to make an effort to keep some of them going. Make time to go out with friends without your baby and show an interest in their lives. Keep talk of your baby to a minimum and focus on what you have in common. Your friends are no less worthy if they fail to share your passion—try to remember a time when you yourself were not interested in diapers and teething!

Your friendships will continue to evolve in the future, and you may one day find that you can play a supportive role when friends go on to have their own babies. Keep things simmering away for now, and remember that this is a phase that will eventually be resolved.

ASK A PEDIATRICIAN

My baby has started to suck their thumb. Is this a problem? About 80 percent of babies suck their thumbs or fingers, which causes their brains to produce endorphins ("feel-good" chemicals) that soothe and calm. Thumb-sucking is a sign your baby is learning to comfort themselves, which is a useful skill. Don't worry about their teeth. As long as you discourage the habit by the time their baby teeth fall out (at about five years of age), there won't be lasting damage. Most suck their thumbs much less by the age of three.

Your baby from
4 to 6 months

MONTH

4

MONTH

5

MONTH 4: ENCOURAGE
YOUR BABY TO ROLL

Your baby may learn to roll over
with surprising speed. Most
babies roll from tummy to back
before mastering the more
difficult back to front roll. Not all
babies roll over—some skip this
stage and go directly to sitting
and crawling.

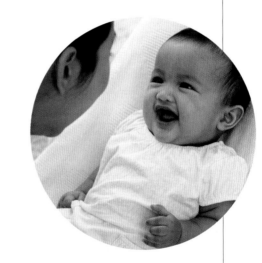

Full-out belly
laughs may
appear around
five months
of age.

MONTH 5: SUPPORT
YOUR BABY TO SIT UP

Toward the end of their fifth
month, your baby can hold
their head up well and is able
to sit upright with plenty of
support. While sat up, your
baby will enjoy taking in the
world around them.

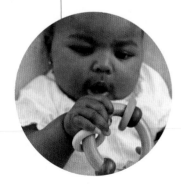

Your baby will **grasp** and
inspect an object that interests
them, before instinctively
putting it into their mouth
for further exploration.

> " Your baby is exploring, laughing, and interacting more with you as well as gaining mobility and coordination. "

MONTH

6

MONTH 6: TIME TO WEAN YOUR BABY

By six months your baby is ready to move to solid foods that will complement their milk diet. Gradually, your baby will have fewer milk feedings as they get used to eating more solid food and enjoying new flavors and textures.

By experimenting with new sounds, your baby is developing their **language skills**.

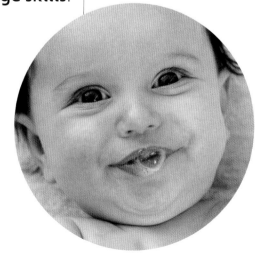

Your baby should be able to **reach out** and **grab things** with greater accuracy.

4 months

BABIES' BABBLING AT THIS AGE SOUNDS THE SAME, NO MATTER WHAT LANGUAGE THEY HEAR.
Your baby should enjoy tummy time more now that they are stronger. If they haven't already, they're about to push up on their arms and support the weight of their upper body—if only briefly. They'll be using a wider variety of sounds, and perhaps even joining syllables together.

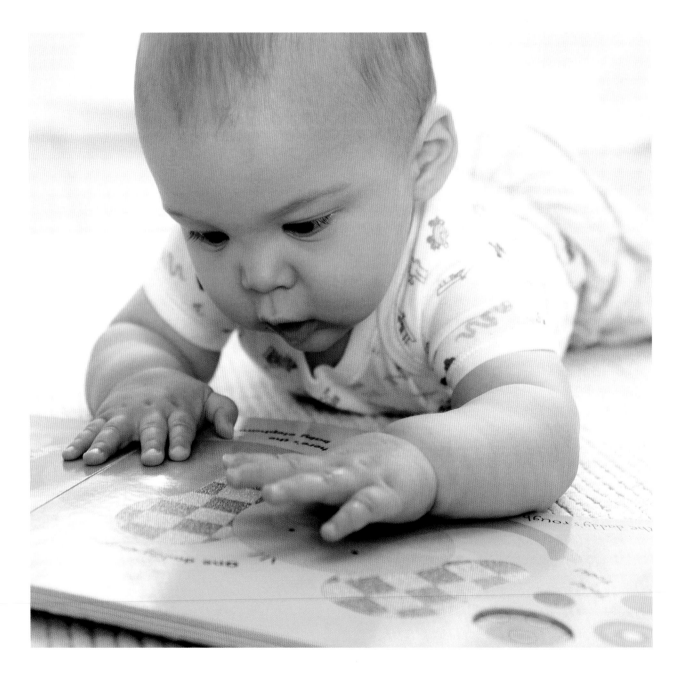

Look who's "talking"

Your baby may start combining sounds and syllables so they sound like "words," but they don't have any meaning just yet.

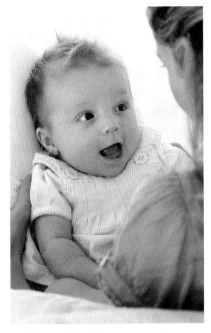

Facial expressions Have a conversation with your baby, encouraging them to talk by imitating your sounds and words.

This week, you may notice that, as your baby practices their vocal skills, many different vowel sounds have crept into their "language," and that they are making more sounds when playing on their own. They may growl and gurgle, and even squeal and shriek unexpectedly. The occasional consonant may now sneak into their vocabulary, and they may create some peculiar words, such as "ibcooo" and "gipgooo." Your baby may also begin to recognize that the way your mouth moves affects the sounds you make, which is more or less lip reading!

You can encourage development of your baby's verbal skills by answering them when they make little noises. They'll be learning the rudiments of language and conversation, which includes both speaking and listening. They were exposed to language in the womb, and were born with a very basic understanding of speech patterns and different sounds. Now, they will attempt to replicate those patterns and sounds, and you may find that they mimic the high- and low-pitched voices you use when you speak to them, and also that their babbling and coos sound much more like language.

Bilingual baby

If more than one language is spoken in your household, don't hesitate to use both languages regularly. Research suggests that being exposed to two languages early on affects brain development, making babies receptive to new languages for a longer period. This is especially true if a baby hears both languages in the first year of life. Also, speaking more than one language helps your child's learning. Speak to your baby in whichever language feels comfortable to you. One of you may speak the first language while the other uses the second, community language. Your baby will adapt and learn to use them individually as they move between home and community.

Sometimes it's thought that children who learn two languages will have delayed speech. This isn't usually the case, and such an assumption can mean that a speech problem is ignored. If you have any concerns about your baby's speech, consult your pediatrician.

DEVELOPMENT ACTIVITY: ROCK, SWAY, AND SWING

The part of your baby's brain that senses motion and balance is known as the vestibular system. As this system matures, it helps them keep their head upright and, eventually, keep their balance when sitting and standing up. Rocking, swaying, and swinging your baby up and down, both gently and more playfully, will encourage the development of this system, and they will love the activity. There is good research to suggest that these types of movements help improve a baby's sense of balance, gross motor skills, and perception of movement in advance of crawling and walking. Try to make movement part of your regular playtime.

Your parenting style

Around this time, you'll have developed your own ideas about raising your baby, but it's good to keep refining your thinking.

Whether to take others' advice is a tricky area for parents. One set of grandparents frowns on the use of a pacifier, your sibling thinks your baby should be potty-trained pretty much from birth, while your best friend thinks that even young babies should be "sleep trained" to last through the night. Not your philosophy? Try not to worry. Establish a culture of respect— you do it your way, I'll do it mine. It's always worth listening to the ideas of others, but if you and your partner are in agreement about how to raise your baby, you are perfectly within your rights to keep doing what you're doing.

The basis of your parenting should always be the provision of a warm, responsive, and loving family. It is too early for rules, but it is the right time to discuss with your partner your joint approach. Talk about how each of you was parented, which will shape your own attitudes. Discuss dos and don'ts: one of you may prefer to bestow rewards, while the other thinks smiles and praise are enough. Find a compromise that suits you both.

FOUR-MONTH VACCINATIONS

It's time for your baby's four-month immunizations around now (see p.103). At four months, they are due for a second dose to protect against rotavirus (RV); diphtheria, tetanus, and pertussis (DTaP); Haemophilus influenzae type b (Hib); and the Pneumococcal vaccine (PCV) and inactivated polio vaccine (IPV). If you haven't already made an appointment, contact your pediatrician now to ensure that your baby's immunizations are up to date.

Growing appetite

Your baby may be hungrier than usual around now, and they may demand the bottle constantly or spend long hours at the breast.

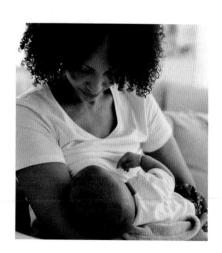

Your increasingly active baby needs more fuel to keep going, which may be why they're hungrier right now. If you are breastfeeding, feed on demand. If you are bottle-feeding, an empty bottle is your cue to give an additional 1 fl oz (30 ml) of formula. If they drain the bottle again and are still dissatisfied, give another 1 oz (30 ml). You may want to give some cooled boiled water between feedings to make sure they aren't thirsty instead.

Your baby's nutritional needs are still being met by milk, so don't be tempted to introduce solids yet; the digestive system won't be ready. If you are considering starting solids before six months, your pediatrician can help you decide if the baby is ready (see also pp.154–155).

More milk Your baby may feed more around now to fuel their increasingly energetic play and their rapid physical growth.

The importance of play

Playing with your baby supports their development in many ways, and promotes healthy communication with you in the years to come.

Playing with your child supports their emotional health—for example, by encouraging self-esteem and trust. Play is an essential component of healthy development in babies and children, providing opportunities to develop motor, cognitive, perceptual, and social skills. It encourages creativity, imagination, and self-sufficiency, and it helps babies discover new things, solve problems, and, above all, relax and enjoy themselves.

Play allows your baby to learn about the world around them. Whenever they hear, see, touch, taste, or smell something, messages are sent to the brain, prompting important mental connections to be created. So when you play with your baby, you're helping to shape their brain. Giving your child a variety of activities to experience will result in more brain connections being made, and repeating these activities will make these associations stronger. Physical play encourages gross motor skills, spatial awareness, and much more; while books, shape-sorters, rattles, cause-and-effect toys, and "conversation" promote cognitive development, hand-eye coordination, and fine motor skills. Mixing different types of play will allow your baby to grow into a healthy, stimulated child.

However, don't fall into the trap of thinking you need to stimulate your baby constantly, or make every play session a learning opportunity. Play should be relaxed, spontaneous, and

DEVELOPMENT ACTIVITY: PLAYING WITH HOUSEHOLD ITEMS

Your baby doesn't need expensive toys; in fact, babies tend to enjoy playing with the things you use and copying what you do. Plastic cups are great for stacking, then knocking over. A clean wooden spoon (keep it light so it won't hurt as much if the baby inadvertently bonks themself on the head) and an empty plastic mixing bowl are great for banging and "stirring." Crumple up a large piece of paper to investigate the texture and crunchy sound it makes. Even a cardboard box or plastic measuring spoons can be fun for your little one to play with. Avoid hazardous items, such as plastic bottles with screw lids that baby might choke on.

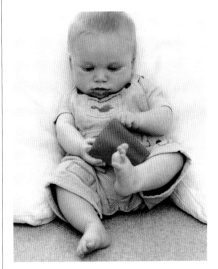 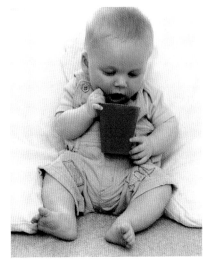

Fascinating new world Things we would consider ordinary are positively exotic to your baby. Almost anything can make a good plaything, as long as it is safe for the task.

fun. Your baby will learn just as much from a tickling game as from expensive, developmentally appropriate, high-contrast flash cards being dangled in front of them. Play never needs to be structured—just do what comes naturally, simply encouraging your baby to attempt new feats, enjoy your company, explore their environment, relax, and have fun. Most importantly, give your baby your time: you will encourage their emotional well-being by simply being there for them.

Weaning

It's no wonder that new parents are often baffled by starting solids—differing opinions and contradictory advice about the process abound. So here's a straightforward guide to what it is, how to decide when to start, and what you'll need to get going.

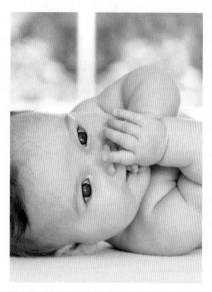

Finger sucking A baby who is ready to move on to solids may demonstrate the classic telltale sign of sucking their fingers or fists.

What is weaning?

This is the gradual process of introducing foods other than milk into your baby's diet It doesn't mean encouraging your baby to stop drinking formula or breastfeeding; milk will continue to be a mainstay of your baby's diet. However, as your baby becomes bigger and more active, they'll need the extra nutrients from solid foods to ensure healthy growth and development.

When should we start?

Over the next couple of weeks, your baby might start showing signs that make you think they're ready for some solid food. Perhaps they are consistently hungry and normal feedings seem unsatisfying, or they've started waking at night to be fed when they previously slept through. Perhaps other babies you know have started solids already, and you're wondering if you should, too. Or an older family member may have told you that starting solids happened much earlier in their day. All of these factors can prompt parents to start weaning—but is it really the right time?

The American Academy of Pediatrics and the World Health Organization (WHO) advocate waiting. They recommend exclusive breastfeeding (or bottle-feeding) for the first six months of life. The practical reasons to wait until six months are that it makes the process considerably easier if your baby is able to sit in a high chair, take food easily from a spoon, and/or pick up and hold food to feed themself.

However, some experts disagree that waiting until six months to start is a good idea. There is a growing body of evidence that this increases the risk of iron deficiency in babies, as well as the risk of allergies. Babies' iron reserves begin to run down at six months, so if they are only just starting on fruit and vegetable purees at this time, they're unlikely to get all the iron they need. Some experts believe breastfeeding for six months is a desirable goal, and that starting solid foods should begin by six months at the latest, but not before four months (or 17 weeks). Also, breast- or bottle-feeding should continue throughout beginning solids, particularly in the early stages.

SOLIDS EQUIPMENT

• A high chair or a seat that clips onto your dining table. Look for a sturdy high chair, ideally with molded corners and crevices to make cleaning easy, a harness or five-point belt, and an insert to hold younger babies snugly. A detachable tray is a plus (see p.206).
• A splash mat for under the chair.
• Two or three small plastic bowls, preferably with a suction cup at the base for stability.
• Two or three plastic or soft rubber baby spoons with a small, easy-to-use "scoop."

• A plastic cup or sippy cup with a spout; choose a "slow flow" one.
• Easy-to-clean bibs.
• A food processor or immersion blender. An electric grinder is useful for foods that become glutinous in a food processor and foods with tough skins, such as peas.
• A flexible ice-cube tray with a secure lid, and mini containers with lids to freeze larger quantities of your baby's favorite purees.
• Stick-on labels so you can note the type of puree and the date that you make it.

There is also research that indicates that introducing foods containing gluten between four and seven months while breastfeeding may reduce the risk of celiac disease, type 1 diabetes, and wheat allergy. Furthermore, high-allergen foods, such as eggs and fish, don't need to be delayed until after six months. Other research suggests that babies who start solids before six months are more likely to enjoy a wider variety of flavors and textures than those who started solids at or after six months.

The right time

Before you begin, be certain that your baby is absolutely ready to take this step. Every baby is different, physically and emotionally. If your baby is healthy, happy, and growing well on their milk-only diet, there is no need to start solids for the sake of it.

The earliest you should introduce solids is at four months, or 17 weeks. Before this time, your baby won't have the digestive enzymes required to digest and extract nutrients from solids; the jaw and tongue won't be sufficiently developed to "chew" and swallow food; and the kidneys will not be mature enough to deal with solids. The baby needs to have lost the "extrusion reflex" (which causes a baby to push out anything that goes into their mouth), and to have the motor capacity to move food from the tip of their tongue. Once your baby is at least four months old, they may be ready for solids if they are doing some or all of the following:
• sitting up unaided, which encourages digestion and helps avoid choking.
• showing interest in your food, and perhaps reaching out to grab it.
• hungrier than usual, and often dissatisfied after the usual feedings.
• waking up at night for an extra feeding after previously sleeping through.
• double their birth weight.
• able to control head movements.
• attempting to put things into their mouth, and "gumming" them rather than pushing them out with the tongue.
• making "chewing" motions.
Talk to your pediatrician, who'll be able to reassure you whether it's the right time and give you advice.

The right pace

If you start your baby on solids before six months, you can take the whole process at a relatively leisurely pace. If you wait until the recommended six months, you will need to progress swiftly from fruit and vegetable purees and rice cereal (see p.210 and pp.216–217) to dairy, meat, fish, eggs, and cereals and grains (Stage 2 solids, see pp.236–237). This is because by then, your baby will need the additional iron contained in protein-rich foods. By the time your baby is 10 months old, you'll have introduced texture (lumps and bumps) as they move toward a balanced diet (pp.286–287).

SOLIDS AND A PREMATURE BABY

If your baby was born prematurely (before 37 weeks), it may be advisable to start solids later than usual. According to the American Academy of Pediatrics, most pediatricians recommend starting a premature baby on solid food 4 to 6 months after their original due date, rather than the actual birth date. The reason is that premature babies often have developmental delays, including swallowing difficulties, and a baby that cannot swallow solid food properly may have problems being introduced to solid foods early. In fact, some premature babies are given a special diet to follow by their doctor, based upon their needs, so it's important to check with your pediatrician before making the call yourself about the best time to introduce those first solid foods—and which solid foods—to your premature baby.

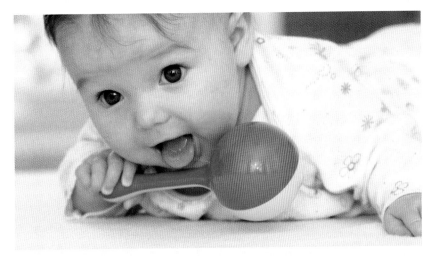

Gumming Frequent "chewing" on objects can be a sign that your baby is approaching the time when they are ready for solid foods to be introduced into their diet.

Sleeping through the night

By now, most babies' tummies can fit enough food to allow them
to sleep longer at night, but your baby may have other ideas!

If your baby is still waking int he small hours, it's likely for comfort rather than food. Ensure they have a good feeding and are burped at bedtime, so you'll know they're likely not hungry or uncomfortable

Then, rather than offering a middle-of-the-night comfort feeding, offer an alternative comfort. Stroke their back, sing to them, and reassure them that you are there. This may be enough for him to settle back down to sleep. Because they have become accustomed to "snacks" at night, and to being picked up and held at regular intervals, they may be a little resistant to this approach at first. Pick them up, but don't feed them unless they appear ravenously hungry.

You can start to encourage them to self-soothe. Go to them when they calls so they know they can trust you. (Leaving them to cry may exacerbate things—they'll learn not to cry eventually, but that doesn't mean they'll be secure and happy.) If they are secure that you are there and will offer comfort if they need it, they will begin to learn to settle themself back to sleep. See to their needs and, over the next few weeks, you can expect them to go longer between waking up until they sleep through the night.

Feeling rundown?

A busy life and sleepless nights may have left you feeling lackluster. You may
need to make small lifestyle changes to get back in the swing of things.

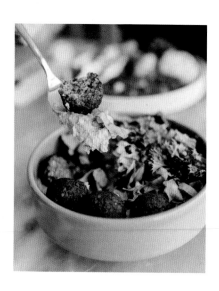

Healthy diet Try to eat three balanced meals a
day, including fruits, vegetables, and whole grains,
with some dairy, fish, and unprocessed meat.

Lack of energy is often related to a lack of sleep, exercise, or decent nutrition, so if you're feeling under par, you may need to do something about one, or more, of these areas. Getting out in the fresh air will help you feel more energetic and could help you sleep better.

It's just as important to eat well. Parenting a new baby is so busy and exhausting that it can be easy to forget to eat properly. Eat healthy food that provides you with a sustained source of energy, such as a baked potato stuffed with tuna, or homemade vegetable soup with a whole grain roll. Eating well when breastfeeding is especially important as milk quality is influenced by diet.

Take time to unwind before bed. If your baby wakes up at the crack of dawn, consider adjusting your own schedule to sleep and wake earlier. If you feel debilitated with exhaustion, see your doctor. You may be suffering from low iron (causing anemia), an underactive thyroid, a low-grade infection, or postnatal depression.

Getting ready to crawl

Although the average age to begin crawling is eight to nine months, your baby is already practicing the moves!

Over the coming weeks, your baby will start to lift their head during tummy time, dig their toes in to see if they can propel themself forward, and push up with their arms. They'll also be getting ready to roll, and in a few cases may flip from front to back. Each time your baby moves, they are learning where parts of their body are and figuring out how they can move together.

During tummy time, they may move arms and legs in a "crawling" motion, and, although they can't boost forward, they might rock forward on their tummy. This helps develop the coordination needed to crawl. They might wiggle their torso to achieve some movement, and will look around with their head raised and chest pushed up using forearms or hands. They are interested in the world around them, but though eager to be mobile, they won't crawl until they can sit well without support, some time after the sixth month.

The agile "one-arm-in-sync-with-one-leg" crawl is quite a sophisticated development in terms of coordination and gross motor skills, so most babies won't have this down pat until they approach their first birthday. Don't worry if your baby doesn't crawl—some babies skip this step and go straight for walking, pulling up on the furniture instead of shuffling around on all fours.

It's interesting to note that, since SIDS guidance that babies sleep on

DEVELOPMENT ACTIVITY: GET THAT TOY

Move a toy just out of your baby's reach when they are sitting upright or during tummy time to encourage them to practice hand-eye coordination and the skills necessary for crawling. Make sure you set it at an achievable distance; if the baby can't reach it, despite their best efforts, move it a little closer and encourage them to try again, so they don't feel frustrated and give up.

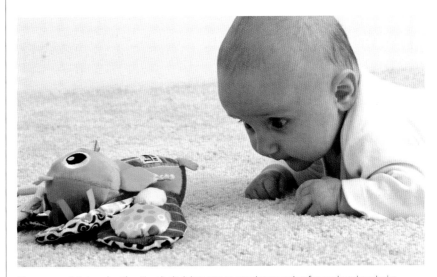

The power of determination Your baby's impetus to crawl may spring from a burning desire to get ahold of something just beyond their reach. You'll be amazed at their perseverance!

their backs came into play around 1994, crawling has begun much later in many babies. It's likely that, because they spend more time on their backs, they aren't getting as much practice time on their tummy, and so crawl later.

You can encourage your baby to spend time on their tummy and enjoy moving their legs by lying

down with them and entertaining them during tummy time. Also, when your baby is on their back, dangle toys above to encourage kicking, or gently "cycle" their legs. These activities will assist crawling when they have developed the balance, strength, and coordination to do so in a few months' time.

Baby gymnastics

Your baby now has greater strength and coordination, so they can bend their body to explore parts they couldn't previously reach!

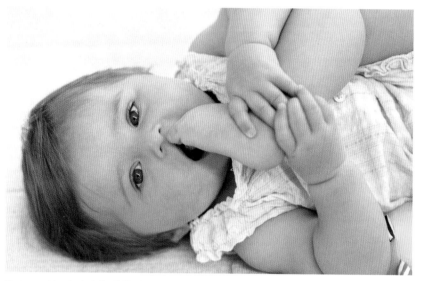

Tasty toes Your baby's flexibility is innate at this stage, so you may see them perform yogic feats of bendiness that would be difficult for an adult to achieve.

Babies are born flexible, but up until now, they haven't had the strength or sufficient control of their gross motor skills to do anything much with this innate flexibility. However, around this time, their ability to perform circus-like contortions develops swiftly. You can encourage their flexibility by holding their legs together, then gently moving them apart to say "peekaboo." Stretch up their arms in a cheer, too.

Strength and coordination

Your baby's muscles are significantly stronger now: their neck muscles are fully supporting their head, and their chest and back muscles are enabling them to sit with support for up to 15 minutes at a time. Babies learn to control the muscles closest to the torso first. For instance, your baby learns to move their arm at the shoulder before figuring out how to bend it at the elbow, then at the wrist. Skillful manipulation of the fingers, or fine motor skills, comes last. Now, your baby will probably be reaching out and grabbing an object with both hands. They'll wrap their hands around it, study it, and most likely put it right into their mouth.

With stronger back and neck muscles, they will love "pony ride" games, such as "Horsey, horsey, don't you stop".

VITAMIN D

Formula contains vitamin D, and breast milk has vitamin D passed on by moms who obtain it through food such as oily fish and fortified cereals, as well as by manufacturing it when their skin is exposed to the sun. However, babies born to Black or Asian parents (dark skin hinders absorption of vitamin D through sunlight) can suffer from a lack of vitamin D, and there have been recent concerns that breastfed babies may not be getting enough vitamin D. A lack of vitamin D can cause rickets, which weakens bones.

Current advice is that full-term breastfed and partially breastfed infants should be supplemented with Vitamin D beginning in the first few days of life. Mothers who fully breastfeed should take vitamin D supplements of 10 micrograms a day from one month after birth. All non-breastfed infants who are consuming less than 32 ounces per day of Vitamin D-fortified formula should receive Vitamin D supplementation. Premature breastfed babies are given supplements from birth; premature formula-fed babies receive vitamins in special formula, but should start supplements once they move to a regular formula.

Running commentary

Tell your baby what you're doing and describe what goes on around them to help them connect your words with objects and concepts.

As you go up the stairs, count the steps; count the toys as you put them back in the basket, and count your baby's toes in the bath. Show them the cat's tail and the leaves on the plant. Point out their tummy, eyes, fingers—and yours. Give them the names of all the things around them to be filed away in their brain. Before long they will have the developmental ability to access and use it.

Repetition is by far the best way to cement your baby's learning. If they have heard you count 1, 2, 3, 4 as you climb the stairs dozens of times, they will find counting that much easier when they are older. Every time you dress your baby, give them the names for all of their body parts. You may find that they start to imitate the basic sounds of the words you use. They won't understand them yet, but they are beginning to associate sounds with objects.

Talking to your baby about what you are doing helps them understand how things work; the order of events; and how activities such as cooking, cleaning, and shopping unfold. Tell them what you are making for dinner, show them the faucets that fill the bathtub, and the light switch on the wall, and demonstrate how it works. Explain what you are doing as you clean up and put things away. Talk to them about what you are going to do each day, and who you'll see.

Describing emotions

Help develop emotional intelligence, too. You can describe the emotions you think your baby is feeling: if they are crying, say "sad." If they are laughing, say "happy." Many of their emotions are felt as physical sensations. Make sure you soothe them when strong feelings are evident to help them learn that you and they can deal with these feelings together.

ASK A CHILD PSYCHOLOGIST

My baby wants to be picked up all the time. Is this normal? Your baby is used to plenty of physical comfort in your arms and still needs that comfort and reassurance from you. However, you can begin to teach that they can cope for a few moments without you holding them. Gently encourage them to play with toys; for example, get down on the mat with them, and spend time showing them how things work. Move a short distance away, but come back if they want you, stroke their back, then move away again. Over time, move farther away, talking to them as you go, so they are reassured by your voice. They'll soon realize that, even if you aren't in their immediate vicinity, you are still there and will come when they need you. If they get distressed and you can't pick them up right away, reassure them with your voice. In a soothing tone, tell them you are there: they'll start to cope better longer and need fewer pick ups.

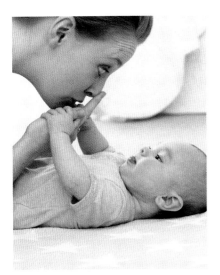 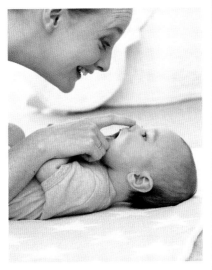

Learning words Point to your nose and your baby's and say the word "nose." Bring his little hand to your nose, repeating the word. Soon, he will point to it himself when you give him a cue.

YOUR BABY IS **FOUR MONTHS OLD**

YOUR BABY MONTH BY MONTH

Building self-esteem

Even at four months, your baby is building up a self-image that will affect their self-perception and perception of the world for the rest of their life.

The most important way in which you can let your baby know that you value and love them is to respond to their needs as soon as you can. If they are hungry, offer food; if they are cold, wrap them up; if they have a dirty diaper, change it right away. Come to them when they need a cuddle, and play when they need to play. Overwhelming evidence suggests that babies whose needs are met quickly grow up to become secure and self-assured individuals.

Your baby needs to know that all the minuscule things they learn to do every day are worth celebrating (and, therefore, doing again). When your baby bats the baby gym and makes a sound, cheer in appreciation to reinforce that this is a success. Kisses, cuddles, clapping, and cheering for even seemingly minor achievements let babies know that they are a successful little person who can do things worth celebrating, in turn developing a sense of self-worth.

ASK A PEDIATRICIAN

I need to go back to work. Can I breastfeed part-time? Yes, you can. You may even be able to continue exclusive feeding of breast milk if you have access to a pump at work and can get your milk home in a cooler. Or substitute formula for the feedings you can't give, and nurse your baby at night and in the morning. Your milk production will adapt as needed. See p.185 for more information on breastfeeding while working.

Playing alone

It's important for your baby's development that they learn to occupy themself for short periods of time and discover ways to entertain themselves.

Babies need moments on their own to gradually understand that they are independent from their caregivers.

Look for occasions when you can place your baby under a baby gym or on a blanket or rug on the floor with some soft toys within easy reach. Leave the baby there for a short time to explore the environment and learn to be alone and amuse themself momentarily. Over a few weeks, try to stretch the amount of time your baby has to themselves. Keep watch and read the signals: pick your baby up before they start fussing. For safety, keep

your baby within sight—they can just as easily learn to amuse themself while you sit nearby. Being able to sense your presence is likely to make your baby feel happier, and willing to play by themself for a little longer.

Learning to occupy themself paves the way for a much easier toddler, who will be more able to find a toy and play with it without always needing your help or participation.

Developing self-sufficiency Give your baby lots of opportunities to play on their own.

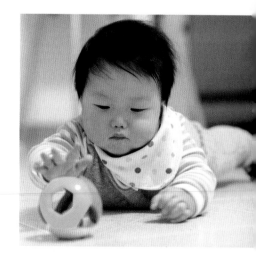

Nature versus nurture

Being aware of how your baby's character is shaped by environment as well as by their genes can help you give them the best possible start.

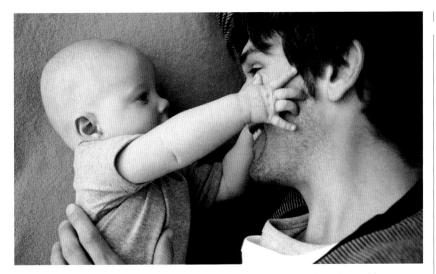

Natural ability Whether your baby seems naturally curious or particularly active, positive interaction with you on a daily basis can help them thrive and develop new skills.

Nature versus nurture is an age-old debate. Whereas in the past, views tended to be polarized, today it's more widely accepted that it's the interaction of genes and upbringing that determines how we develop. Your baby's environment and everyday care are crucial components in how they interact with you and others, and learn new skills. This is especially true in the early years, since it's thought that the care and stimulation a baby receives can affect how the brain develops. The caregivers' vital role in a baby's positive development is undisputed.

While your baby's genes may favor them having certain traits, for example being particularly dexterous or musical, they need to be in a stimulating and secure environment provided by you for these traits to flourish. At this stage, they are learning new skills at a rapid rate, and their senses are constantly bombarded with new information. Your job is to help them make sense of each new experience and ensure that they are sufficiently stimulated without being overwhelmed. It's thought that positive interaction with your baby on a daily basis actually enhances brain development, and responding to their needs will help them thrive. On the other hand, failing to respond to your baby and/or limiting the time you spend interacting can make them feel less secure, and more likely to act out negative character traits.

While talking to, playing, and

ASK A CHILD PSYCHOLOGIST

Do girls and boys develop differently in the first year? Boys and girls do have differences in their development but these tend to show as they reach the toddler years onward. In this first year, if you compare a boy and a girl, you will notice plenty of variation in personality and development, but this is the natural outcome of being two separate individuals, rather than related to their sex at birth.

There is one significant difference between boys and girls in the first year that is useful to know about. Studies have found that boys are more vulnerable to stresses in the family, such as adult conflict and parental depression. Boys are more likely to react to this by being sad or showing withdrawn or aggressive behavior, compared to girls, who tend to be more resilient and less distressed by it. The reason behind this difference is not clear. If you are depressed or have family tensions, getting help will benefit your children, especially your son, as well as yourself.

interacting with your baby are crucial nurturing skills, it's important, too, to be in tune with your baby's needs, recognizing when they have had enough, and letting your baby develop at their own pace. That way, they will have time to process each new piece of information, and consolidate each new skill with you providing support on cue.

Tooth care

Some time between four and seven months, your baby will cut their first tooth. As soon as they have it, you need to start taking care of it.

Your baby's first tooth might come through any time now, and it will usually be one of the two lower front teeth, which tend to appear first (followed by the upper front teeth). Although baby teeth eventually fall out (a process that usually begins at around six years of age), they are important because they enable your baby to speak and eat (chew) properly. For these reasons, you need to take care of them as soon as they appear to avoid infection and promote good dental hygiene habits that will hopefully last throughout your baby's childhood and into adult life.

There is no need to use toothpaste while your baby is so little. Instead, use a little water on a very soft infant toothbrush or piece of clean gauze, and sweep it lightly over the tooth in the morning and evening.

Change your baby's toothbrush or gauze regularly. Avoid allowing your baby to fall asleep with a bottle in their mouth or to nurse while sleeping because formula and breast milk contain sugars that will remain on the teeth all night and can lead to tooth decay. Offer cool water as a supplementary drink rather than diluted fruit juice, which contains high amounts of sugar.

Picking things up

Not too long ago, your baby could only just curl their fingers around objects, but now, at 4 months old, they hold on to them confidently.

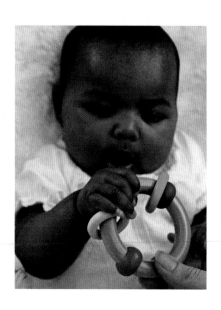

Developing skill As your baby's grasp develops, they can hold onto objects for longer periods.

While your baby still uses the broad "palmar" grasp, a reflex present from birth that causes them to grasp anything placed in their palm and which remains until around six months of age, they are able to hold onto objects longer now and shake a toy as they hold it. Giving them rattles, cups, and other objects will help them develop their handling skills. Blocks are great for learning to pick up and hold.

Your baby might love to hold a ball and then release it on the floor and watch it roll away (make sure the ball is too large to fit in their mouth). Many baby balls have specially designed grip holes that they will be able to fit their fingers into.

Interestingly, babies at this age are not as competent at letting go of objects as they are at picking them up, and will release something they are holding only when they feel the object is up against a hard surface, such as the floor.

Whatever your baby picks up will end up in their mouth: keep choking hazards well out of reach.

Fun baby classes

From the age of about five months, fun baby classes abound! They are good for your baby and also provide a way to meet other babies and parents.

Look online or in local magazines to see what's happening in your area. While some activities can be expensive, others, such as those at the local library, are often free of charge. Among frequent offerings are:

Baby gymnastics

From four—and certainly six—months, classes are designed to build up babies' core body strength, using exercises such as forward rolls.

Sensory development

These aim to give babies a wide range of visual, auditory, and tactile experiences to encourage learning. Fiber-optic light shows, bubbles, bells, musical fun, baby signing, and puppet shows are among the attractions. With so much variety, these classes might be good for babies who are easily bored!

Music

There are lots of courses aimed at introducing young babies to music, most of which involve singing songs and nursery rhymes, dancing, and playing percussion instruments. Babies do enjoy listening to new sounds, but at this age they have a short attention span, so parents might enjoy them more than baby.

Baby yoga

Yoga classes are said to be great for helping babies sleep. A typical session involves stretching and movements such as swinging, rolling, and lifting that will all help strengthen a baby's muscle tone and encourage coordination and flexibility. Some classes enable parents and babies to exercise together.

DEVELOPMENT ACTIVITY: UP AND DOWN

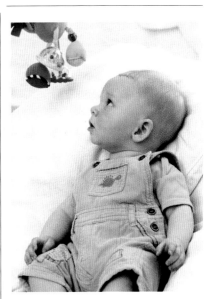

Vertical tracking Being able to watch an object as it moves up and down is a skill that develops after horizontal tracking.

Your baby is now able to follow objects with their eyes as they move vertically. To hone this ability, move a brightly colored toy up and down in front of them. Hold the toy still to begin with, until you see them focus on it, then slowly move it down, watching their eyes as they track the movement. Once you have reached the bottom of their field of vision, slowly move the object back up again. Describe what you are doing as you go. Move slowly at first, so their eyes have a chance to keep up with the object.

PARTNERS GET THE BLUES, TOO

While postpartum depression (PPD) in women is well documented, it's less well-known that around 1 in 10 partners suffer depression after the birth of a baby. Although the hormonal triggers are not present for non-birthing parents, many of the other triggers that contribute to PPD are relevant, such as sleep deprivation, isolation, and changes in their relationship. These factors can be compounded by additional financial responsibilities, and worries about combining the demands of work and parenthood. They may also feel resentful if partners, maybe unwittingly, undermine their baby-care skills. Symptoms can include exhaustion, anxiety, irritability, poor concentration and appetite, and worries about the future. It's important to seek professional help if feelings persist, and to talk to family and friends about feelings.

Milk matters

If your bottle-fed baby seems ravenous all the time now, you might consider using a formula specially designed for hungry babies.

First-stage formula is specially designed to reflect the composition of breast milk closely and be easily digestible. It's fine for your baby to stay on this formula for the entire first year. However, if your baby is no longer satisfied after a feeding, even when you've offered some more, you may want to consider using a special "hungry baby" formula, which contains more casein than regular formula, making it less easy to digest. This supposedly keeps your baby feeling fuller for longer, even though the calorific content is the same. Ask your pediatrician for advice before changing, but if you do change, follow the manufacturer's instructions exactly. Be aware, too, that the transition may cause constipation. In that case, offer some cool water in addition to the usual feedings.

FLU SHOTS

The Centers for Disease Control recommend that all children, from 6 months on, get a seasonal flu shot annually. Children under age 5 have a higher risk for serious complications from the flu. Babies under 6 months old have the highest risk, but the flu vaccine is not approved for such young children.

Action rhymes

Action rhymes provide a fun way in which to enhance your baby's coordination, memory, language—and even social—skills.

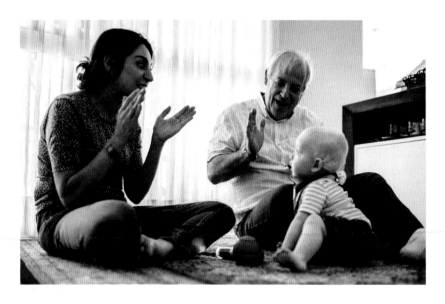

Singing to your baby helps them identify different sounds, timbres, pitches, and patterns of language, and engages them in a way that speech may not. "Itsy bitsy spider," "Patty-cake," "If you're happy and you know it," and "This little piggy" all encourage singing along and practicing the actions. Show your baby how to move their hands in time, and repeat the rhymes to help with memory.

Rhyme time Get a friend or relative to recite a favorite rhyme—it's familiar to him, but also novel because someone else is doing it.

Making sense of sounds

Your baby is now able to make connections in their brain between what they see and what they hear. They're recognizing more sounds every day.

Your baby is now making and becoming familiar with more sounds. They are accustomed to the noise of their rattle, the sound of your voice, and the creak of the door opening and shutting. They are also beginning to associate objects and sounds, and the ability to anticipate is just emerging: they may respond with squeals when they hear your voice since they know your arrival will follow.

Their hearing has been good since birth, but they may have now made the leap to processing what they hear and linking it to what they know about the world in a more complex way. He may expect you to sing "Patty-cake" when you set them up for their clapping game, because they have learned to associate this song with the movements that always accompany it, and may be surprised if you clap but don't sing when they're expecting to hear the familiar words. Your baby will also watch your tongue and lips intently now as you speak: they are starting to link the sounds you make with the movement they see in your lips. Let them see your face when you talk and sing to them to encourage this skill.

While loud or sudden noises may distress your baby, they will be soothed by familiar sounds, so you can calm them in bustling, noisy environments they find disturbing by quietly singing a familiar song; they will be able to focus on your voice and relax more easily. It is likely

DEVELOPMENT ACTIVITY: ANIMAL NOISES

Nothing fascinates a baby more than unusual sounds, and animal noises are ideal for stimulating your baby and helping them understand that different animals make different sounds. Show them pictures in a book and explain that the cow goes "moo," the sheep says "baa," the chicken says "cluck," and so on. Exaggerate your voice and let them see your lips so they can see how you shape your mouth to form sounds. Point to the picture of the animal—or show them a plastic or soft-toy version—so they make the association. While they won't repeat animal noises until they're into their first year, they will have fun listening and learning in these early months.

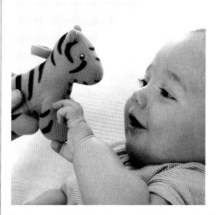 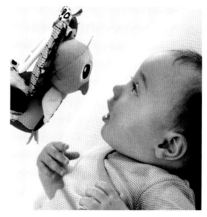

Seeing and listening As you mimic the sound of an animal, show your baby a toy or picture of that animal, so they can make the association between the animal and the sound it makes.

that your baby associates their favorite lullaby with rocking, so if you want to calm them by singing them the familiar lullaby, you'll need to rock them, too.

Interestingly, recent subtle changes in their hearing mean that your baby also understands more about the tone of your voice. When you are happy, they will respond in kind; if you are stressed, they will pick up on this and may become anxious. Using positive body language—turning to face them and making plenty of eye contact when you talk to them—will enhance your communication.

Bundle of laughs

First your baby got the giggles—now they're really ready to laugh. The simplest things can make them chuckle over and over again!

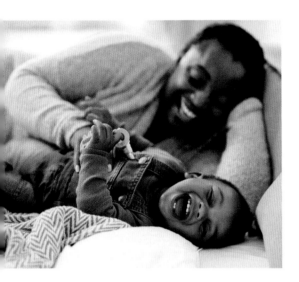

Pop-up toys, silly faces, gentle tickles under the chin or arms, and hiding your face behind your hands before revealing yourself with a "boo" may well invoke a fit of laughter. Your baby is just gaining the cognitive ability to anticipate what happens after a certain event. As this ability emerges, your baby may, for example, laugh the moment you put your hands over your eyes, or when you press down on their pop-up toy.

Fun and laughter Incorporate fun into your daily routine so your baby has plenty of opportunity to enjoy laughter with you.

This marks a key developmental milestone that shows your baby's socialization and language skills are developing. They have learned to communicate by crying, cooing, and grunting, and are now learning to interact by giggling and laughing. Sometimes the best distraction for a fussy baby is to bring out a silly hat or pop a favorite toy out from a blanket to play peekaboo.

Laughing produces chemicals in your baby's brain that will make them feel happy and secure.

Falling asleep on their own

If your baby is used to being rocked to sleep, or to being picked up during a night waking, you'll need to teach them how to go to sleep on their own.

Encouraging your baby to go back to sleep without you there will help them quickly drift off by themselves whenever they wake and, therefore, have a better sleep.

This does not mean you should leave your baby to cry, rather that you should try to put them down while still awake, allowing them to begin to associate the crib with falling asleep.

Lay your baby down snugly after their feeding or story. Dim the lights

and offer a soothing hand on their back. Say goodnight in a calm voice, or choose a phrase you will always use to settle your baby so they learn to associate it, with sleep. Leave the room and see how your baby does. If they resist, return and stroke them again, speaking gently to reassure that you are there. Come to your baby every time they call, but, if possible, try to comfort them without picking them up and rocking them to sleep.

Eventually, they'll get the message that it is safe to sleep, secure in the knowledge that you will come when they need you. However, if your baby really isn't settling and simply continues crying, then do pick them up for a reassuring cuddle before settling them back down.

If your baby cries every night having previously been easy to settle, they may be in pain or unwell. Consult the pediatrician.

Diaper leaks

A leak every so often is to be expected, but if you're mopping up on a regular basis, you might need a different diaper.

Leaking diapers are a rite of passage for all parents. But, if leaks happen all the time, you need to investigate.

First, check that your baby is wearing the right size of diaper. Diapers are sized by weights, but these do overlap and vary between brands, so you may need to experiment. The right diaper should fit well around your baby's legs, without digging into the flesh, and fit snugly around the waist with no bunching or gaps. If the diaper is leaking urine, try going down a size; if poop is the problem, the diaper is probably too small.

Second, check that you're changing your baby's diaper frequently enough—about every two-and-half hours during the day now. However, if your baby looks uncomfortable or the diaper feels full, change it more regularly. Change a poopy diaper immediately so the acid in poop doesn't harm the baby's delicate skin.

Your baby's bladder is larger now, so it can hold a lot of urine and, as a result, your baby will urinate regularly during the night. If your baby is waking with soaked pajamas and bedclothes, you can try adding a booster pad to the diaper (disposable or reusable) to absorb the excess urine. Alternatively, you could try using ultra-absorbent nighttime diapers. Also, if you use disposables, it may be worth trying another brand, if only for use during the nighttime, to see if it prevents leaks more successfully.

ASK A DOCTOR

My baby has diarrhea. How can I help?
Diarrhea in babies can have a number of causes, the most common are gastroenteritis and, less often, milk intolerance. It can also be a temporary problem after antibiotics. Diarrhea can be dangerous in babies, quickly causing dehydration. Call your pediatrician if your baby has a few loose stools in a day, especially if they vomit or refuse to be fed, have a fever, are floppy, sleepy, or pass blood in their stool. Your doctor will decide on the best treatment and whether they need a stay in the hospital if dehydrated. Meanwhile, breastfeed on demand, and continue to give formula if you are bottle-feeding: it's important that your baby gets as much fluid as possible.

My baby coughs a lot at night—what should I do? The most common cause of a cough is a cold. Secretions from the mouth trickle down the back of the throat, causing irritation and a cough. Raising the head of the mattress a bit may bring relief. Another cause of a persistent cough that is often worse at night is narrowing of the airways caused by an infection such as bronchiolitis. Some babies need a short stay in the hospital to help their breathing. See your pediatrician if your baby struggles for breath, rejects feedings, has a fever, is sleepy, sick, or coughs for over a week. Follow your instincts: if you're worried, take them to the doctor.

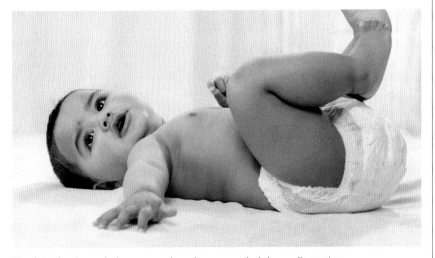

The right size As your baby grows and requires progressively larger diaper sizes, make sure the diaper fits snugly around the leg and waist, without either bunching or digging into your baby's flesh.

Your baby and infections

Babies do get sick, but symptoms are a sign that your baby's immune system has kicked into action, and is fighting the infection.

It's normal for babies to become more prone to infections in the first year as the immunity they gained in the womb wears off. Breastfed babies have immunity for longer from the antibodies in breast milk. Babies' own immune systems are immature at birth and develop over the first year. Try not to worry if your baby seems to catch one infection after another. As long as your baby continues to gain weight, is happy, content, well between illnesses, and developing as expected, they should be fine. With every infection, your baby's immune system becomes more mature and efficient and, in future, will be far better at quickly fending off low-level illness. If you're concerned, though, talk to your pediatrician.

The very best way to prevent illnesses is to not expose your baby to cigarette smoke. Do not smoke and do not allow anyone else to smoke in your home or near your baby. Also, avoid large groups of people, and ask that all family members and friends wash their hands before play.

If you are breastfeeding, continue to do so as normal while your baby is ill. Breast milk boosts your baby's immunity while providing them with your own antibodies.

Restful sleep is also important for a strong immune system, so don't be tempted to skip the naps or keep the baby up too late; your baby still needs at least 15 hours of sleep in every 24-hour period. Finally, when your

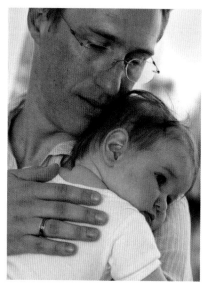

Signs of illness Disruption in your baby's usual patterns of feeding, sleeping, and responses will alert you to any changes in their state of health.

baby begins solids, make sure that everything you give is fresh, healthy, and nutritious. You'll be giving only little tastes at the outset, but every vitamin and mineral will contribute to overall health and well-being.

Seeking advice

If you think your baby is ill or you are unsure about how to care for them, consult your pediatrician first. If the baby stops feeding, develops a rash, or has a fever, do not delay in seeking help as babies can deteriorate quickly.

IS MY BABY SICK?

Many parents instinctively know when their babies are sick. Babies who are inexplicably tearful, more tired and clingy than usual, fractious, not smiling or playing, and experiencing a change in feeding patterns (for example, appearing uninterested, or feeding poorly) may be sick. Being aware of the signs of illness will ensure you respond promptly and seek help if needed.

Obvious signs include:
- A fever (over 102.2°F/39°C)
- Diarrhea or vomiting.
- A rash or spots, or bruises.
- Pale, clammy, or mottled skin.
- A weak or high-pitched cry.
- Being unusually quiet.
- Blood in the stools

Less obvious signs include:
- Unusually long sleeps.
- Not sleeping.
- Failure of your baby to smile when they normally do.
- Irritability or clinginess.
- Excessive drooling

Always seek medical help immediately if your baby:
- Develops breathing problems.
- Has a convulsion.
- Seems blue around the mouth.
- Feels floppy or limp.
- Has a bulging or depressed fontanel.

Keeping up with exercises

It can be tempting to let your Kegel exercises slip, but it's worthwhile continuing them to keep these important muscles in shape.

Strengthening your pelvic floor (see p.65) and increasing your abdominal exercises will really benefit you now. Carrying even the smallest baby for long periods can strain your back and cause discomfort, but you are less likely to suffer if your core is strong.

If you haven't exercised yet, it's not too late to start—they will not only help improve your posture and reduce minor back pain, but will also improve your circulation and help your pelvis "knit" back together where it meets in the front. Your ligaments, including those in your pelvis, became more elastic during pregnancy to allow for the birth of your baby, and regular exercise is necessary to bring your core muscles back in line.

Kegel exercises practiced every day will strengthen the muscles supporting your womb and bladder. This will get you back in shape for subsequent pregnancies, and help prevent urine leaking when you laugh or cough.

There's no time limit on how long to continue these exercises; in fact, it's worth continuing indefinitely.

Continue to practice your pelvic tilts to help your abdominals. Sucking in your tummy and holding for a few seconds will help flatten it and encourage correct posture—which helps avoid back pain. Aim to perform pelvic tilts 8-10 times once or twice a day—perhaps while your baby is occupied under their baby gym.

Touch and feel

Your baby's senses are continuing to develop. The sense of touch, in particular, teaches babies a great deal about their environment.

Show your baby how to stroke their soft toys, feel the crunch and crackle of scrunched-up paper, and experience warm water running through their fingers. Books, play mats, and toys with different textures come into their own at this age. Let your baby roll in the grass, and feel the texture of their soft blanket. Use words to describe what they're feeling: soft, rough, hard, smooth, and so on. This helps your baby learn more about their world.

Stimulating your baby's sense of touch can improve curiosity, memory, nervous system development, and attention span. They'll also develop confidence in unfamiliar situations, since curiosity rather than fear is piqued by the things they can feel around them. Soon, they'll be introduced to solid food—a whole new world of textures. If they've had experience of textures in the lead-up to this, they'll feel less daunted by a squishy avocado or vegetable puffs.

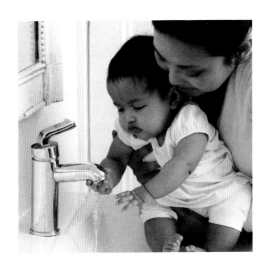

Water play Wash your baby's hand under a running faucet. They'll enjoy the feel of water flowing through their fingers.

Taking a tumble

No matter how careful you are, accidents can and do happen. Try not to worry where minor tumbles occur, though—babies are remarkably resilient.

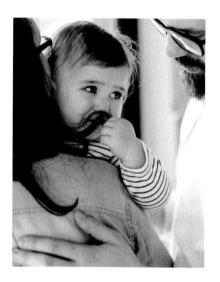

No matter how minor, most parents feel mortified when their babies take a tumble, and suffer paroxysms of guilt and anxiety over what harm the baby may have come to.

However, fortunately, most babies emerge from minor incidents almost entirely unscathed. So, while not downplaying the importance of keeping your rolling baby safe at all times, and being careful when you hold or carry them, try not to feel too

Kiss it better A comforting hug and plenty of kisses will help your baby get over the upset of a minor accident more quickly.

anxious if your baby has a small fall or knock. If they cry right away, or almost right away, all is likely to be fine, especially if they smile soon afterward and calm down quickly.

However, get medical advice if your baby has a sizable bump after a fall, especially on the head; cries for more than a few minutes; has trouble moving a limb; or has significant bruising. If your baby vomits or becomes unusually sleepy, or you have any other concerns about the severity of the fall, consult your pediatrician urgently.

A parenting team

Adopt a team mentality to tackle the sink full of dirty dishes, towering laundry pile, and caring for your baby's every need.

The simple truth is that you and your partner are probably never going to see eye to eye on every parenting issue or household responsibility. Try to develop a strategy that gives you both an opportunity to shine at the things you like and are good at, and allows relaxation time for all.

Different parenting styles are not grounds for a clash. Everything that you and your partner bring to Team Parents will provide important gifts

and opportunities for your baby. Avoid criticizing each other—there is no single "right" way to raise and take care of a baby. Respect and celebrate your differences and be prepared to compromise from time to time.

Attack that to-do list together. Make a list of everything that has to be done around the house and to care for your baby. What do you enjoy? What jobs does your partner enjoy? What does each of you loathe? Where

you're both vying for the good stuff and trying to shake off the unenjoyable, agree to take turns or split the good, bad, and indifferent equally between you. There are always compromises, as long as you are willing to communicate and plan. Resolve these issues now to avoid any buildup of frustration, which could affect your relationship. As a team, you can give your baby the best possible home life.

Body language

Until your baby is able to communicate verbally, you can rely on the way they move their body to figure out what they're trying to tell you.

With every day that goes by, you and your baby are getting to know each other a little better, and not only is their body language becoming more clear to you, you are getting better at interpreting it, too. Learning to read your baby's cues (see p.118) can be an invaluable method of anticipating mood changes and diverting their attention before a meltdown.

Yes, I am bothered

Babies can get annoyed and frustrated just as much as adults can. They may narrow their eyes, lower their eyebrows, and grimace or purse their lips into a square shape. If your baby's facial expression seems to darken, think about what may be bothering them. You may be offering the wrong set of toys or playing the wrong game; equally, your baby may think it is not the right time for a diaper change or to undress for a bath. A little distraction and the usual tricks that make them laugh should be enough to ease them gently out of the mood.

Babies also sometimes wrinkle their noses to show an aversion. Your baby may not want that silly rattle game again; they may not want to be held by someone unfamiliar; they may not want what you just had for lunch via their breast milk. Watch your baby's nose!

If your baby arches their back and flexes their fingers and toes, with eyes open wide, they may be in pain.

Burp them to see if trapped air is the culprit. Or, if they're bottle-fed, think about the last bowel movement— it's possible that they could be constipated (see pp.371–372).

Party on or party over?

If your baby is purposefully averting your gaze, fidgeting, and turning their head away when you are playing, they may simply need time away from stimulation and interaction and are ready for a break. This is a good moment to try a quieter activity to help them unwind: pop your baby into the crib under a mobile, or on the floor under the baby gym, and let them have a little "alone time." You may also notice that they cover their eyes with their hands, which is their way of avoiding excess stimulation and loud noises.

If your baby is kicking up a storm, however, and breathing rapidly, they're probably excited and happy, and boisterous games and tickle time will definitely be appreciated! Similarly, if their hands are clasped at the front of their chest, they are ready for playtime.

DEVELOPMENT ACTIVITY: DO WHAT I DO

Your baby is a natural mimic and will learn emotional expression and control of their face, mouth, and tongue muscles by copying what you do. Stick out your tongue at them, then put it back in slowly. Repeat, and watch them try to do the same. Make sure you applaud their efforts—they may not even know they've succeeded. Open your eyes wide and make a funny face. Continue to repeat it until you see that they're trying it, too. Your baby will soon start this game on their own when they settle down to play with you.

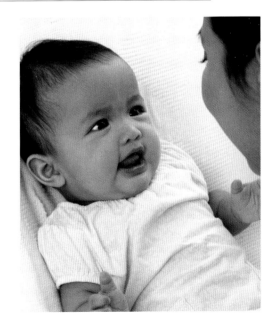

Copycat Make faces and expressions and watch as your baby tries to copy them.

5 months

BABIES WILL COPY FACIAL EXPRESSIONS, WHICH HELPS THEM LEARN HOW TO EXPRESS EMOTIONS. Learn to read your baby's signals for when they are up for noisy toys and physical play and when they are more in the mood for a quiet "chat" with plenty of smiles and eye contact. Getting to know their body language will help you understand what they're in the mood for.

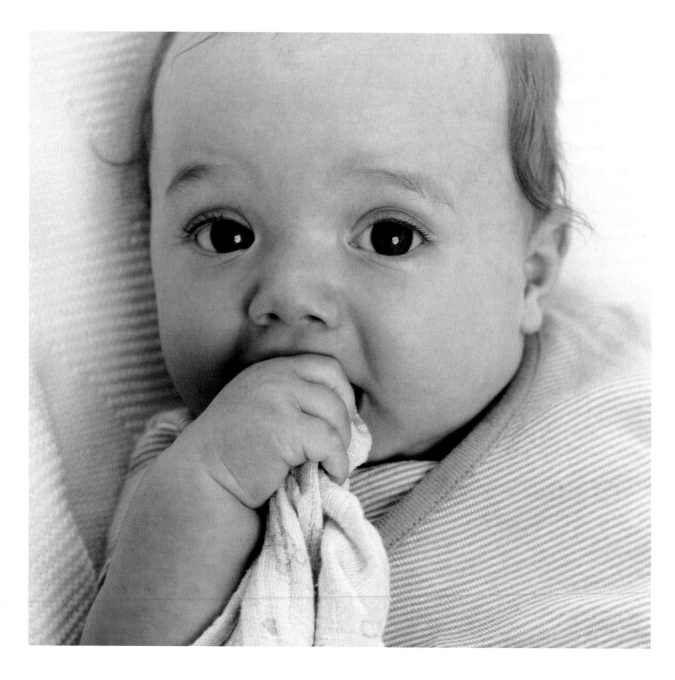

Competitive parenting

Child rearing isn't a competitive sport even if some parents treat it that way. All babies grow and advance at the right pace for them.

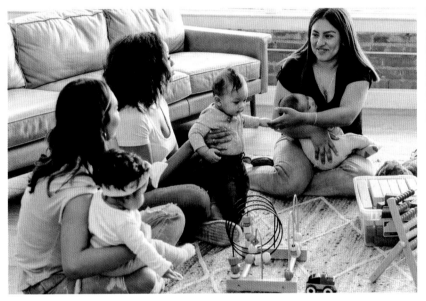

Enjoying groups Being with other parents and babies can be valuable for you and your baby, as long as you don't feel bad if another baby sleeps longer or reaches a milestone earlier.

PREMATURE BABIES AND TWINS

Consider your premature baby's corrected age when reviewing whether or not they are meeting milestones at appropriate times. Little ones who had an early start can take much longer to catch up, but that doesn't mean they don't! In the vast majority of cases, premature babies catch up by school age, and go on to succeed at the same level as their peers.

Similarly, try not to compare your twins to each another; it's common for one twin to leap ahead a little on the developmental front, which is the legacy of sharing resources and space in the uterus. Again, celebrate their unique characteristics, personalities, and achievements, and give each of them the support they need to be the best they can be at the time that is right for them.

Being with other parents whose babies are a similar age provides an opportunity to socialize and access to support. However, occasionally, a hint of competitive parenting emerges. It is natural to talk about and compare milestones, and positive for a parent to be proud of their own child, but watch out if there are suggestions of superiority if one baby is a little ahead of the others. Avoid being drawn in—remember that your baby will develop in their own time. Choose friends well, avoiding those who undermine confidence. If, though, you are worried about your own baby's milestones and if there is a clear, consistent difference between your baby and others the same age, seek advice from your pediatrician. For the small number of babies whose development is delayed, early help is most effective.

Your baby is unique; they will develop, learn, and grow at a rate that is right for them, and shine in some areas more than others. Moreover, early crawlers or talkers don't necessarily go on to be "early" achievers later on. Celebrate your baby's individuality and personal milestones at their unique pace.

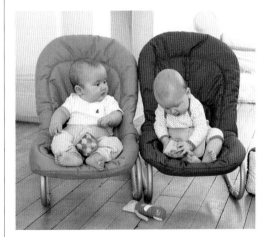

Individuals It's easy to forget that twins pick up skills at different rates. Enjoy their individual achievements.

Are you listening carefully?

By five months, your baby may be using sounds to try to tell you something. You just have to figure out what it is.

It's common for babies to create their own sound vocabulary in advance of real words. Sometimes your baby might be experimenting with sounds by copying. For example, if you always say "Gooood baby" when changing their diaper, they may start to make an "oooo" sound when they're being changed. At other times, they may use a sound to say that they're tired: grunting is common, as is a slightly whiny, fussing sound. They may try to let you know they're hungry by smacking their lips and plaintively "babbling" while trying to maneuver themself into a feeding position. If they're in the mood for fun, they may coo, gurgle, or squeal. Throughout, it is important to respond by listening, replying, and seeing to those needs.

Getting the message

As well as the different sounds your baby makes, their tone and body language will also give clues. When you respond to them quickly and "read" their sounds, expressions, and movement, they know you understand. Respond with words of your own and wait for them to react: they are learning the turn-taking and listening skills vital to conversation. Listen to their babbles and you will hear sounds repeated over and over: respond and encourage, and they will want to communicate even more.

If sometimes it's hard to figure out what your baby is communicating, look at their body language, follow their gaze, and point at things they might want, then watch. If you've got it right, you are bound to get a smile of appreciation. Name objects, activities, and even feelings. You are filling your baby's memory with words to retrieve when their verbal skills develop. These first conversations are an important step in their cognitive and speech development, and, as they reach the 12-month mark, you'll be rewarded with their first words.

10 GOOD THINGS ABOUT BEING A PARENT

When you're feeling exhausted, remind yourself of some of the reasons why being a parent is so fantastic!

• The immense pride you feel at having created a life from a single moment.
• That lurching feeling when your baby first returns your smile.
• Reliving your own childhood. Even while they're so young, it's exciting to anticipate all the things you can share.
• The realization that this is forever is scary, but amazing, too! Putting another's needs first is liberating.

• That intoxicating baby smell, and that incredible cuddling!
• Looking at things as though for the first time through your baby's eyes.
• Rediscovering the art of giggling—you never realized how infectious your baby's giggles could be!
• Enjoying a new sense of closeness with your partner.
• Watching your parents fall in love with your baby, too.
• The first time your baby says "mama" or "dada"—that's you!

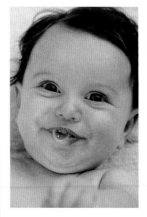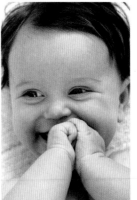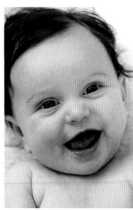

Baby love Raspberries, gurgles, and giggles—a baby's endearing attempts to communicate are enough to melt any grown-up heart, but particularly those of their parents.

Daytime play

The more your baby enjoys playtimes during the day, the more they'll learn and the stronger your bond will become.

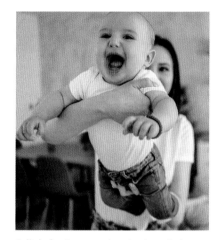

Built-in fun Every good routine has a little time set aside for playing together.

Daytime play sessions expend some of your baby's exuberant energy, and encourage them to use their muscles, practice coordination, and increase awareness of how their limbs move. They also provide opportunity for learning and development in a relaxed, fun way. Plus, they nourish and support your bond.

Your baby will anticipate your play times with pleasure. Think of different ways to keep them entertained and stimulate or challenge them a little; for example, you could sway and dance with them in your arms, hold toys out for them to bat or kick, or blow bubbles for them to swipe at (make sure they don't pop in their face). Try giving them some different smells to sniff—rubbing a little lavender or cinnamon on your hand, for example.

Keeping playtime fun and upbeat is important, since they will learn best in a calm, happy environment. Some parents worry that their baby is not reaching developmental milestones as quickly as others, and use playtime to push them to achieve skills before they are ready. Avoid falling into that trap. Play should be about stimulation and fun in a supportive environment.

Your baby's role models

Adults are not just your baby's first caregivers, but also role models who set an example and teach positive lessons for life.

As a parent, you and your partner are already sensitive to your baby's needs, providing both the day-to-day care and the love that are the cornerstones to healthy emotional development. In addition, the other adults in your baby's life—their grandparents, aunts, uncles, cousins, godparents, and close family friends—provide extra role models.

While it may seem too early to be setting a good example for your baby, they are learning all the time, so it's important to start demonstrating now all the qualities you want to see in them as they grow up. All of the adults in your baby's life can teach them fundamental qualities such as empathy, good manners, fostering a positive outlook, responsibility, and healthy social interaction. Your baby will observe positive characteristics and, eventually, copy these and use them in their own life.

Your baby is learning all the time, and absorbs the most about their world—and how to interact within it—from the people around them. Supplying them with strong, responsible, and loving role models will give them a support network and influences that will guide them through childhood and into adulthood.

Daytime naps

Some babies may be ready to drop a nap now—probably the late-afternoon one—while others continue happily with three naps a day.

Your baby still needs around 15 hours of sleep in every 24, broken into naps during the day and a longer nighttime sleep. They may be ready to have two longer naps during the day, rather than three or four short ones. They're likely going longer between feedings, which means that naps can now last a little longer. Often, the late-afternoon nap is first to go, and babies of this age can manage on a midmorning nap followed by a longer sleep after lunch. However, babies are naturally more playful at this age, so don't assume your baby is ready to drop the nap just because they're harder to settle down to sleep. They may need a pre-nap routine to encourage sleep. If your baby isn't sleeping, but playing, they probably don't need to be asleep.

There's no reason they can't spend some quiet time in their crib—a little solo play will relax them and give them (and you) a break.

When you first drop a nap, it may be a struggle to reach bedtime without your baby becoming cranky, so it's a good idea to push bedtime forward by half an hour or so, until they make the adjustment.

Receiving affection

At this age, your baby loves attention from you—but is also learning how to return your love and affection. Enjoy!

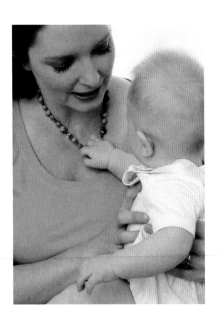

The simple exchange of physical affection between you and your baby is a potent way to express your relationship. At first, affection is largely one way as you offer cuddling, hugs, massage, and stroking. Now, though, as your baby gains control over their body, they will respond. Give and take will begin as they put their arms around your neck when you hold them, or squeal in delight when you tickle them. Very soon, they will reach out their arms to invite you to pick them up or give them a hug.

Reaching out Your baby loves to be held close and will begin to reach out for you—if you're wearing jewelry, they might want that, too!

This early gesture is important in their developing ability to communicate. Responding to their gesture shows them that they have successfully communicated their need, and will encourage them to continue communicating with you.

Your baby also displays affection when they snuggle into your body, and, in turn, feels safe when you hold them against you. Support their head and let them nestle into your shoulder, allowing them to take a good look at the world from the security of your arms. Keep interacting positively with your baby, giving them plenty of attention and responsive communication.

Using initiative

Your baby needs brief periods each day for experimentation on their own, to play without your direction and explore at their own pace.

It is certainly time to give your baby brief periods when they can play unaided. Your role is to make their toys available, whether attached to the stroller, or beside them on the rug, then supervise, but don't interfere for a few minutes. Solo play allows your baby to direct their attention without prompts, so they can spend as little or as much time as they want feeling, mouthing, and watching their toys or mobiles. This should not be their main form of play, however, since they gain most when you talk to them about their world, and play and interact together.

When your baby does play on their own, set them up so they are either well supported by cushions, lying on their back on the rug, or securely strapped into the stroller or bouncy seat. Place a selection of toys within reach, but not so many as to overwhelm them. They may enjoy a basket of small, easy-to-grasp, noisy toys to grip and explore texture and sound as well as bring them to their mouth. Provide toys that they can work themself, such as pop-up toys and fixed items, such as those on a baby gym, that won't roll out of reach and frustrate them.

When they play without your intervention, they'll keep trying to reach their goal, whether kicking upward to hit a toy dangling from the play gym, or pushing buttons on a stroller toy. They may try a bit longer when you aren't there, but can also get frustrated, so intervene if needed. If they become distressed or get into an awkward position, be ready to help out immediately. Solo playtimes should be of short duration, and you need to be nearby and attentive, even though you are not involved.

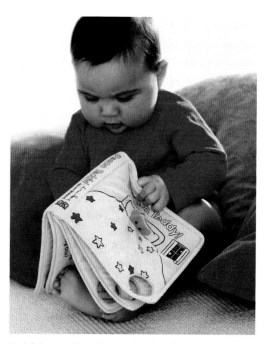

Satisfying toys To make solo play fun, give your baby toys that are easy to use, such as textured fabric books that squeak easily.

CALM AN OVERSTIMULATED BABY

It's important to help your overstimulated baby gain some peace when they need to have the volume on life turned down. You'll have to follow their lead to figure out what they need to calm down. Sometimes "alone time" can be just the thing. Try lying your baby in their crib on their back. Turn on the mobile and let them watch it go around, or put a few easy-to-manage (or chew) books in the crib and let them lie quietly.

Alternatively, your baby may need some comfort. Hold them on your lap and sing their favorite nighttime song or recite a familiar rhyme that has calming associations. Speak quietly and stroke their back. Physical touch has a calming impact on their nervous system, so a gentle touch is always soothing.

Babies who are overstimulated often respond positively to a cool, dark environment. Pull down the blinds and turn down the heat, open a window, or undress them a little to help them cool down (but keep checking them since they can quickly become too cold).

Your baby's first foods

So you've decided that the time is right to start your baby on solids? Going about it the right way from day one will help make the whole experience more enjoyable for you and your baby and encourage them to try new flavors.

Choose a time when your baby is alert and not too hungry. About an hour or so after being fed is a good time to

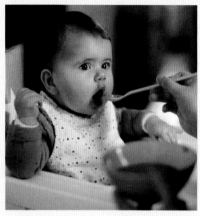

New flavors Choose healthy and tasty foods for your baby, using an immersion blender or food processor to puree them.

start. Put the baby in the high chair or bouncy seat, and have everything prepared so the baby doesn't need to wait. The puree should be lukewarm—test a little on the inside of your wrist, as with milk.

Offer the spoon

Use a spoon to scoop up a little puree and, coming from the side, put the spoon against your baby's lips. If they open their mouth, gently insert the spoon. In the beginning, your baby will "suck" the food from the spoon, rather than use their lips to remove it. Hold it there until it's gone; if the baby doesn't do this, gently scrape the spoon against the upper gums so the puree is left in the baby's mouth. Your baby may look a bit shocked, or spit

the food back out again. (If spitting happens repeatedly, your baby may not have lost the "extrusion" reflex, in which case you may have to wait a couple of weeks and try again.) If your baby doesn't open their mouth, rub a little puree on their lips. Their tongue will eventually appear to lick it up.

Clean up any puree on your baby's chin with the spoon and scoop it back into their mouth. Then start with a fresh spoonful. Most babies will only have one or two spoonfuls on the first few occasions, so be patient. If your baby seems reluctant, stop.

Social mealtimes

Talk to your baby as you offer the spoon, and open your own mouth to show what to do. You may even take a taste from a different spoon to make it clear that it's delicious. Let your baby play with the food—this is part of the process of learning to eat. Your baby may dip in their fingers and suck them, or try to scoop up some of the food and eat it themself.

At the beginning, offer just a spoonful or two per day, usually in one sitting. Offer a new food every three days. If they don't like something, introduce it again a little later. For more information on how to progress, see pp.216–217.

Baby-led weaning

Over the past 15 years, this approach has become increasingly popular. From the age of six months, babies are

GOOD BEGINNINGS

All babies start with simple fruit and vegetable purees, as well as a little cereal, such as baby rice, which can be mixed with your baby's usual milk. Start with vegetables—babies who begin on fruits tend to develop a sweet tooth and then later resist anything more savory. Try a variety of vegetables of different colors—orange, red, white.
- **Vegetable purees:** Potato, carrot, butternut squash, parsnips, turnips, pumpkin, sweet potato, spinach, broccoli, avocado.
- **Fruit purees:** Apple, pear, banana, peach, nectarine, mango, papaya.

- **Baby rice or oatmeal:** (Can contain gluten, introduce after four months).
- **Consistency:** First purees should be liquid, then gradually thicken them as your baby gets used to pureed food.
- **How often:** Once a day for the first week or two if starting solids earlier than six months, or for the first few days if after six months.
- **Best time:** After a milk feeding so your baby is calm and not ravenous.
- **How much:** 1–2 tsp at first; you can give more once your baby becomes accustomed to purees and if they want more (see pp.216–217).

encouraged to feed themselves. To date, there is little empirical evidence to support this method and more research is needed to assess its impact on babies' nutrient and energy uptake, and on their eating behavior and weight.

Keeping a food journal

Make a note of every new food you introduce, when you introduce it, and any reactions your baby has. Introduce new foods in the morning or at lunchtime, since this makes it easier to monitor your baby's reaction to it during the rest of the day.

MAKE PUREES

To make first purees, steam your chosen vegetable or fruit until it is soft. (Vegetables such as carrots can be boiled, or cooked in the microwave.) Use either a tiered steamer pot, or a steamer basket that fits in a regular pot. (Some purees, such as ones made with very ripe peach, papaya, mango, and banana, don't need to be cooked.)

You can puree a large batch of baby food in a food processor, or use a small bowl attachment for little amounts. Alternatively, use an immersion blender or food mill to achieve the correct consistency. First foods should be semi-liquid and almost milklike in consistency to make them easy to swallow. You can add your baby's usual milk or a little cool water to thin purees if they are too thick.

Prepare batches of purees, then chill them right away, and freeze them in portion-size, freezer-safe containers. Ice-cube trays produce ideal baby-size portions. Batch cooking helps you give your baby a variety of tastes every day, and provides you with a series of great stand-by purees when you're busy. To preserve nutrient content, cover ice-cube trays or freezer pots. Fill them almost to the top and put them in a freezer at –0.4°F (–18°C) or below within 24 hours. You can keep purees in the freezer up to a month.

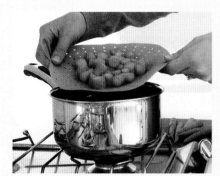

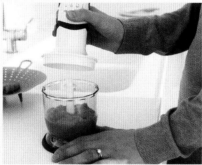

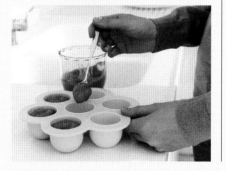

Light steaming Peel and dice your chosen vegetable and put it in a steamer basket inside a pot containing a little boiling water, or in a tiered steamer pot, and steam until the dice is soft (above). **Pureeing** Put the steamed dice in a bowl to cool, then blend with an immersion blender, food processor, or food mill to achieve the correct consistency (top, right). **Freezing** Divide the puree into portion-size containers, cover, label with the date and contents, then freeze (right).

Can I give my baby fruit juice when starting solids? No. Bottle- and breastfed babies do not need juice before they begin eating solids. Until one year of age, their main drink should be their normal milk or plain water. Drinking juice won't help them learn to chew while swallowing, nor will it help in the development of the jaw and tongue muscles. Furthermore, juice given in a bottle can damage a baby's emerging teeth because it "swirls" around their mouth before being swallowed.

Is there anything my baby shouldn't eat under the age of six months? Recommendations have recently changed to encourage the introduction of some of the more allergenic foods early, at 4-6 months of age. These include eggs, dairy, soy, fish, and peanut products. Check with your pediatrician about how and when to give peanut products.

It is important to avoid any foods that might be a choking hazard, such as nuts or seeds, hot dogs, popcorn, or hard foods. (See p.217 for foods to avoid under a year.)

Can I reheat purees in the microwave? Yes—but stir it carefully and test the food yourself before serving since it may have hot spots. You can also use the microwave to defrost foods. Defrost thoroughly, then heat them well in a little boiled water and allow to cool to the right temperature.

Safe rolling

Some five-month-old babies can roll—often at speed—right across the room. Now is the time to babyproof your home!

If your baby can roll themself along the floor, you might be surprised at how much ground they can cover within just a few seconds. Make sure there is nothing that could harm them along the way.

Most importantly, check your floors thoroughly and remove anything that you don't want them to put in their mouth. Also, remove anything that, if grabbed, could cause something to topple over and hurt them, such as loose wires attached to lamps. Your baby's perspective is much lower than yours—get down on your tummy to see what dangers lurk beneath sofas. Keep an eye out for small toys older children may leave lying around.

When you change your baby's diaper, dry them after a bath, or get them dressed, do so on the floor so they can't roll off an edge. If you have no choice but to put them on a raised surface (say, when using a changing table in a public bathroom), keep one hand on them at all times.

ASK A PEDIATRICIAN

Do I need to sterilize my baby's toys?
You may choose to sterilize bottles, nipples, and pacifiers, and you can decide to sterilize mouthed toys, too. However, since your baby needs exposure to some germs to build immunity, common sense is the key. If the dog has licked a toy, or a sick sibling or adult has touched it, clean it in a hot dishwasher or washing machine, or in a sterilizer before letting them play with it again. Otherwise, use common sense.

Frustrated baby

Some babies are determined to get ahead in life—and want to do more than they are physically capable of. No wonder they're frustrated!

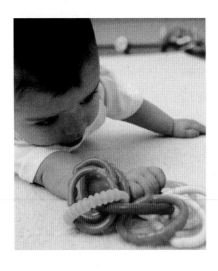

While some babies are content to sit back and watch the world go by, others really do want to run before they can walk! If yours is the latter, you are going to have to expect tears of frustration when your baby sits up and reaches forward to support themselves on their arms, but then collapses; and anticipate a meltdown if they become "stranded" on their tummy. Although it might be difficult to witness on a daily basis, just accept that this is an essential part of the learning process—without it, your baby would be content to sit still. You have a baby who will likely be much happier once they are able to crawl.

Of course, if your baby begins to get very upset and frustrated, sometimes it's best to step in. If they are reaching for a toy, gently stretch them toward it so they can grab it themself; if it is being stranded on their tummy that is upsetting them, move in and reposition them gently, praising their efforts as you do so.

Striving and success Your baby's frustration will be alleviated when their goal is achieved.

Feeling connected

Parenting is both wonderful and stressful. At times, the road ahead seems tough, but there are lots of resources you can tap into.

Connecting with other parents can be invaluable, not just for new parents, but also for parents with older children. By sharing experiences and advice, you can find and offer reassurance on parenting issues and concerns that can be difficult to deal with in isolation.

If you are a new parent, and not many of your existing friends have started families yet, local parent-and-baby groups are a great way to meet other families. Groups are often run at community centers, places of worship, or libraries, so take a look at notice boards in your area, your pediatrician's office, or support forums on social media for details. You can also search online (see also the resources section of this book, pp.384–385). Some birthing centers run "stay-and-play" sessions to enable parents to socialize with other new parents and babies.

Community-run family services

Many local places of worship and community centers offer help and guidance to parents. Some may offer advice on different aspects of parenting, from the health and well-being of your baby to self-care. Others may offer free classes for moms and babies, so you can meet and socialize with parents who have babies the same age as yours. Check your local resources for the type of free classes that may be given. Some might be parent-and-baby exercise classes, where you use your baby as resistance, while others might be playgroups or story time at libraries.

Local recreation centers or national chain gyms offer fun classes for parents and babies, where you can introduce your baby to different types of movement, rhythm, and group participation. You'll need to register and pay for classes, but you might enjoy interacting with your baby in a social group of like-minded parents.

Internet resources

Social networking has boomed in recent years, and among the many chat rooms and blogs lie parenting websites that offer invaluable advice. Many facilitate live chat and give advice on topics from feeding to sleeping, and information about local groups and activities.

Several online communities can connect you with local listings, advice, and opportunities to log on and share experiences. Above all, they can provide a sense of community, and, if your baby does something that worries you, or doesn't achieve a key milestone, you will find other parents who have gone through the same thing and can offer practical advice, or at least a reassuring voice. However, if you remain concerned about any aspect of your baby's health, seek professional medical advice from your pediatrician.

SINGLE PARENTS

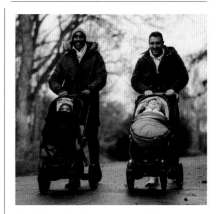

Good times Both you and your baby may benefit from socializing with other families.

From advice on finding appropriate child care to arranging contact with your baby's other parent, single-parenting websites help you negotiate the particular twists and turns of taking care of a baby on your own. Many provide extensive advice on rights and benefits, in addition to case studies and guidance on how to deal with the challenges of juggling work and taking care of a baby on your own. Downloadable fact sheets, help lines, and email advice are just some of the services they provide, and, if you become a member, all tend to offer an online chat forum so you can share your concerns and successes with other single parents.

Brain development

Your baby's experiences build up to create trillions of neural networks in their brain, forming the basis of their understanding of the world.

Babies are born with all the brain cells they will ever have but, at first, there are only a few connections between them. With every passing week, whatever your baby sees, hears, touches, smells, or tastes creates unique connections or neural pathways. These complex connections lay the foundation for thinking, feelings, and behavior, and are responsible for your baby's many mental milestones. Your care and your baby's environment play into how these connections are formed. The more experiences you provide, the more your baby's brain will absorb: talking helps form language pathways; attending to your baby's needs helps develop the emotional intelligence, and so much more.

BRAIN CELLS

Your baby's brain has 100 billion brain cells, or neurons; their brain is shaped by experiences taken in by the five senses, which help form connections between these cells. By the age of three, your baby's brain has formed approximately 1,000 trillion connections.

Diversion not discipline

You can't explain anything to a baby, so if yours is doing something they shouldn't, the best tactic at this age is to divert them.

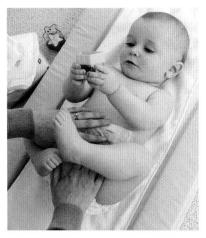

Diversion tactics Occupy your baby with a favorite toy to keep them calm and cooperative when doing less than welcome tasks.

Your baby does not yet have the capacity for naughtiness—the mistakes they make the result of a supremely inquisitive mind and investigations into cause and effect. There are safety lessons you'll want to reinforce, but at the moment, one of the most effective ways to do that is through diversion. If they pick up and chew something they shouldn't have, offer a safer object and remove the original object from their grasp. If your baby reaches for something you don't want them to have, simply move the object away and divert their attention with a toy. Babies are fickle—you'll probably find that they switch with barely a blink.

Try to limit the times you use the word "no" to those with the most serious consequences for the baby. Instead, correct them using positive statements of redirection as much as possible. Be consistent about activities that elicit a "no" from you, so your meaning is clear.

Finally, never become angry with your baby and, above all, avoid physical discipline. They are more likely to learn in a safe, loving, nurturing environment, and listen to you if they trust you. If you yell, they will cry, but if you are calm, consistent, and firm, they will begin to understand the boundaries.

Instant energy fixes

It's important to keep your energy levels up, so if you're feeling drained take time out to review your diet and routine and make a few quick fixes.

Eat breakfast

Try to make time for breakfast every day—a bowl of oatmeal, yogurt, or a smoothie will keep hunger at bay. If you don't have time to eat at home, pack a banana or energy bar to eat on the go. Aim to drink eight glasses of water a day (more if breastfeeding). In addition to water, herbal teas, decaffeinated drinks, soups, and fruit and vegetables all count. Avoid high-sugar or highly processed snacks; instead, have a bowl of unsweetened muesli, or plain yogurt with fresh fruit to get a more sustained release of energy. Opt to home cook family meals as much as possible. Choose simple, freezer-friendly batch cooking recipes that you can prepare ahead of time.

Get some exercise

A brisk 30-minute walk (at a pace that gets you breathing hard) will push your heart rate up and boost your circulation and energy.

Take some deep breaths

Deep breathing allows a more efficient intake of oxygen, making you feel energized. Sit back on your heels and rest your hands on your knees. Sitting upright with your head facing forward, breathe in slowly and deeply through your nose, then slowly exhale, forcing the air out of your lungs. Repeat these deep, slow breaths in and out three to five times, then return to normal breathing again.

Take a cold shower

If you can bear it, try alternating the shower temperature between hot and cold. This technique is said to speed up your metabolism and boost circulation, increasing the oxygen flow to the body, making you more alert.

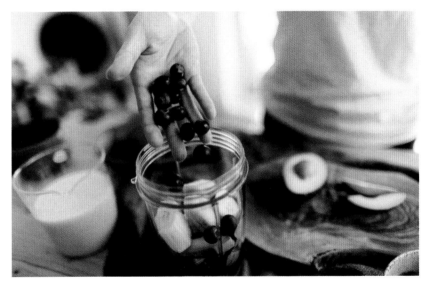

Super foods Healthy food choices will give you the nutrients and energy to stay strong and motivated.

ENERGY NAPS

Being a parent is a great excuse to revive the siesta! Research shows that the body is designed to have a short rest in the afternoon, and that doing so improves energy levels and cognitive function significantly. When you put your baby down for their afternoon nap, take the opportunity to take a nap yourself. A longer nap of about an hour or an hour and a half should put you through a full sleep cycle, which has excellent restorative effects on your energy levels for the afternoon. However, if you also have jobs to do while the baby is sleeping, try to take a 20 minute nap, which will be enough to refresh you, but not send you into such a deep sleep that you wake up feeling groggy. Set an alarm so you don't have to worry about judging the time.

Milk still rules

Even after your baby starts on solid food, milk should remain the mainstay of their diet throughout their first year.

Your baby's diet will change during the next month or so as you introduce new tastes, textures, and foods. This coincides with their ability to master the skills necessary to chew, swallow, and digest. However, that doesn't mean that milk feedings become any less important. In fact, milk is still the most important part of their diet.

When your baby first starts on solids, they'll have only a few spoonfuls of very liquid purees (see pp.178–179). Although these should be nutritious and healthy, your baby will rely on their usual milk to supply them with key nutrients, fats, proteins, and carbohydrates.

As your baby progresses from their first tastes toward regular meals (see pp.286–287), you can reduce the number of milk feedings you give, or the amount of time you spend feeding (and, therefore, the amount of milk they receive). But you'll also need to play it by ear—if they're hungry, they'll need to be fed.

Until they are a year old, babies need at least 17–20 fl oz (500–600 ml) of formula or breast milk per day, and that means regular feedings. Formula or breast milk added to purees will count toward your baby's overall milk intake, too.

Comfort feedings

Aside from needing the nutritional value of their usual milk, your baby also enjoys the familiar comfort that sucking offers. At this age and beyond, babies still require lots of physical touch to nurture their emotional development. Also, by continuing to breastfeed or bottle-feed your baby, you are helping them establish positive associations between food and feelings of love and security.

There's no doubt that some babies are a little reluctant when eating solids commences. However, they soon begin to accept the difference and enjoy the new tastes and textures. They will feel reassured that milk—their old favorite—is still available.

It's better to wean your baby gradually from the breast or bottle since this helps both you and baby adjust both physically (the sense of physical closeness) and emotionally to the change.

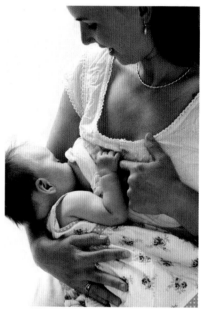

Staple diet Milk, whether in the form of breast milk or formula, continues to constitute the greater part of your baby's diet.

ASK A PEDIATRICIAN

When will I be able to tell whether my baby will be right- or left-handed? You'll have to wait until your baby is at least 18 months before you notice any marked preference, and, particularly if your child uses both hands equally, it might not be until 5 or 6 years old that they make a final choice. Right- or left-handedness is determined as one or other side of the brain becomes dominant; if the right side prevails, your baby will be left-handed, and vice versa. However, babies rarely show a preference for using a particular hand in the first year. They tend to grab with the hand nearest to what they want, rather than twist to use a preferred hand.

About 10 percent of people are left-handed, a trait that is thought to be influenced by genetics. If both you and your partner are left-handed, your child has a 45 to 50 percent chance of being left-handed, too. Try not to influence a preference since this may affect psychological well-being and interfere with writing later on.

Breastfeeding while working

Returning to work doesn't have to spell an end to breastfeeding. With careful planning, your baby can still receive your nourishing milk.

If you are returning to work soon and hoping to express your breast milk, you will need to plan for this at least several weeks before you return. You should inform your employers in writing before you return to let them know your intention so they can provide a safe environment for you to express your milk. Employers are advised to provide a private, clean, comfortable area for you to express (bathrooms are not suitable), and to help you plan dedicated time out during your day for you to do so. How often you will need to express will depend on the age of your baby and the frequency of their feedings, so discuss this with your employer when planning your working day. They should also ensure there is adequate refrigerator storage space for your milk.

Try to start expressing your milk at least several weeks before your return so you can practice and perfect your technique. You will also need to make sure your baby is comfortable taking your milk from a bottle. Again, introduce a bottle gradually several weeks before your return date.

If you are planning to partially breastfeed, and for your baby to receive formula from their caregiver during the day, you will need to reduce your breastfeedings gradually to avoid having your breasts become engorged. Drop one feeding every four to five days until the remaining feedings fit around your working day. You may need to stick to this routine as much as possible on the weekends and holidays so your milk supply remains consistent.

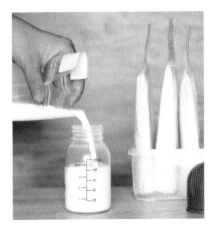

Getting organized In addition to your pump, you will need sterilized bottles or bags to store your milk, and ice packs to transport it home.

CREATING A MEMORY BOX

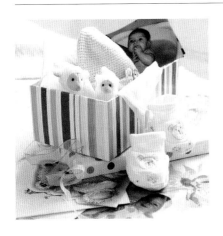

Collecting memories Start a collection of items that will help you remember your baby's infancy. Include a scrapbook in which you can jot down accounts of memorable milestones.

Your baby's hospital wristband, a lock of hair, pictures from your pregnancy scan, a recording of coos and giggles, a book noting down their "firsts," and even a print of their hands or feet can form the basis of your baby's memory box, which you can build over the years to produce a perfect record of all of those memorable moments. Pop in anything that will evoke memories, such as their first onesie or rattle, when they've outgrown them. Keeping special mementos in one place will allow for a wonderful trip down memory lane in years to come.

Little wiggler

With so many things to do and new skills to practice, it can be difficult for your baby to stay still. It's time for a little distraction!

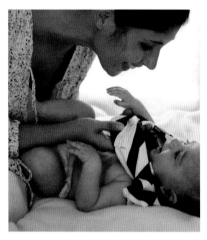

Distraction skills A bit of fun is often all it takes for your baby to forget for a while that they dislike having their clothes changed!

Changing your baby's diaper or clothing and feeding them can become more challenging as they wriggle a bit more, and become distracted by their surroundings. This normal development can last for a few months, so parenting tactics are key.

Try catching them unawares. Change them or get them ready for the bath in a new spot. A little break in routine may intrigue them, and they may forget to try their escape techniques. Put a mobile over their changing table and a few toys nearby to attract their attention. Sing and talk to them, keeping eye contact. Count their toes, tickle their tummy,

blow a raspberry on their neck, buy a new bath toy, talk about the colors of their clothing, and, meanwhile, do your job as efficiently as you can!

If they wiggle when you feed them, move to a place with no distractions. Set up a "feeding association" that imparts pleasure, comfort, and relaxation, such as a new lullaby. Sing it to them when you settle them down to be fed; they'll soon realize that it signals the time to be calm and enjoy close, quiet time with you. When they are eventually reintroduced into noisier, busier environments, their feeding lullaby will help them concentrate on the job at hand.

Weight-gain checks

It is normal to be concerned that your baby is putting on the right amount of weight, and growing at the right rate for their age.

With the focus on childhood obesity, you may worry your baby is too chubby and could have a weight problem; or if small, you may be concerned they're underweight and will always be small. Most parents are reassured by regular weight checks, and generally if your baby remains close to, the "percentile" line (a line showing the expected pattern of growth) on which they were born, they're doing well.

If you are breastfeeding, your baby is less likely to have weight problems. If they seem too small or thin, chances are that regular weight checks will pick up potential problems. As long as they're alert, active for periods during the day, sleeping well, and feeding and filling diapers normally, all is well

A bottle-fed baby may be more prone to weight gain, simply because they can be overfed more easily.

During weaning, reduce their milk appropriately. Babies can be reliant on milk for comfort as well as nutrition and hydration. So, cut out feeds slowly over the next few months so your baby has plenty of time to adjust physically and emotionally.

If you're concerned about your baby's weight, your pediatrician can check their weight and height and reassure you.

Early rising

Just when your baby begins to sleep through the night, and you think you may get some rest, they begin to wake early—to play!

Babies this age vary in the amount of sleep they need, with a few managing 11 hours a night, some 8 hours, and many still waking for a night feeding. If your baby is going to bed at 6:30 p.m., and rising again, fully alert, by 5 a.m. , try putting them to bed a little later. Don't be tempted to cut down on their daytime naps, though, as this will not encourage them to sleep longer at night, and your baby still needs two to three naps. Instead, try timing their naps to ensure that they don't sleep past 4 p.m.

Think about whether they are waking early because they are being disturbed by something in their environment. Morning light, perhaps. If so, consider installing a black-out blind. Are other family members getting up early and rousing them? Try to keep noise to a minimum.

Make sure your baby is physically active in the day, with plenty of playtime and stimulation. If they're regularly sitting in their chair or in the back of the car for too long (which is inadvisable anyway), they simply may not be physically tired enough to sleep for long periods. A good balance of stimulation and rest will ensure they are tired enough to fall and stay asleep, and will give them more information to "consolidate" at night.

If your baby is happy to play on their own for a short period when they wake up, leave something to look at, such as a cloth book or soft toy.

If you think they're stirring rather than waking, try your usual techniques, such as rocking, stroking, singing, humming, or simply patting them as they settle themself. Avoid feeding them in the middle of the night, as this could become an unwelcome habit very quickly.

If all else fails, take turns getting up with them and enjoy their high spirits, even if you would rather be tucked up in bed!

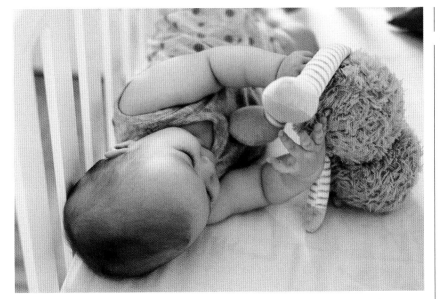

Early riser If your baby is waking up earlier than usual, you may need to make some slight adjustments to their routine to encourage them to wake up at a more sociable time!

FOCUS ON TWINS: WAKE-UP CALL

Even if both twins are sleeping through the night now, at some point in the next few weeks or months you can expect one of them to wake up earlier and disturb the other. Perhaps one twin needs more sleep, or has adapted more readily to a regular sleep pattern. Although it is important for them, and for you, to synchronize their sleep patterns as much as possible, if one of your babies is waking up a lot earlier, it's easiest to separate them. If your twins are still sharing a crib, it might be time to explore separate cribs.

Small is beautiful

As your baby's eyesight improves, they'll take an interest in the tiniest things—dials, knobs, little flowers, and even your smallest earrings.

Around this time, you may find your baby looking with interest at the polka dots on their pants, the eyes on their teddy bear, or the clip that fastens your diaper bag. The smallest items will now capture their attention, and they will reach out to touch them and try to pick them up using a whole-hand grasp. This practice develops fine motor skills.

By now, your baby can also stretch out with one hand to grasp toys and other objects, and can hold them, examine them, and will probably lift them up to suck.

Encourage your baby's curiosity by giving lots of different objects to look at and pick up. Transparent plastic balls with "surprises" inside, toys with fine design details, and activity boards with buttons, dials, and knobs will all fascinate them.

However, beware and keep everything smaller than their fist out of reach. Ensure that buttons are firmly sewn onto clothing (theirs and yours), and avoid leaving your bag or anything that may contain potential choking hazards near your baby.

Fast learner

Your baby's development continues to surge ahead. You'll be amazed at your baby's ability to learn and remember new things.

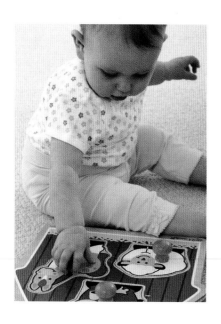

Repetition is the best way for your baby to learn about their physical and social environment. Developing the ability to reason (figuring out patterns for things and learning about how the world operates) requires repetition for your baby's neural pathways to process information well. While social interaction is best for stimulating their senses and building emotional security at this stage, your baby will also enjoy some independence to explore things at their own pace,

Ring ring Your baby won't make a connection between pushing buttons and hearing noise yet but they might if they do it many times over.

fathom how things work, and experiment. If you pick up their toy each time they drop it, you won't be giving them a chance to retrieve it independently, and so learn a number of valuable skills, including hand-eye coordination, fine motor skills, and, some self-sufficiency.

Give your baby toys they can play with on their own without too much help—it won't speed up their development to give them toys intended for older children. In fact, mastering skills with familiar toys helps reinforce new pathways in their brain and will give them the confidence to move on to more complicated toys when they're ready.

Into the big bath

If your baby is getting too big for the baby bath, it might be time to introduce them to the full-size tub.

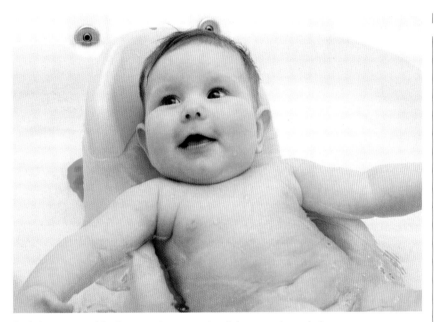

Bath time support A bath support leaves your hands free to wash your baby. It prevents your baby from slipping, and keeps their head out of the water.

WASH A RELUCTANT BABY'S HAIR

If your baby, like so many babies, does not like having their hair washed, squeeze warm water over their head during bath time so they become used to the sensation, and distract them with a toy as you wash their hair unobtrusively. While supporting them with one arm, place a drop of shampoo on their hair, then press a damp washcloth to their forehead to prevent water or soap from entering their eyes. Massage the shampoo into their hair and scalp, then wet a second washcloth or sponge and squeeze it over their head. Continue until the suds disperse. If they still resist, consider buying a special rinse cup, which has a lip to prevent water from reaching their face or eyes. While you wash their hair, make soothing noises to help them relax.

Some babies take to a big bath right away and enjoy the freedom of being able to splash around; others are daunted by the expanse of space, and need to get accustomed to it gradually. You know how your baby is likely to react, so if you think they'll be fearful, pop the baby bath into the big bath a few times before taking the plunge. Or you may want to get into the bath with your baby to help get them used to it.

When you do put your baby in the big bath on their own for the first time, make sure they're safe. Use a nonslip mat for the base of the tub. Get the water temperature right, around 98.6°F (37°C)—run the cold water first, then add hot water until the temperature is just warm. Keep a small washcloth over the hot faucet while your baby is in the bath to catch drips and prevent them from being scalded. Always supervise them in the bath—don't leave them even for a second.

Make bath times as fun and relaxing as possible: place favorite bath toys within easy reach, and add some exciting new ones. Show baby how they bob on the water or how the water runs through them. Speak quietly and gently; your voice will probably echo around the bathroom, and if they show any sign of distress, sing a familiar song.

Bath supports

You may want to use a bath support suitable for young babies, which holds them securely, leaving your hands free to wash them. Sit-up bath seats aren't suitable for babies under six months old, as they need to be able to sit without support so they don't slip down in the seat. Look for ergonomic bath supports that recline and are molded to support a baby's head, shoulders, and back, which are suitable for babies who can't yet sit upright very well.

Introducing a cup

If your baby can sit steadily with support, you might want to let them experiment with a sippy cup now so they don't resist it later on.

The longer a baby drinks from a bottle, the more difficult it tends to be to get them to drink from anything else. Sippy cups can be useful for breastfed babies who refuse to drink from a bottle. While the advice is to start babies on sippy cups at six months, some babies readily accept them at five months. The main prerequisite is that your baby is able to sit up with support. If they're not sitting properly upright, there is a risk they may choke on the fluid. Giving your baby a cup doesn't mean giving up the breast or bottle entirely; it is simply an additional means of giving them fluids.

The right cup

Choose a sturdy plastic cup with a lid that won't break when dropped to the floor. Try experimenting with a few different cup styles until you find a combination of handles and spout that your baby finds comfortable. Some babies prefer to hold a cup with no handles between their palms; others like a handle to grasp. Babies who have been bottle-fed sometimes prefer soft spouts, which are more like bottle nipples, while breastfed babies often prefer the harder, flip-up spouts, which release liquid more easily. Many babies are frustrated with spouts that require a strong suck. Keep in mind that a slow-flowing spout is a good way to start on a cup, since the first few times they use a cup, your baby may gag.

What to put in the cup

You don't need to start expressing milk into a cup; nor do you need to switch to giving your baby his formula in a cup if you are bottle-feeding. Instead, put a little water in and allow a few sips at a time. Once they start on solids, you can offer a cup at mealtimes and stick to the bottle or breast for milk feedings. Babies don't need juices or fruit drinks because the sugars can damage newly erupting teeth.

HANDLING A CUP

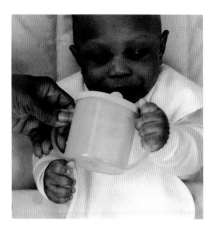

Taking hold You will need to hold the cup for your baby at first, but as they become more dexterous, they will be able to hold it themself.

• Put only tiny amounts of fluid in the cup to begin with, because your baby won't be able to take too much at a time. It will also make it easier for them to learn how to handle the cup.
• Teach your baby how to bring the cup up to their lips and tip it back to enable them to take a sip.
• Put them in a bib. Your baby is likely to swallow only small amounts of the liquid they take into their mouth, and the rest will run down their chin and onto their bib, if you're lucky, or their clothes, if not!
• If they can't hold the cup for themself effectively, give them a helping hand, supporting the bottom as they take sips.

• Once your baby turns their head to indicate they don't want any more, don't force the issue. Put the cup away and try again tomorrow or next week.
• If your cups are dishwasher safe, the best way to clean them is in the dishwasher. Be sure to take all of the parts apart, including valves and straws, and put them in the dishwasher separately. If the cups become scratched or cracked, throw them away and replace them.
• Never leave your baby unattended while they are learning to drink from a cup, in case of choking.

Learning through imitation

Your activities fascinate your baby. They'll enjoy having their own versions of objects and tools you use regularly—to be just like you!.

Babies learn by imitating their parents and caregivers, and enjoy age-appropriate toys that mimic common household objects they see being used in front of them. Toy keys, mixing bowls and spoons, pots and pans, cell phones, and even a baby guitar can provide hours of entertainment and, better still, your baby will be learning as they play.

Show baby how to stir their bowl. Have a pretend phone call, each on your own phones. Teach them how to bang a drum like their big sibling, or jingle toy keys. Your baby is making sense of the world, and these activities provide the opportunity to experiment in a safe environment.

Choose toy versions, or real household objects, such as bowls and spatulas, that are very clean and easy to handle, so your baby doesn't hurt themself. The more you repeat activities and sounds, the greater their understanding of the world will be, and the larger their memory bank—and their ability to retrieve information from it.

Vocal imitation

From around five months, babies imitate not just movements and facial expressions, but also sounds. You may find that your baby hums while they "stir" their bowl with a spoon, as you do when you are cooking; they may make noises that are louder and more excited than usual when they are "talking" on the phone; they may even "sing" when banging on the drum.

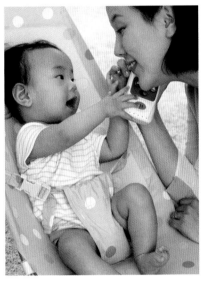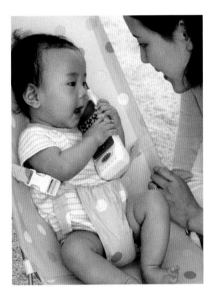

It's for you! Activities such as having a pretend phone conversation will encourage your baby to act out what he sees in real life, which stimulates his imagination and enhances his creativity.

Your baby's vocalizations take on a similar tone and energy to yours when you perform certain activities. For example, they may coo in a quiet, melodious way at bedtime, just as you are likely to talk softly; shout and squeal during playtime; or murmur in the bath if they are used to you soothing them while they splash.

Interestingly, too, you'll find that your baby is beginning to mimic your tone, so their vocalizations with you will differ from those with their deeper-voiced relatives as they copy each of you. Imitate the sounds your baby makes so they will, in turn, imitate you.

ASK A CHILD PSYCHOLOGIST

Should I say "no" to my baby? Yes, you can say "no," but use the word judiciously—save it for times when your baby may be in harm's way. Babies reach an understanding of the concepts of "yes" and "no" when they are around 9–12 months old. Start using these words now and you are preparing them well to reach this milestone. As you pair the word "no" with an action, such as holding your baby back from touching the hot oven, you teach that the word "no" means they should stop. They want your approval, and "yes" and "no" will soon become clear signals as to what you do and don't want them to do.

Creating memories

Your baby's memory is developing quickly. They remember sequences of repeated events, and anticipate what comes next.

You'll notice that your baby's face lights up when they see a familiar book or favorite toy. They may quiet down when you snuggle up with a book at bedtime as they recognizes this as part of the evening routine.

The things your baby will retain first are those that are most frequently repeated and those that most engage their interest. They will remember and imitate actions that they've seen you do many times. Through repetition, they'll know where their toys are, or how to activate sounds on a favorite book with buttons. Repetition is the most effective way of encouraging your baby to learn; don't expect them to recall things after just one try. Your baby's memory skills are still rudimentary. They may show recognition with a very familiar story, but not with one they have heard only a few times; and will master more quickly a regularly presented toy. This need for repetition means they may delight at seeing a grandparent who regularly cares for them, but be less willing to accept a cuddle from a relative who visits less often.

Emotional baby

Your baby won't hesitate to express their emotions, and you may find that they're capable of picking up on and expressing your moods, too!

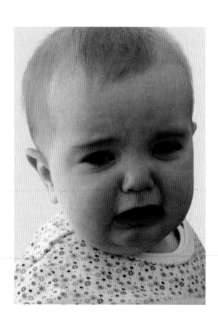

Your baby may throw a toy in frustration, or become angry, tearful, and anxious when you leave the room. They may be excited and happy one moment, giggling and squealing as they play with an older sibling or are tickled by your partner, then annoyed and angry the next, when the games stop or they've had enough. They aren't able to control or understand their emotions: they are simply there and can feel overwhelming. Knowing this can help you feel less frustrated by your baby's emotional outbursts.

High emotions Your baby can't understand or control their emotions yet, and may be happy one minute, and crying the next.

From a very early age, your baby has been sensitive to your emotions, too, and often responds to things in a way that's similar to your responses. If you are stressed and anxious, you may find that your baby becomes tearful or fractious; if you are happy, they may exhibit a sunny, smiley demeanor.

It is important therefore to try to keep calm. Research suggests that children not only pick up on stress, but also become stressed as a result. If your baby is regularly stressed by your emotions, their ability to learn and remember can be affected and they may become oversensitive to adverse experiences, making it hard to respond well to stress in later life.

Good nutrition for babies

Your baby's nutritional requirements are different to yours—so it's good to know the basics before you begin to introduce food.

Now is a great time to think about what the essentials are for your baby's diet, in preparation for the time when you begin to wean your baby. Naturally, their diet will be different from your own, as they have particular needs; their diet must include adequate nutrients and energy to support healthy growth and development. There are four main constituents that should feature, in varying proportions, in a balanced diet—fats, proteins, carbohydrates, and vitamins and minerals.

Fats

Your baby has high energy needs in relation to their size, so breast milk or formula provides a high proportion of fat, which is a concentrated source of energy (calories). When you start to introduce solid foods to your baby (see pp.178–179), it is a good idea to combine them with a little breast milk or formula as the flavor will be familiar to your baby and may encourage them to try new foods. Small amounts of cow's milk can also be mixed with food, but not given as a drink until your baby is 12 months old. You can introduce full-fat dairy products, such as plain yogurt or low-sodium pasteurized cheeses. Avoid highly processed foods, such as fries, chips, cakes, and cookies, opting instead for whole foods in which fat is naturally present, such as avocados and nut butters when your doctor recommends them.

Carbohydrates

Lactose, or milk sugar, is the main carbohydrate in breast milk, which is why it is sweet. Formula also provides lactose. As your baby's diet widens, they will encounter starches and other natural sugars in fruits, vegetables, grains, and potatoes. Although not as concentrated a source of energy as fat, carbohydrate-rich foods contain different vitamins, minerals, and protective plant chemicals (phytonutrients). Your baby's diet should gradually become lower in sugars and higher in starches as more foods are introduced and milk plays a less dominant role.

Proteins

Every cell in the body contains protein, and milk is a great supply. However, it's important to introduce other protein-rich foods into the diet because they also provide important minerals and vitamins. Red meat, for example, provides essential iron and zinc. Vegetarian sources of protein, such as tofu, are easy to mash or puree and are a good source of iron and calcium, too.

Vitamins and minerals

These are essential. Fruits and vegetables are excellent sources—the more colorful, the better. Include green vegetables such as broccoli and spinach early so your baby gets used to their flavors.

BABY'S BALANCED DIET

Below are foods from each of the four main groups to include in your baby's diet after beginning solids.

- **Fats:** especially for babies 10 months and older: vegetable oils (such as olive and rapeseed), fish (such as salmon), cheese, yogurt, butter, eggs, avocado, and nut butters.

- **Carbohydrates:** Baby rice; potatoes; yam and sweet potato; cereals and foods containing gluten such as wheat, rye, barley, and oats (usually after six months); followed by pasta, bread, and unsweetened breakfast cereals.

- **Vitamins and minerals:** Fresh or frozen vegetables, including cooked (soft) carrot sticks, green beans, and baby corn. Fruit may be fresh, frozen, or canned in natural unsweetened juice. Good choices are sliced banana, pear, avocado, soft summer fruits (peeled and cut into bite-size pieces), grapes, and blueberries (both halved to avoid choking).

- **Proteins:** Lean red meats (cooked through); chicken or turkey (opting for the darker cuts, which contain more iron); white fish fillets and oily fish such as salmon, or canned fish in oil; lentils, beans, and peas cooked as dhals; low-salt hummus; eggs.

Playing alongside others

Although it will be a long time before your baby is able to play properly with other babies, at six months they will play happily side by side.

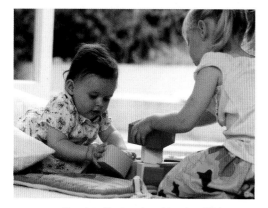

Play date Playing alongside other children helps your baby discover new activities and toys, and they may get their first view of sharing.

Your baby is fascinated by faces, and will probably watch other babies and children with amazement. Your baby will learn new skills by watching and mimicking others. Babies of this age copy other babies, for instance by picking up a rattle if that's what another baby is doing. Your baby may cry when another baby cries, and smile and "talk" to other babies. Regular play dates with other babies or play with older siblings will provide your baby with opportunities for social interaction, which builds the foundations of future social relationships. Although it is far too early for them to absorb social skills, they will see all sorts of relationships in action.

Your baby is likely to absorb themself in their own play, even in the company of other babies. Your baby is not necessarily shy. Their behavior simply reflects their developmental stage. Furthermore, new faces and experiences involve a period of adjustment. Once social experiences become familiar and they remember them as fun, they will be eager to repeat them.

Who's that baby?

It will be many months before your baby understands the concept of "you" and "me." For now, their identity is inextricably linked to you.

Your baby is experimenting all the time with how their body moves: they will begin to copy you and others in simple ways, deeply interested in their interactions with you. Your baby does not yet recognize, or see, themselves as an individual. Put your baby in front of the mirror and you'll find that they are excited by the "new baby" they can see, completely unaware that it is a reflection of themself, even if they recognize you and know that they are in your arms.

You may find your baby looking back and forth between you and their reflection and wanting to reach out and touch both.

It will not be until your baby is around 16 months old that they will begin to recognize themself as a separate individual, a stage of development called differentiation. At this point, they will finally realize that they are a separate individual able to make their own choices, which may begin with saying the word, "No!"

ASK A PEDIATRICIAN

Should I discourage my baby from thumb sucking? I'm worried it will become a habit they won't be able to break?
Thumb sucking is very comforting for babies and gives them a convenient way of soothing themselves without your help. There's no harm in it, so let them suck away. Most children do grow out of the habit and, provided that it ceases by the age of five, there's no evidence that it does any harm to the alignment of teeth.

You're not only a parent

No matter how much you love and enjoy caring for your baby, it's normal to need a little time without them to just be yourself.

All parents need a little time to themselves to pursue their interests, enjoy some adult interaction, and reestablish a sense of self outside of parenthood. In fact, creating a satisfying life alongside your life with your baby will not only make you more relaxed and happy, but will probably make you a better parent, too. It won't be helpful for you or your baby if you feel isolated and never take the time to recharge your batteries.

While it is important not to overload yourself with new projects and activities that can leave you tired and frustrated, it is beneficial to achieve a balance in life that allows you some space to follow your own interests and maintain your identity as an individual.

Your baby is approaching six months old, so can be left with a family member, trusted babysitter, or friend for short periods of time. In fact, if your baby is weaning, they'll probably be able to go a little longer between feeds and be happy to take a spoonful of puree to keep them satisfied while you are away.

You may enjoy using social media and staying in touch with friends via your smartphone, but it's important to enjoy time away from technology, too. Take time out to curl up with a book or magazine and relax, or maybe you want to plan some regular trips to the gym. If you have career aspirations, or are thinking about changing careers when you return to work, you may want to consider investigating the opportunities available to acquire new qualifications. Even time out with friends whose focus is not on babies and children can be rewarding and remind you that, while your role as a parent is paramount, there are other aspects of your life that are valuable and need to be nurtured.

Talk to your partner about making time to pursue individual interests. You could also discuss things you can do together without your baby to help to cement your relationship. It isn't selfish to ensure you are appropriately stimulated. Ultimately, you are a role model for your baby. If you show them how to live a balanced, satisfying personal life, in which individual interests and family both play an important role, they are much more likely to follow your lead as they grow, and develop friendships and interests.

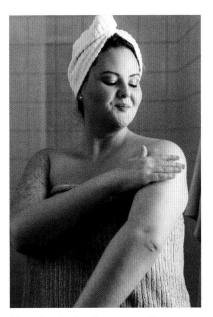

Alone time Having time to yourself to relax and see to no one's needs but your own will refresh you so that, when you return to your baby, you'll be that much more ready for action!

ASK A CHILD PSYCHOLOGIST

My baby makes a big fuss when I pay attention to my other children. Is this normal? You are the center of your baby's world and, at this stage, they will naturally think you belong to them. They won't understand that you have other responsibilities or grasp the concept of sharing time yet. Involve them when you are with your other children; talk to your baby and encourage your other children to do so as well. As long as your baby is getting attention, they'll probably be content. If you are playing with another child, set your baby up with some toys nearby so they can have fun while you're occupied. Show affection to all of your children regularly so your baby becomes used to sharing your time. Sharing will then become natural to them in time.

6 months

IF YOUR BABY LOST THEIR HAIR IN THE FIRST MONTHS AFTER BIRTH—WHICH IS VERY COMMON—IT MAY LOOK PATCHY FOR A WHILE BEFORE IT STARTS TO GROW BACK. Your baby may be increasingly mobile and will make good use of developing hand skills to reach out and grasp objects. They are also experimenting with cause and effect, and learning fast that when they push a ball or roll a toy they can make it move away.

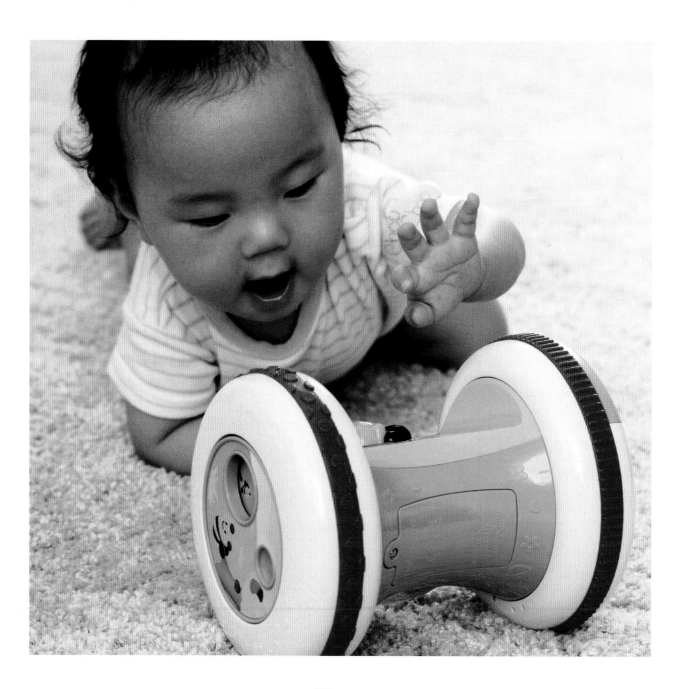

Six whole months

Can you believe how grown-up your baby seems? They're on a roll now—or rather onto much more purposeful moving around.

Your baby is already halfway through their first year. You have probably settled into your roles and grown more comfortable and confident with the responsibilities of parenthood. Can you even imagine now what you did with your time before your baby was born?

Your six-month-old baby is more sociable than ever, and loves to be with people. They'll be smiling and laughing with gusto in company—but may be a little more selective about whom they want to engage one-to-one with. Take advantage of their sociability to introduce them to a variety of people and encourage them to say hello and wave goodbye.

There is a sudden burst in awareness. Your baby is curious and wants to explore everything. They also appear to make decisions when choosing which toys to play with. They will love playing face to face with you, and their sense of trust and confidence is growing. They'll enjoy studying faces, touching, poking, and pulling them to understand their separateness from other people.

Big and beautiful

Most babies have doubled their birth weight by six months so; having filled out nicely, they're probably looking particularly adorable now.

Your baby may be able to sit without support, and be capable of bearing some weight on their legs

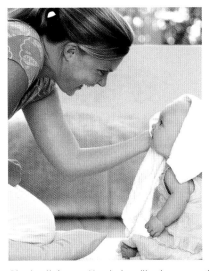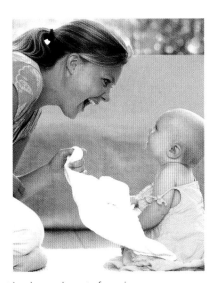

Giggle all the way Your baby will enjoy games that involve an element of surprise or silliness. Hide them under a blanket and then "discover" them. They'll be amused and burst into peals of laughter.

and bouncing when held upright. They'll use their entire hand to rake over a small object and then pick it up, and will purposefully grasp, shake, and bang items. If they drop things, it probably won't be deliberate yet (that will appear around nine months).

BABY WALKERS AND BOUNCERS

It's best to avoid these toys. Baby walkers can be dangerous as they give your baby extra height, allowing them to reach out-of-the-way hazards, and can tip over, causing distress, and injury if they collide with something. There are more accidents with these than with any other toy. Moreover, your baby needs to learn to sit, roll, crawl, and play on their tummy to gain the skills needed to walk, and baby walkers prohibit these activities. Baby bouncers are no longer recommended as they put too much pressure on bones, joints, ligaments, and muscles at too young an age. Also, accidents can result if they're not attached properly.

Your baby's teeth

Your baby's teeth started developing in their gums in early pregnancy—
now the first of their 20 primary baby teeth may begin to come through.
Some babies experience discomfort, while others sail through teething
with barely a dribble.

Most babies begin teething between 4 and 8 months old, although some can start as late as 12 months.

The bottom incisors (bottom front teeth) are the first to come through, followed by the top incisors a month or so later. At 9 to 12 months come the top lateral incisors (either side of the top front teeth). The bottom lateral incisors emerge about a month later, then the canines (the pointy teeth on either side of the bottom and top incisors) at about 16 months. Molars (back teeth) might appear before the canines; and second molars, at the back, may not appear until after 20 months. By the age of about 3 years old, all 20 of the primary teeth will be through.

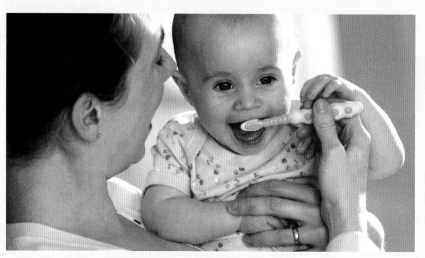

Brushing their teeth Make brushing fun for your baby, and start to get them into the habit of brushing each morning and evening now, so it becomes a familiar part of their routine.

Caring for primary teeth

As soon as your baby cuts their first tooth, clean it regularly (see p.162). Once they have three or four teeth, move on to a toothbrush designed for babies, with super-soft bristles and a small head that can reach gently into the corners of your baby's mouth. Use a tiny speck of children's lower-fluoride toothpaste (1,000 ppm) on the brush. A small amount of fluoride strengthens tooth enamel and helps prevent tooth decay. Don't allow your baby to eat the toothpaste.

Wait at least half an hour after feeding before brushing to allow the antibacterial properties of saliva to get to work first. Brush gently in a circular motion, cleaning the area around the gums in particular, as this is where plaque can build up.

If your baby resists having their teeth brushed, make a game of it. Count their teeth when you brush them, and give them the toothbrush after brushing so they can experiment on their own. You'll need to brush their teeth for them until they are about seven years old.

Seeing the dentist

Take your baby with you to your dental appointments, to familiarize them, then expect your baby's first full appointment to be at around 6 to 12 months old.

ASK A DOCTOR

Is it normal for my baby to have diarrhea when teething? Although there is no reason why your baby should experience a runny stool, some parents do report that their babies tend to have looser bowel movements during teething. If the diarrhea is short-lived, there shouldn't be anything to worry about. However, it should never be assumed that teething is the direct cause of diarrhea. If your baby's diarrhea becomes persistent, they seem at all unwell, or they have a temperature, call your pediatrician just in case.

Tearful parenting

It's often said that once you're a parent, tears tend to flow at the slightest provocation. Read on and don't weep.

A distressing story on the news, a poignant picture, even a troubling episode of your favorite show can have you feeling extra-sensitive, particularly in all matters concerning children. It seems to come with the territory of being a parent. Perhaps this change has to do with becoming more empathetic. Feeling intense love for your own child makes you more aware of other people's—especially children's—suffering. If you talk to other parents, you'll probably discover that they are just as sentimental as you are.

However, if you're breastfeeding and your propensity for tears is accompanied by severe premenstrual syndrome (PMS), and you are in the process of weaning, your feelings may be a result of hormonal changes. When you stop breastfeeding, prolactin, which helps you feel calm and relaxed, declines and progesterone and estrogen levels increase, triggering symptoms. The feelings of aggression, or anger, or low mood associated with PMS should lift once your hormones settle. If your low mood persists, see your primary care physician—you may be experiencing postnatal depression.

Hands free

Once your baby can sit propped up, they'll be able to practice using their hands more, and will soon use them more effectively and efficiently.

Having two hands free allows your baby to practice their hand–eye coordination more readily and to develop the ability to pass a toy from hand to hand. They may also choose a toy for each hand and bang them together, or examine them both with interest before dropping one to concentrate on the other.

The ability to use both hands together to manipulate an object is known as bilateral coordination, which usually evolves and develops throughout your baby's first year. Any two-handed activities provide good practice. Toys with dials to turn, strings to pull, and buttons to push, as well as busy boxes, activity boards, shape-sorters, stacking blocks, and toy rings are all ideal.

Not every baby develops this skill quite so early, so if at six months your baby can grasp an object and put it into their mouth, bring their feet to their mouth, hold smaller objects, and even release objects purposefully from time to time, they're on track with the developmental milestones necessary for bilateral coordination.

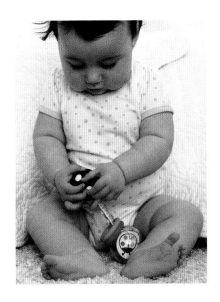

Two-handed exploration Give your baby toys that require them to use both hands to develop their "bilateral" coordination.

That looks yummy, mommy

Your baby is looking longingly at your food and reaching out to grab a taste, but can they have it yet?

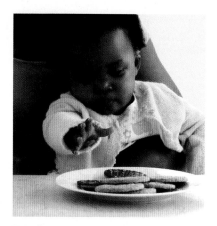

Tempting It's best to avoid introducing certain adult foods, such as cookies.

ASK A NUTRITIONIST

Will weaning my baby early make them more prone to allergies? Your baby's digestive system can cope with solid foods from about 4 months, but weaning is generally recommended from 6 months. Talk to your pediatrician if you plan to introduce solid foods earlier. It is now recommended that you aim to introduce common allergenic foods, such as wheat, dairy, egg, peanuts and other nuts, shellfish, and fish, around 6 months of age to induce tolerance and lessen the risk of allergies. Studies on this topic are ongoing. However, if your baby shows signs of intolerance, such as swollen lips, face, tongue, eyes, or itchy skin rashes or abdominal pain or vomiting seek urgent medical attention. See pages 225 and 376 for more information on food allergies.

Watching you eat and looking interested in foods is one of the developmental signs that your baby is ready to start solids, or "complementary feeding." However, not all foods you eat are going to be suitable for your baby in the early months, and some are best avoided. To introduce your baby to family foods, you will need to adjust your meals so they are suitable and safe for them to eat. Adult food often contains ingredients that are not suitable for babies.

Too much salt Many foods—especially highly processed foods—contain salt. Babies' kidneys are not fully developed, so can't cope with more than 1 g of salt (sodium chloride) per day before the age of one year. That includes the salt naturally found in vegetables and grains, and through your breast milk. An average bag of savory snacks contains at least 0.5 g salt, and a few baby-size pieces of pizza could easily exceed your baby's recommended amount—a good reason to avoid processed foods.

Too little fat Your low-fat yogurts are great to help you with weight control, but they do not contain sufficient fat, and therefore calories, to support your baby's growth and development. Full-fat dairy products, including cow's milk used in cooking, are useful additions to your baby's diet up to the age of two, with a gradual reduction recommended up to the age of five.

Too much sugar Your baby is born with an innate preference for sweet food, hence the importance of introducing vegetables and savory foods early on. Foods with added sugar can encourage a baby to choose sweet foods over savory, which not only causes a dietary imbalance, but also increases the risk of tooth decay once teeth have erupted.

Too much bulk Avoid giving your baby too many high-fiber foods. It's fine to encourage your baby to eat fruits and vegetables, but not to the exclusion of other higher-calorie foods. Vegetables, fruits, and grains tend to be filling, so it can be easy for a baby to feel full without having eaten many calories. It is a good idea to mix your baby's first solids with their usual milk, and move on to other higher-calorie foods. You'll probably know if you are giving your baby too much fiber to eat because the number of diapers you change will increase!

Sweeteners Sugar substitutes were developed to help adults and older children reduce their intake of added sugar. They are not suitable for babies or toddlers, so drinks and foods that contain sweeteners should be off limits.

Alcohol Some adult desserts may contain alcohol. Be very careful not to allow your baby to taste these.

Repetitive sounds

You can encourage your baby's recognition of sounds and words by talking to them constantly, and naming everyday objects.

At this age, your repetition of words and sounds is a vital component in your baby's language development. They will constantly be babbling and running strings of sounds together. Your baby is busy improving their control of their mouth, lips, and tongue to form sounds. Your job is to keep talking to them, to show natural gestures, and to be responsive to them by listening to their babbles, repeating them back, then waiting and listening while your baby responds.

You can gradually develop your baby's understanding of language by regularly demonstrating in your everyday speech that words can be labels for an object. So repeatedly saying "teddy" when a teddy bear is held out is an excellent way to build the connection between something or someone and the name for them.

Familiarizing your baby with sounds will assist them with word recognition later on, helping them take the next developmental leap.

ASK A PEDIATRICIAN

Is it safe for my baby to play in the playground sandbox? As long as they are supervised, they will probably enjoy this experience and learn a lot from watching other children, feeling the texture of the sand, and seeing how it moves in their hands. Choose a pit that is protected from dogs and cats and cleaned regularly. Ensure they don't put sand in their mouth, and wash their hands afterward.

MONTHS 4–6

Nature trail

Whether your baby is lying on a rug in the yard or enjoying a wildlife tour in your arms, they will love the sights and sounds outdoors.

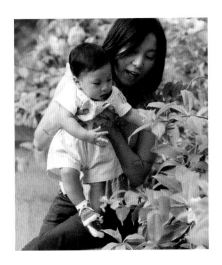

The great outdoors can be a source of fascination for babies. Pop your baby on a blanket in the shade in your yard, or in a safe area of your local park, and let them experience the fresh air and the wealth of stimuli that surrounds them. Point out a squirrel leaping between trees, a fragrant flower, a colorful bird, and a quacking duck in a pond. Encourage your baby to touch the soft blades of grass, some gritty sand, and the coarse bark of a tree. Take your baby's socks off and place their feet into a children's sand pit. Each new experience will stimulate their senses and expand their knowledge.

All the while, continue to add to your baby's memory bank of words. Tell them the names for everything around them, and give them words such as "rough" or "soft" to describe the different textures they encounter.

Environmentally friendly Help your baby explore all the exciting sights, smells, and textures of the great outdoors.

Story time

At this age, your baby begins to anticipate story time with pleasure and will want to become actively involved in the process, too.

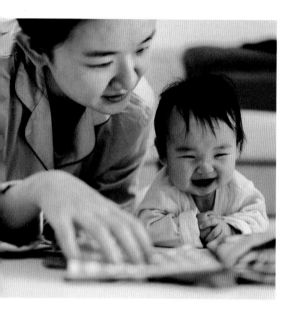

Your baby will love familiar stories and shows anticipation about what comes next. They may pat or try to grab the book to show interest, and show unhappiness with a frown or crying if you stop reading or put the book away. In addition to the enjoyment they get, reading to your baby introduces them to a wider vocabulary, different tones and pitches of speech, their first experience of looking at letters and words, and following a sequence of events. All of these assist speech development, and are good preparation for the future

Involved reader Encourage your baby to explore books by getting them to help turn pages, lift flaps, and stroke textured areas.

when they start to read themself. If you've got twins, you can probably manage to read to both of them from time to time while they're settled on your lap. However, it's good, too, to read to each baby on their own, to give each an opportunity to have one-on-one time with you and develop their own reading preferences. Prop up one baby on the floor with their own books and toys while you read to the other, or ask your partner to read to one while you read to the other.

While it can be tough for over-stretched parents of multiples to allocate reading time for each child, this really will benefit their language and learning skills, particularly if they were born prematurely.

Building independence

When your baby finds a task difficult, resist the temptation to leap right in! Give them a chance to learn by trial and error.

Babies learn best through repetition, trial and error, and your guidance through new activities as they slowly but surely master the skills necessary to achieve their goal. Your baby may repeatedly drop a toy, or be unable to get their little fingers into just the right position to make their pop-up animals pop, and they may fumble as they try to turn the pages of their book.

However, try to resist doing everything for them. On the first attempt at a new movement or activity, guide them through the actions: you might hold their hand or support their body in the right position as they try. Next time, give less, or no, help as they try independently. Make positive sounds of pleasure when they attempt something new, and a cheerful

"not quite" or "uh-oh" when they don't quite manage it. If they become frustrated, do step in and help.

If they get attention for trying, and are encouraged from the sidelines to carry on trying, they are much more likely to continue their efforts. Their problem-solving skills will be enhanced, and so will their confidence, effectiveness, and, of course, pride.

Learning by experience

Now that your baby is more interested in their surroundings, and feedings are easier to plan, you might enjoy venturing farther out.

Your baby is now more aware of what's going on around them and is very receptive to new experiences. For your part, it's probably much easier to anticipate what they need and when they need it. This means that you can be a bit more adventurous and enjoy longer outings occasionally, because you'll know when to take a pit stop to feed or change them while you are out and about. So perhaps now is the time to visit that friend or relative who lives a bit farther away, organize a day out with other moms and babies, or spend a day at the beach with the family.

Visits to grandparents help your baby get to know them better: the more familiar they and their homes become, the easier it will be to plan short stays for your baby with them in the future.

Babies at this age love the great outdoors and so will be fascinated by parks, playgrounds, and beaches (as long as they have some shelter from the sand, heat, and sunlight). Your baby will also enjoy activities where there are other children to watch, such as soft play areas where there are separate designated areas for babies, or visits with your own siblings who might also have children—the bond between cousins can often become quite special.

If you are planning to use public transportation with your baby, it's probably worth checking in advance what the facilities are for strollers. For example, check if you will be able to push your stroller onto a bus rather than having to fold it up; and whether there are elevators at the station.

BEING PREPARED

Outings with your baby can be great fun for both of you, especially if you are prepared for every possible situation. Nothing can spoil an outing more effectively than running out of clean clothes for your baby if their diaper leaks, or not having enough toys to distract them if they become fussy. Ensure you are armed with everything you'll need, and a little more, in the event of an unexpected change of plans. Make sure your diaper bag is fully packed, and that you have enough diapers, baby food (if you are starting solids), formula (if you are bottle-feeding), toys, a comfort item to help to soothe them, and changes of clothes for you both.

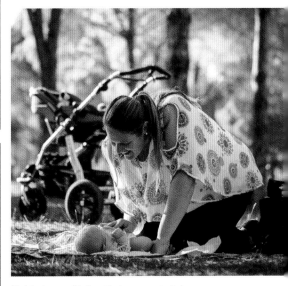

Quick change Clothes that are easy to take off and put on make for hassle-free diaper changes when you're on the go.

ASK A PEDIATRICIAN

A friend has come down with chickenpox. We saw her recently—could my baby have caught it? It's possible, but unusual, for young babies to contract chickenpox. This is because most babies get antibodies against the virus from their mothers while in the womb, giving them immunity for the first few months. After being exposed to chickenpox, symptoms usually appear within three weeks and last for between 5 and 10 days. If your baby has caught it, they may be tired, less hungry, and a bit feverish. You may notice small red spots, typically on the trunk, and sometimes on the face. Chickenpox in babies tends to be mild, so is not usually a cause for concern. If you think your baby has chickenpox, consult your pediatrician.

Legs bearing weight

Your baby may love to bounce when held upright, which strengthens their leg muscles in preparation for crawling and walking.

Now, when held in a standing position, your baby's legs may be able to bear most of their weight. This position helps strengthen their bones and muscles. It's important not to force a baby to stand who is not ready. It's worth noting that some babies prefer to shuffle on their bottoms. These babies tend to be later walkers.

Many parents share a few common concerns when they start to hold their babies upright, such as whether encouraging them to stand will make them bow-legged. Here, you'll find answers to issues that might arise now.

Bow-leggedness

Holding your baby as they stand and bouncing them won't give them bow legs. Most babies have legs that curve outward from the hip, then in again around the ankle, giving them a "bow-legged" appearance. In the womb, the legs take on this shape to make the most of the space they have available.

When your baby begins to stand, and eventually walk, new bone grows and is remolded in order to support their weight. The result of this is stronger, straighter legs. By the age of three, your baby's legs should be as straight as they will be in adulthood. If you have any concerns, call your pediatrician.

Slender legs

Parents of slim-framed babies with slender calves and thighs often worry that their babies' legs are not physically strong enough to bear their weight. If,

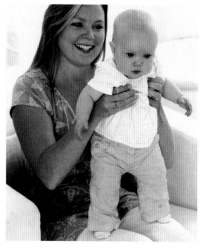

Learning to stand Bounce your baby on your lap to help them develop balance and build their lower-body strength.

when held upright, your baby is strong enough to bear their own weight, they're fine. Leg muscles develop through movement and play. Try placing your baby on their back and cycle their legs, then hold their hands to encourage them to pull themselves up. Tummy time will help strengthen your baby's arms and hands, helping them propel themselves forwards.

Flat feet

All babies appear to have flat feet, partly because of "baby fat," which masks their foot arch, and partly because the arches don't develop until about the age of two, once they have been walking for about a year.

ASK A PEDIATRICIAN

One of my baby's legs looks shorter than the other, and I can't get them to put any weight on that leg when I hold them upright. What could be the reason for this? Your baby could have a condition known as developmental dysplasia of the hip (DDH). This occurs when there is an abnormality in the shape of the head of the femur (thigh bone), or in the hip socket or supporting structures. The abnormality may be mild, where there is incomplete contact between the femur and the hip socket, known as subluxation; or it can be more severe, where there is no contact, known as dislocation. DDH affects 1–3 percent of newborns, is more common in girls, and runs in families. It also occurs more in breech and multiple births, and in babies with clubfoot (talipes).

All babies are checked at birth for DDH, and throughout the first year, and those at high risk are also given a hip ultrasound. However, because it can develop after eight weeks, consult your pediatrician with any concerns, including if your baby won't take weight on one or both legs by about seven months; if their legs seem to be different lengths; or if they always turns one foot outward when taking weight on their legs. After four months, a pelvic X-ray can be used to confirm a diagnosis of DDH. If treatment is given early enough, the prognosis is excellent, and most babies with DDH do not walk late.

Sensing something's wrong

Your baby is affected by your feelings, so it's important to try to shield them from negative emotions and accentuate the positive.

You may find that your baby watches you carefully if they hear a note of sadness or frustration in your voice; if you make an angry phone call, they may stop what they are doing and turn to check that everything is okay. If they see that you are sad, distressed, stressed, or angry, they may cry and hold out their arms to be held. They don't understand your change of moods, but want you to be happy because it makes them happy. They still feel very much an extension of you, and your emotions will guide theirs. When you are sad and anxious, they will become clingier and

in need of reassurance and comfort. Of course, this is a paradoxical situation because the very last thing you need when you are feeling dispirited or distressed is a fractious baby; however, what they're doing is reminding you that they are there. Some experts believe this "antennae" is a primitive instinct that helps a baby ensure their mother doesn't become too preoccupied and ignore them!

Your baby is becoming more sensitive to your moods and in tune with them as they learn about their world. They are watching you and

picking up clues about how to react in each new situation. If you become angry or frustrated in different situations, they will learn that this is the correct and appropriate response. If you are happy and cheerful, and sociable with others, they'll be more inclined to adopt this frame of mind, too. Although no one can be even-tempered all the time, try to make an effort to keep your voice and your facial expressions bright and positive. Your baby will feel much more secure as a result, and will learn to react positively in difficult situations.

Safety first

It's exciting to see your baby's interest in exploring their world, but ensure you keep potentially dangerous objects out of reach.

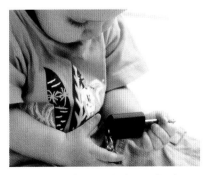

Fascinating objects Your baby may be drawn to dangerous objects such as scissors and keys that have sharp or pointed edges.

A major hazard is button batteries, which are used in a variety of portable devices around the home such as toys, remotes, watches, musical greeting cards, and indoor lights. These tiny batteries are bright and shiny, which make them attractive to young children, and they can become a choking hazard if placed in the mouth or can become lodged if poked up a nose or into an ear. When these batteries get wet, the acid in the battery can break down and become

corrosive, causing burns or serious internal injury if swallowed. Call the pediatrician immediately if you think your baby has swallowed a battery.

Babyproof your home and try to take sensible precautions. Avoid storing cleaning products in low cupboards where they're within easy reach of a curious baby. Household objects such as scissors, string, and glue present the risk of choking, strangulation, or injury. Sharp objects in handbags also present a risk.

Speech development

At around six months, your baby repeats sounds and uses more consonants. They'll begin to try out sounds such as "ma ma ma" and "da da da."

Much as you may want it to be, your baby's first "mama" or "dada" will not be said with meaning: they just happened to get certain sounds in the right order. But your excited response will encourage them to repeat it, and when you answer their call, they'll eventually (in three or four months' time) learn that Mama is you!

Don't be surprised if "Dada" is your baby's first recognizable word. Hard consonants, such as D and B, are learned before soft ones, such as N and M, so Dad may get the honor of being named first.

Your baby will love it when you repeat their babbles back to them, and benefits when you name objects and people, as this strengthens the concept that they can be represented by words, something they'll start to grasp over the coming months. At this point, speaking is a game, and your baby is experimenting with using their vocal cords, tongue, and teeth to make many sounds. Babies have similar patterns of speech development and babbling vocalization regardless of their native language, so around the world there are babies making sounds like yours! They'll make sounds that they find interesting and fun, and repeat them when they provoke a response, or just because it feels good!

High chairs

Your baby's high chair will help them master their eating skills, and make them feel part of the family as they join in the fun of eating together.

A high chair can be a considerable investment, so be armed with a list of requirements before you buy one.

Practicality

Your baby's chair should be easy to clean (a detachable tray is easier to wash and dry than a fixed one) and be suitable for the size of your kitchen. If space is tight, you may prefer a model that folds, or one that can be pushed up against a table and, therefore, doesn't require a tray. Some models can be raised and lowered, which can be useful if you don't have a kitchen table, in which case you can lower the chair and push it up to a coffee table. Or you may prefer a model that adapts to become a table and chair for toddlers.

Comfort

The seat should preferably be padded or able to hold a padded insert that supports your baby in an upright position. Removable, washable padded inserts are best—buy two, so there's always one available while the other is being laundered. A chair with an adjustable footrest and seat heights may prove useful as your baby grows.

Safety

Make sure the base of the chair is wide, so it can't topple over without considerable force. The high chair should also have a five-point safety harness, which should be used each time your baby is in it—babies have an astonishing ability to slither out of high chairs. Finally, ensure that a foldable seat has a safety latch and won't trap your baby's fingers or collapse while they're in it. Secondhand chairs are perfectly fine, but ensure their restraint systems conform to US Consumer Product Safety Commission requirements.

Changing your baby's feedings

You might be thinking about stopping breastfeeding, or you may wish
to mix breast- and bottle-feeding, or try a new formula now.

If you have been breastfeeding and are going back to work, you can arrange to express and store your milk during your workday (see p.185). Though Mom's milk is best for babies for at least the first year, you may decide to mix bottle- and breastfeeding in a way that works for your schedule and your baby's needs.

If you have difficulty getting your baby onto a bottle, try smearing the nipple with a little of your usual nipple cream, or mix formula and expressed breast milk to make it more palatable. Also, try changing nipples, or offering formula in a lidded cup.

PLANNING TO STOP BREASTFEEDING

If you have a date in mind in the next few weeks for stopping breastfeeding, you may wish to start replacing a session with a bottle-feeding now. This is because it's not a good idea to stop abruptly, as your baby is likely to be distressed by the withdrawal of their main source of comfort and sustenance. Also, stopping suddenly can cause your breasts to become engorged and may result in mastitis. Instead, you need to cut down the number of breastfeedings your baby has and slowly replace them with bottle-feedings over a period of a few weeks. The advice is to drop one feeding every four to five days.

You may want to start by dropping the early evening feeding. If your partner or another caregiver can feed the baby in another room so they won't smell your milk, so much the better. Usually the last feedings to go are late evening and morning, which your baby will associate with security, cuddles, and contentment.

If you do have to stop breastfeeding suddenly and your breasts become uncomfortably engorged, you'll need to express some milk. Express just enough to relieve the discomfort; if you express too much you will produce more. It can take up to a couple of weeks before your milk completely disappears. (For more information about planning to stop breastfeeding, see pp254–255.)

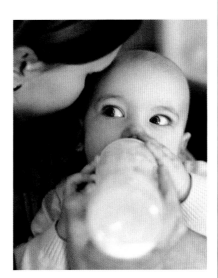

New experience Switch from breast to bottle slowly so your baby has time to adjust.

A new formula

It's not necessary for your baby to move on to follow-up milk as they can remain on their first formula until the age of 12 months. However, whether you have been breastfeeding and are moving onto formula, or have been bottle-feeding, and your baby seems to be hungry even after a good feeding, another type of formula may be more appropriate. The idea of follow-up milks is that there is more nutrition in a smaller amount of formula—in particular, there may be more iron, which babies will increasingly need.

However, your baby will be slowly and gently weaned off their regular milk as they eat more solid foods, and, if you are careful to provide your baby with a variety of healthy foods, they'll undoubtedly receive an increasing amount of vitamins and minerals from solids and become less dependent upon milk for their nutrition.

That said, if your baby is fussy and slow to take solids, consider milk designed for older babies—not only because it often contains more calories and is, therefore, more satisfying, but also because it's designed to provide more iron, omega oils (EFAs), and vitamin D.

Whatever milk you choose, it should satisfy your baby and they should continue to put on weight as normal. Talk to your pediatrician for advice on formula milks and feeding.

Rest and recharge

Your baby's eyes are working together to form a three-dimensional view of the world and all the learning and consolidating as a result is exhausting!

Your baby needs their daytime naps more than ever now—learning so much about the world and their early attempts at moving about will use up lots of energy and tire them out.

As your baby becomes increasingly mobile they will make good use of their developing hand skills to reach out and grasp objects. They are also experimenting with cause and effect, and learning fast that when they push a ball or rolling toy they can make it move away.

Your baby may be able to bear some weight on their legs if you hold them in a standing position, but don't force them to if they're not interested.

Daytime naps Short naps will help your baby reenergize so they are ready for their next adventure!

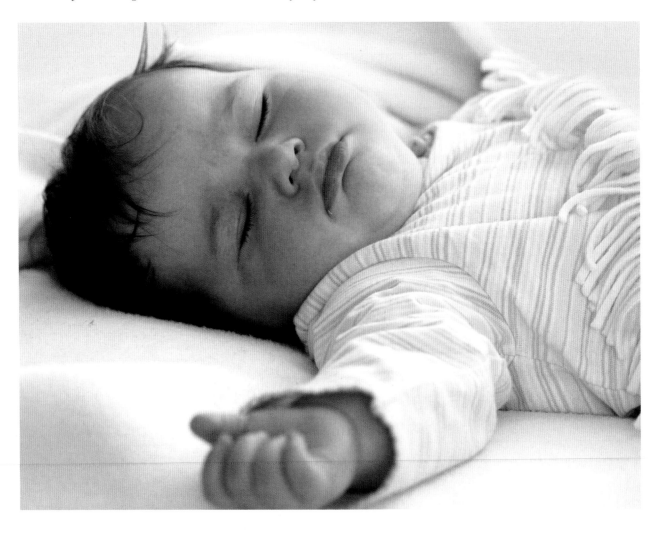

On your mark, get set ...

Your baby is about to get going! Whether rolling, commando crawling, or crawling on hands and knees, they're entering a new mobile phase.

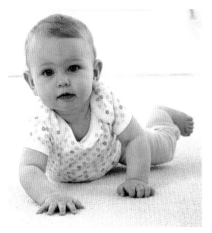 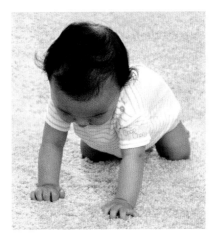

On the move Once your baby begins to experiment with creeping or crawling, carpets or rugs on the floor provide soft cushioning during practice sessions.

It's still early for babies to roll or crawl, but some babies do start to become mobile this early—so it's just as well to be prepared.

Babies learn to maneuver themselves in different ways. Some babies rock on their hands and knees to move forward or backward; others develop an efficient bottom shuffle and never make it onto their hands and knees. Some babies roll across the floor, wiggle on their bellies, or pull themselves along with their tummy to the ground. Some babies crawl backward rather than forward; others skip the crawling stage altogether and pull themselves up on furniture and try to walk. If you have twins, you may find they move in different ways and, of course, in different directions!

Road to independence

The way in which your baby moves is not as important as the fact that they do move. Mobility is a step toward emotional and physical independence, and a developmental milestone that must, obviously, be reached before your baby is able to walk. It allows them to explore their environment at their own pace, satisfy their curiosity, entertain themself, and develop coordination, balance, and muscle strength. What's more, it exercises their heart and lungs, lifts their spirits, and promotes deep, restful sleep.

Encouraging your baby to be mobile helps them enjoy physical exercise, understand how their body works, and, ultimately, have fun as they pursue what interests them.

ASK A PEDIATRICIAN

Is it OK to use an activity center?
Activity centers foster fine motor and problem-solving skills, imagination, and independence. A sturdy activity center, in which your baby is seated and surrounded by dials to turn, flaps to lift, shapes to sort, and buttons that produce sounds, can stimulate and amuse them. Stationary activity centers are appropriate once your baby can sit unassisted, and many adjust to different heights to ensure they can reach the activities while sitting upright. Once they start to stand or walk, these centers are no longer safe.

When my baby starts crawling, can I put them in a playpen when I want to keep them safe? Once your baby is mobile, a playpen prevents them from doing what they really want to do: get around and explore; so they're likely to protest loudly at being confined. It's important to give them as much freedom as possible to investigate and move physically at this stage of development, so try to make sure that they have a babyproofed area where they can scuttle about freely (under your supervision, of course). On the other hand, there are times when you can't watch them every second, and if you want to make sure that they're safe when your attention is focused elsewhere—while you make a phone call, for example—and you have plenty of space, a playpen can be useful.

Learning to eat solid foods

When you start to give your baby foods other than milk, keep in mind that it takes time to learn to adapt to food coming on a spoon.

At the outset, your baby will enjoy purees of baby rice with fruits or vegetables. The purees should be thinned with milk, so your baby can suck the liquid from the spoon. As they become accustomed to taking purees from a spoon, you can make them a little thicker by adding less milk, or by adding more baby rice. Baby rice on its own is also a good starter food because it is bland, easy on your baby's digestion, and most brands are fortified with vitamins and minerals.

Depending on when you start the process and how well your baby receives foods, you'll probably find that for the first few days your baby will only try one or two spoonfuls at one meal a day. However, if your baby seems to want more, allow them to eat more. They will turn their head, get upset, or close their mouth when they've had enough. If reluctant to try altogether, simply stop and wait until the next day to try again.

It is important to make mealtimes pleasant and upbeat so your baby establishes a healthy association with food right from the outset. Ensure, too, that you offer a variety of foods, even ones you don't enjoy. Don't be tempted to add salt or sugar to foods to make them taste better, neither is healthy or necessary.

First foods should be nutritious. One of the most important parts of weaning involves introducing your baby to the flavors and textures of whole foods. The earlier your baby learns to eat

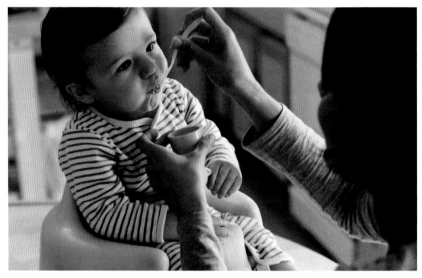

New tastes and textures Eating solid food from a spoon is an entirely new experience for your baby, and they will need time to adjust to it.

vegetables, for example, the more likely they will continue to eat them throughout their childhood and into adulthood. So, giving in and offering your baby their favorite apple puree because they refuse the broccoli puree will not encourage them to enjoy broccoli. Remember your baby may respond to your cues about food, so your dislikes may become theirs. Offer your baby one new food every day or so. If they refuse, try again another day. It can take up to several encounters for a baby to consider a food to be familiar, and it may well take that long for them to take to something that was previously refused.

TIPS FOR SUCCESS

To help the process of introducing solids get off to a smooth start for you and your baby, try the following:
• Find a time when your baby isn't too tired or too hungry—a good time is often after a small milk feeding.
• Be relaxed and happy yourself.
• Expect a mess, be prepared for a range of reactions, and don't allow yourself to become flustered.
• Give praise and encouragement for each mouthful.

Sleeping alone

If you're planning to move your baby into their own room, start getting them used to the space now, before you make the transition.

From the age of six months, it's safe for your baby to sleep alone. Help them make the transition from your room to their own room. Settle them down in their own room for naps at first, so they can become familiar with the feeling of falling asleep in this new environment. Slowly increase the number of naps they take in their own room before you take the plunge and put them there for the night.

You may find that your baby sleeps better in their own room because they won't be disturbed by your nighttime coughs and movements. Alternatively, your baby might wake more often because they miss the rhythmic sound of your breathing, and may feel a little lonely and frightened at first. If they cry in the night, go and soothe them so they learn that you're still there if you are needed.

Give them a comfort object to help them settle. Being able to see, touch, and smell something familiar can help soothe them to sleep. Don't forget to remove objects from their crib overnight.

You may wish to invest in a baby monitor for your own peace of mind. Many parents experience sleepless nights when their babies first sleep in their own rooms. You may find yourself waking repeatedly to check on your baby. If you can hear their cries and their breathing, you will feel reassured that it's safe for you to fall asleep. If you can find a monitor that allows your baby to hear your voice, too, they may also sleep better with a few whispered words from you, or listening to a gentle lullaby.

Tip and tilt

Gently tipping your baby or changing their position gives them a whole new perspective on familiar surroundings.

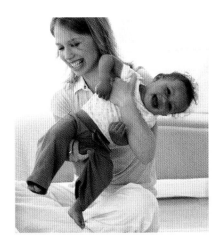

When held in different positions, your baby benefits from sensory feedback. While supporting their neck, tip them back so they can look at the ceiling; lay them on their back over your knee and tickle, or blow raspberries, on their tummy or neck. Your baby may wiggle with pleasure or remain still as they take in this new perspective. Hold your baby's body firmly, rather than by their limbs. Try tipping back their stroller seat when you are out so your baby can look up toward the sky.

This type of play stimulates a baby's vestibular system (which controls balance). Your baby will rely on different muscles, and the coordinated effort to maintain balance and support. Being held in different positions will give your baby new and exciting perspectives, which benefit both your baby's muscles and neural development.

A new perspective Tilt your baby's body to give them different sensory feedback about how their body moves.

Eagle eyes

Their eyesight has greatly improved. Your baby will watch you like a hawk, and notice the subtlest of changes around them.

Babies first develop depth perception between the ages of three and five months, and by now your baby's brain can efficiently interpret the images from each eye to create a sophisticated three-dimensional view of the world.

Depth perception requires visual experience, good eye–muscle coordination, and sufficient maturity of the nerve cells in the eyes and brain. At this stage, your baby's level of vision is approaching that of an adult's, and by the time they are about eight months old it will be almost perfect. Although objects at close range will interest your baby most, they can now see and recognize things from across the room. They'll notice the curtains stirring in the breeze, a toy lodged under the sofa, and your purse tucked away in the corner. Once they can make out these objects, they'll be determined to get to them because now they're attracted by novelty, whereas previously they were probably more interested in looking at familiar objects.

AS A MATTER OF FACT

Studies of depth perception in babies involved a "visual cliff"—a glass surface with patterns creating the illusion of a drop. Babies crossed the "shallow" side, but most reacted with fear of the "deep" side, suggesting that most babies who can crawl have depth perception. This won't keep them safe though, so precautions (e.g. baby gates) are vital.

Sunshine and vitamin D

Vitamin D is important for you and your baby. It is needed for the development of bones and teeth, and for immunity and cell growth.

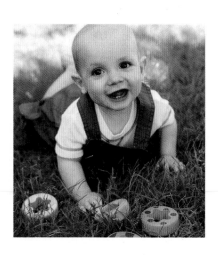

Ideally, we should all get at least 10 minutes of sunlight a day (without sunscreen) to maintain vitamin D levels, which the body manufactures when the skin is exposed to sunlight.

Natural sunlight in the shade is as effective as direct sun, so in the warmer months, pop outside for a brief spell of shady play without sunscreen, each day if you can, avoiding the hours between 10 a.m.

Outdoor play Ten minutes per day in the shade allows your baby's body to produce vitamin D.

and 3 p.m. when the sun is strongest. For the rest of the day, protect your baby's skin with a high factor (30-50) sunscreen outside, even in winter. Some babies are vitamin D deficient, so it's appropriate to give a vitamin D supplement; for example, for breastfed babies and for babies with darker skin (such as those of African, African-Caribbean, and South-Asian origin), because their bodies are not able to make as much Vitamin D naturally (see p.158). Ask your health-care practitioner for advice.

Separating gently

If you plan to go back to work, try to ease your baby into the idea of separation, and give them confidence in the fact that you'll be back.

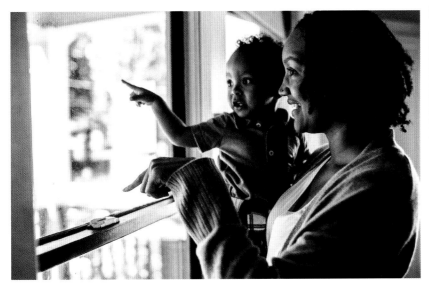

Happy goodbyes Make the separation as easy as possible for both of you by ensuring your baby is familiar with their surroundings and the people who are caring for them in your absence.

Use the following strategies to make the parting easier on you both. Introduce your baby to their caregiver, and have a few sessions together so your baby can get to know their new caregiver in the security of your presence. The first time you leave your baby and their caregiver alone, do so only briefly (say, for 15 minutes).

Avoid leaving your baby if they are tired, hungry, or unwell. The happier they feel, the more likely they are to settle quickly. To help them feel secure, give a comfort object (see p.282) to hold on to while you are gone—something you have enjoyed playing with together, for example.

Adopt an exit ritual—your baby will find security in the routine. Give them a hug, a kiss, and a firm goodbye. Keep your tone positive and expression happy. If they cry, reassure them that you'll miss them, but will soon be back. (Later, you can provide a marker for your return, such as "after lunch" or "after your nap.") Say goodbye again and leave. Avoid the temptation to return to soothe any crying. Instead, put yourself out of earshot. If you are worried, call the caregiver after about 15 minutes to see if your baby has settled down—in most cases, babies are easily distracted.

DEHYDRATION

This occurs when a baby isn't getting adequate fluid, for example through poor feeding because of illness, making them sleepy, breathless, or uninterested in feeding. It also occurs when a baby loses too much fluid, for example through vomiting and/or diarrhea, as in gastroenteritis, or through sweating, caused by a fever or overheating.

Dehydration is a potentially dangerous condition. You should call your baby's doctor if you suspect they might be dehydrated. Continue to feed them as often as possible, offering bottle-fed babies some rehydration solution alongside regular feedings. Rehydration solution, which replaces lost fluids and body salts, is helpful in maintaining their body chemistry.

If left untreated, dehydration can develop into a medical emergency causing brain damage, so if your baby shows signs of lethargy or drops in and out of consciousness, call an ambulance, or, if quicker, take them to an emergency department, at once.

Signs of dehydration include:
- A sunken fontanel
- Listlessness
- Sunken eyes
- Dry mouth, eyes, and lips
- Strong-smelling urine
- Clammy hands and feet
- Fewer than six wet diapers per day.

Showing a preference

Your baby is becoming more aware of themselves, you, and other people.
They may even indicate who they prefer to have taking care of them.

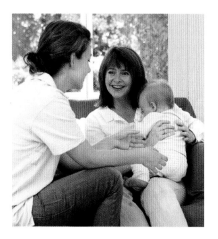

Wary of strangers Your baby may feel shy with less familiar people, and may "nestle in" to a parent for some comfort and reassurance.

While both parents have a role in their baby's life, the primary caregiver is likely to be the one whom your baby prefers when they feel insecure. Equally, the parent who comes home and focuses on play carves a special place in their affections. Try to keep the baby care as balanced as you can when you are at home together. Take turns to put them to bed.

Some parents worry that their baby will come to love a caregiver more than them. There is nothing to worry about on this score. Babies know instinctively who their parents are, and, as long as the time you spend with your baby is spent happily (with lots of play and interaction), your baby will never switch allegiance from you. Try to remain thankful that your baby loves their caregiver, because it would be much harder to leave them if they didn't, and was crying for you.

Sleep at six months

In theory, your baby should enjoy 8–10 hours of blissful sleep each night.
In practice, a good night's rest may still be a distant dream.

Most babies will sleep 12–14 hours out of 24, and for twice as long at night (8–10 hours) as during the day. However, if your baby is still waking for feedings, your nights will be interrupted. Now might be a good time to encourage them to break the pattern of nighttime waking. If your baby is still sleeping in your room, you might be disturbing them. Consider moving them to their own room now (see p.211); this may prove disruptive while she gets used to it, but better for you all in the long term.

If you're breastfeeding and you think your baby is waking in the night because they're hungry, you could try giving extra feedings, known as "cluster feedings," in the early evening before they go to bed. You could also try rousing them very gently, but without waking them completely, if possible, for a drowsy nighttime feeding just before you go to bed, so between 10 p.m. and midnight. You could also try this late feed to help a bottle-fed baby sleep longer at night (but cut out a daytime bottle-feeding

to keep the calorie intake appropriate). These tactics may not work, but they're worth a try.

At six months, your baby might be showing the first signs of separation anxiety (although this generally happens at around eight months), so they may wake up and worry that you're not there. If this is the case, you will need to go in to reassure them and help them settle back down, so they feel secure enough to go back to sleep. For more strategies, see pp.324–325.

Dad's shift, mom's shift

Whether dad stays at home full-time, or you share your baby's care, switching traditional roles can present challenges for parents.

Parents who take a more active role in childcare are known to find it enormously rewarding, regardless of stereotypes. But there are stresses that can develop as a result of one parent being the main caregiver and the other the main "breadwinner." The breadwinner may feel resentful or guilty at being separated from the baby. The parent at home can feel isolated. Even if both parents work flexibly and split baby care more or less equally, it's common for one parent to feel that they shoulder most of the domestic burden.

Do whatever it takes to make sure you are comfortable with your roles and responsibilities. Remember that the baby is forming a relationship with each of you, so parenting collaboratively is essential. Talk about every aspect of your baby's care and make decisions together. Apportion the household chores fairly; plan your baby's menu for the week; make sure you're both consistent about naps and bedtimes; discuss what to do if your baby is upset or won't eat; and check that you're in agreement when it comes to setting boundaries. It's important to make sure that you both are equally involved in your baby's life.

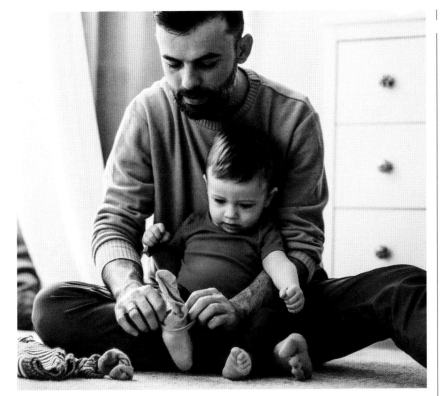

Hands-on Many dads are spending more time at home, building strong bonds with their baby, and enjoying the rewards of playing with them and watching each milestone.

AS A MATTER OF FACT

Studies show that babies who have spent quality time playing with and interacting with their fathers in the first five to seven months of their lives achieve more in school and find it easier to form strong relationships.

Interestingly, it doesn't seem to be the amount of time a father spends with his children that has the most influence in this way, but his immersion in the activity with them during the time he has.

Even if you have only evenings and weekends to play with your baby, studies suggest that if you give your full attention, your baby will grow up to be more self-assured. In addition, your enthusiasm for fun and physical play develops their trust in you and their own confidence. In the coming months, rough-and-tumble play promotes mental and physical strength in both sexes.

Stage one solids—first tastes

If you have waited six months before introducing your baby to solid foods, now's the time to start doing so in earnest. If your baby has already enjoyed their first tastes, now you can start expanding their repertoire.

From six months on, breast milk or formula alone isn't sufficient to meet all your baby's nutritional demands. Additionally, your baby is more likely to accept new flavors, tastes, and textures between five and seven months, so if you've waited until the recommended six months, as soon as they accept food from a spoon, move on quickly using lots of variety.

How to start

Offer your baby single flavors of vegetables, fruits, or baby rice, each mixed with their usual milk. Try each food on its own so you can tell what your baby likes or dislikes and make a note of it. Wait until your pediatrician gives the go-ahead before introducing any potentially allergenic foods, including eggs, cow's milk products, wheat, peanuts, or tree nuts (see p.241 for further information). Your baby is more at risk of a reaction if they have a

family history of atopic conditions—for example, if either your or the baby's other parent or any siblings have a food allergy, eczema, or asthma. If this applies to your baby, it's a good idea to keep breastfeeding while starting solids because this seems to provide some protection against developing these conditions. If you have been using infant formula, don't give any of these foods under six months.

What next

When your baby is happy with a few single flavors, you can begin to offer blends (purees with more than one fruit or vegetable blended together). The more combinations you offer, the more likely your baby is to enjoy different foods.

New routines

Some babies find it hard to adjust to the concept of food coming on a spoon,

SIMPLE STARTERS

As soon as your baby accepts simple single purees, you can blend them to create new flavor combinations.

• **Fruit and vegetable blends** Such as carrot and parsnip; pea and cauliflower; spinach and sweet potato; peach and banana; apple and pear; avocado and banana.

• **Vegetables and meat/poultry** Try carrot and chicken; broccoli and beef; peas and ham; sweet potato and lamb; turkey and sweet potato.

• **Starchy foods with fruits** Try stewed pureed apricots with baby breakfast cereal; mashed banana with wheat biscuits; baby rice and oatmeal (mixed with breast milk). (Slightly older babies can try multigrain and wheat in the same way, but rice and oatmeal are best for younger babies.)

• **Consistency** Semi-liquid purees quickly progressing to thicker purees and mashed foods.

• **How often?** 1–2 meals a day, progressing to 3.

• **How much** 4–6 tsp (more if your baby is hungrier) of 2–3 different foods at each sitting.

• **Milk** At this stage, your baby won't need to drop any milk feedings.

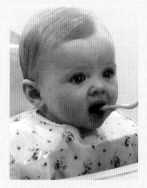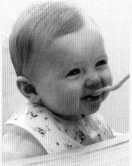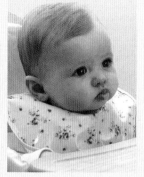

First tastes Gently place the spoon with some pureed food in your baby's mouth. They may take a while to get used to taking food from a spoon, and may push out more than they take in to begin with. Simply scrape it up with the spoon and try again.

BABY-LED FEEDING

Baby-led feeding is a different approach to introducing solids that involves skipping purees and spoon-feeding and allowing babies to feed themselves from the outset.

Some babies who start solids this way may find the transition to lumpy foods easier and manage family meals much earlier. And because they are given an element of choice, some people think that babies who start solids in this manner enjoy the process of eating more than other babies, and are less likely to be picky eaters. There is a risk of choking with this approach, so babies must be supervised when eating.

Some health professionals are concerned at the lack of clinical trials that properly assess the adequacy of nutrition using this method of starting solids or confirm claims that babies eat better as a result. The American Academy of Pediatrics recommends introducing solid foods by spoon-feeding basic foods like rice cereal mixed with breast milk or formula in a 1:4 or 1:5 ratio, then introducing different fruits, vegetables, and other flavors gradually (waiting two to three days before introducing a new ingredient to check for food sensitivities or allergies). The AAP suggests waiting until a baby is eight or nine months before offering finger foods to feed to themselves without choking.

It's also important that the foods babies eat are highly nutritious (see p.210). Finger foods tend to be bulkier than purees and babies may fill up without having adequate calories, so introducing the right foods is key.

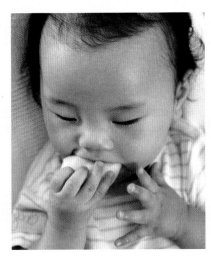

Helping themself At first, a baby may simply play with their food, grabbing chunks of whatever is in front of them, and sucking it.

especially if they are still under six months old. You may want to let them suck some food from your clean finger. Keep offering different foods at regular times, but if they don't want it, don't force it. It might be that they'd prefer to be more in control and feed themself (see Baby-led feeding, above), or need to take things at a slower pace.

Expanding the menu

As soon as your baby is happy eating vegetables and fruits, you can introduce other foods such as pureed or blended meat and poultry. If you're worried that pureed meat will be unappealing to your baby, serve it mixed with fruits or vegetables that they're already familiar with to make it more pleasant. Chicken is an ideal first meat as it is mild-flavored and tender. The dark meat contains twice as much iron and zinc as the breast, so try to give them some dark meat, too. You can also start to introduce well-mashed lentils, split peas, chickpeas, or other pulses; and within a few months, full-fat dairy products, such as yogurt and cheese.

FOODS TO AVOID

Some foods are not suitable for babies until they are over 12 months old, so those listed below are off the menu until then.

• **Some types of fish** Shark, marlin, and swordfish can contain high levels of mercury that could damage a baby's developing nervous system.

• **Salt** Don't add salt to your baby's food—if you are cooking for the family, season your meal after taking out your baby's portion. Avoid salty and processed foods, such as bacon, ham, olives, sausages, ready-to-cook meals, and pizzas.

• **Honey** Because of a tiny risk of a potentially serious food poisoning bacteria (Botulinum), it's safest not to give honey to babies under one year.

• **Unpasteurized dairy products** All dairy products should be pasteurized because of the risk of bacterial infection. Cow's milk as a beverage should not be served to babies until after their first birthday, and cook egg yolks until they are firm.

• **Artificial sweeteners and food colorings** These ingredients are not designed for use in foods for babies, so keep them off limits.

• **Adult foods** It's important to avoid deep-fried foods, chips, fries, or oily dressings; sugar and sweetened foods, such as grown-up desserts; tea and coffee, which contain caffeine and can interfere with your baby's ability to absorb iron; and low-fat or diet foods (see also p.200).

• **Whole nuts** These are not suitable for children under five years because of the risk of choking.

As new evidence emerges, guidance is updated. For the latest dietary advice check online at cdc.gov/nutrition/InfantandToddlerNutrition.

Diaper news

On their milk-only diet, your baby's poop was yellow and mousse-like in consistency. That changes with the introduction of solids.

Your baby's gut can't yet absorb their food fully. This manifests itself in the form of multicolored poop! If you give your baby broccoli, you are likely to find that their poop is slightly green; give them carrots, and the poop will be bright orange.

Consistency

When you start your baby on solids, expect to find some soft lumps in their diaper. If, however, you find that the lumps are dry and hard, it indicates they aren't getting enough fluids and may be constipated. If your baby is eating finger foods, you may find chunks make their way through the digestive tract almost undigested.

Smell

The poop of a baby on solids begins to smell more like adult poop, unfortunately! Where possible, shake the loose poop into the toilet so you can flush it away. If you don't already have a dedicated diaper pail with a lid, now might be the time to invest in one—or, put the soiled diapers into the main trash outside as soon as possible. You will definitely want to invest in some scented diaper bags, too.

Unhealthy poop

Look out for stools that are too hard or too loose, which might indicate either constipation or diarrhea respectively, and speak with your doctor if you spot mucus or blood in your baby's poop. Some believe that babies who are teething have slightly looser stools, but if your baby is also unwell or has a fever, consult the doctor.

Having fun with mirrors

Your baby is developing socially all the time. Babies are natural mimics, and you will often see your expressions reflected in their faces.

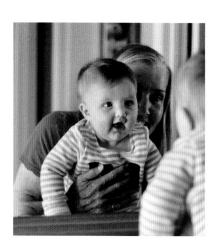

Most experts agree that self-recognition doesn't happen until around 14 months. However, babies love looking at faces—their own and yours—and will respond to the different expressions they see you make, often copying them. This behavior shows they are developing as social beings, learning that they can increase their interaction with you by responding to your expressions with ones of their own, and back and forth on and on.

Build on this interaction by holding the baby up to a mirror and interacting with their reflection. Make a range of faces and expressions— silly faces; a sad face; a happy, smiley face; and a surprised face. Exaggerate your expressions to help your baby read emotions. As well as watching you, your baby will see the delighted response of the baby in the mirror!

Here's looking at you Hold your baby in front of the mirror so they can see you both. Say their name and point to parts of their face.

Vitamins for babies

Vitamins are vital for your baby's healthy development—which is why supplementation of vitamin D may be recommended.

Because of concerns that some babies and children are not getting enough of the key vitamins in their diet, it is recommended that babies are given vitamin drops containing vitamins A, C, and D from the age of six months.

Ask your doctor for advice on supplements and where to get them—some pediatricians recommend other supplemental vitamins. Supplements can also be bought over the counter in pharmacies, but these may contain other vitamins or ingredients, so talk to your pharmacist about which supplement would be most appropriate for your baby. It's important to remember that having too much of some vitamins is as harmful as not having enough. Do not give your child two supplements at the same time.

Vitamin A
This vitamin is essential for the normal growth of different cells and tissues, and plays an important role in the development and maturation of your baby's lungs. A lack of adequate vitamin A can lead to a susceptibility to infection as well as the poor functioning of the lungs and other tissues. Food sources include: egg yolk; butter or spreads; oily fish such as salmon; yellow and orange fruits; and leafy green vegetables.

Vitamin C
Vitamin C is important for general health and the immune system. It also helps the body absorb iron. Good

PLAYING WITH WATER

Babies enjoy playing with water. They'll splash about, soaking themselves in the process. Ensure that they are supervised at all times: play alongside them, and keep their bodies stable and well supported so they can safely lean forward. Half-fill a large bowl with warm water, put in some bath toys, and encourage your baby to fill and empty cups, bob their ducks, swirl the water with a spoon, or simply to splash with their hands. They're used to water at bath time, but this activity teaches how water works in a confined space, and how their actions can cause it to ripple, pour, bubble, splash, and seep. They will also learn how things float and sink. Encouraging water play helps to increase a baby's confidence in water.

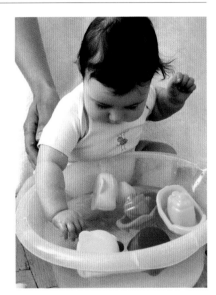

Water play Babies are fascinated by water and they relish the opportunity to pour, splash, or sprinkle.

sources of vitamin C include kiwi fruit; strawberries; broccoli; tomatoes; sweet potatoes; and butternut squash.

Vitamin D
Important for the bones and teeth, inadequate vitamin D can lead to rickets, which causes bones to soften and become weak. It is mostly made in the body by the action of sunlight on skin. Few foods contain vitamin D—oily fish, eggs, and butter among them—but many breakfast cereals are fortified with it.

Iron
The manufacture of red blood cells and the development of the nervous and immune systems rely on iron, which is best absorbed by the body from animal foods. Red meat is the best source, but dark poultry meat, and oily fish, such as canned sardines, are also good.

Tofu, chickpeas, legumes, and dark green leafy vegetables are all good plant sources of iron.

Your baby from
7 to 9 months

MONTH

7

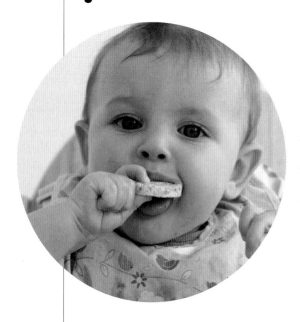

By now, your baby will enjoy **feeding themself** with simple finger foods.

MONTH 7: ENCOURAGE THEIR PASSING SKILLS

There's quite an art to passing an object from hand to hand, because your baby needs plenty of hand–eye coordination and to be able to open and close their grip efficiently. Once they've mastered this skill, they will enjoy practicing.

MONTH

8

MONTH 8: SEPARATION ANXIETY MAY HAPPEN

Around eight months is when your baby is most likely to become anxious about strangers or separating from you, and therefore may need extra reassurance.

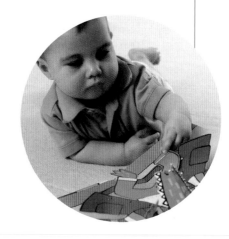

Your baby's **problem-solving** and fine motor skills are developing fast.

" From sitting to standing to doing simple puzzles to trying new foods, your baby is a busy little person. "

MONTH

9

MONTH 9: PRONE TO EMOTIONAL OUTBURSTS

At this age, babies may cry from frustration at not being able to master something, or become sad when you leave the room. Emotions often feel overwhelming, so calm, patient handling is key. In time, your baby will learn how to better regulate their emotions.

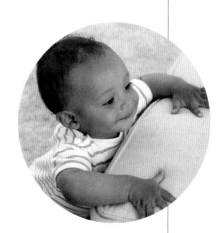

Using a piece of furniture for support, your baby may be able to pull themself up to a **standing position**.

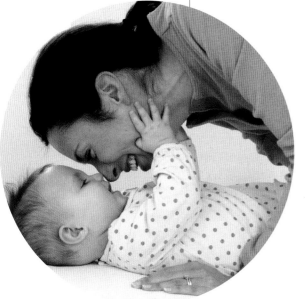

As their comprehension improves, your baby will **want to copy** your sounds and movements.

7 months

EARLY BABBLING IN BABIES USUALLY CONSISTS OF ONE SYLLABLE REPEATED, SUCH AS "MAMAMA."

Your baby may now be able to sit up on their own without support. This means that their hands are free so they can take full advantage of their increasing dexterity. Babies want to play constantly, and enthusiastically explore anything within their reach and beyond!

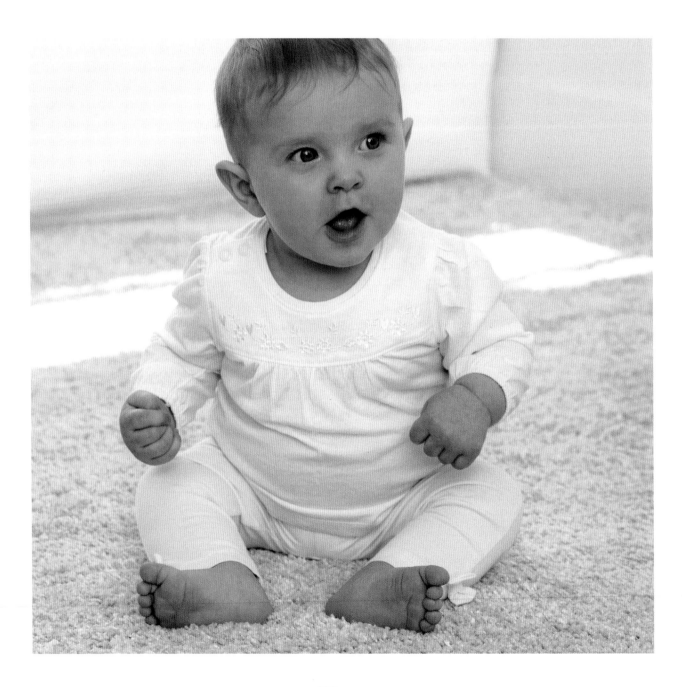

One hand to another

You'll notice that your baby has more control over their hands, and seems quite enthralled by passing things between them.

RAISING AN AVID READER

Make books a part of your baby's daily life to support the development of verbal skills, understanding of language and pleasure in listening, and to promote a habit that may one day become a passion. Select age-appropriate books and get baby to turn pages and lift flaps. Use an expressive, exaggerated voice that will appeal to them, and don't hesitate to read the same book frequently. Repetition will spark memory and help them learn. Look for chunky books that will withstand attempts to explore them. Simple stories are ideal, and books with peep holes will stimulate curiosity. Keep a selection of books around the house, and in your handbag or the stroller to pass the time when you are out and about.

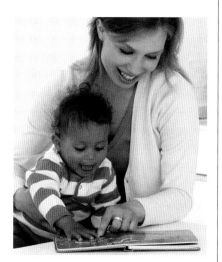

Book fun Make reading part of your routine so your baby anticipates it and develops a positive association with books.

Your baby is developing the ability to transfer objects from one hand to the other, and to accurately place them in a container. They will visually explore whatever they are holding. For example, they might hold it at a distance, then pass it from hand to hand, to find out about its properties. This enables them to learn that objects don't change size when moved closer or farther away, even though they look bigger or smaller.

Manipulative movement

Suitable toys and opportunities for play will support the development of your baby's manipulative movement. This involves the controlled use of their hands and feet—grasping, opening and closing their hands, and waving are all examples of manipulative movement. This type of movement develops throughout childhood, and involves fine motor skills and hand–eye coordination.

Give different sized objects to handle, as well as items with varying textures. Small, soft bricks and blocks are ideal at this age—while your baby won't be stacking or building for a good while yet, they will be able to grasp them with their fist and pass them between their hands, and will enjoy exploring the shape and feel. You may find, sometime between seven and nine months, that they start to clap on their own, as you do, when they hear their favorite action rhyme.

While your baby is keen to discover the world and practice their growing

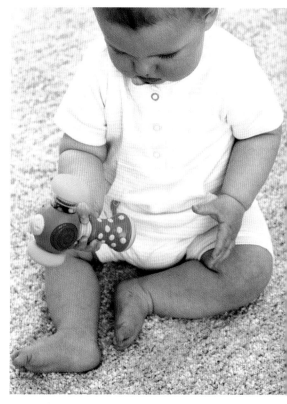

Improved grasp Your baby can now scoop things up with one hand and transfer them to the other. Give plenty of objects, such as soft blocks and toys, to help them practice this skill.

bank of skills, they will also continue to imitate you. You are their role model; so while you move around the room engage them and demonstrate different actions, such as picking an object up or placing it into a basket.

Let me investigate

Babies will attempt to do everything they see you doing to find out all about it, and want to investigate anything that looks exciting.

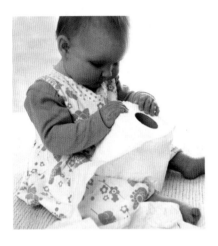

Your baby's growing ability to perceive depth and see at a distance allows them to spot new things constantly, and they'll make an effort to get to them. They may become fixated on objects, such as the potted plant you moved out of their reach, or your car keys, and become quite vocal in their attempts to get to them. They may stretch, reach, and wiggle toward what

Learning touch Your baby's explorations and experiments teach them about the properties of different objects.

they want, so make sure dangerous items are put away out of reach. Watch out for your cup of coffee on the table, fragile ornaments, and small parts from toys left lying around by older siblings. You may need to do frequent sweeps of your home to be safe.

Curiosity leads to learning, and babies respond to sensory experiences with a desire to find out more about the world. Playing with and exploring different textures, tastes, and consistencies all give valuable feedback about the world.

When's a good bedtime?

Your baby doesn't have to be in bed at 7 p.m.; provided they get enough quality sleep, you can adjust bedtimes to suit your lifestyle.

Consistent bedtimes are, indeed, important for babies because they help set their body clock and form part of a good sleep routine. However, putting baby down to sleep at 8 p.m. instead of 7 p.m. is certainly possible, and gives working parents more opportunities to spend some quality time with their babies. If you do go for the later-bedtime option, ensure their room is dark enough to allow them to sleep a little later in the morning. They'll still need 8–10 hours of sleep a night, regardless of when it starts and stops.

Avoid the second wind

If your baby becomes overtired, they may get a second wind and find it difficult to settle. Giving them a late afternoon nap can help prevent this. You may need to experiment a little to work out how much sleep they need in the late afternoon to last until your partner comes home. When whoever has been out all day does get back, make sure they don't overstimulate the baby with exciting fun and games right before bedtime. While it is a happy occasion for all of you to share

this time together in the evening, activities prior to bedtime should be low key and relaxed.

Early bedtime

If you prefer to have some time to yourself in the evenings, and your baby naturally tires at around 6-7 p.m., put them down to sleep at that time and get the rest you need to refresh yourself. The habits you establish now should not be hard to alter later. Babies are generally quite adaptable up until the age of about 12 months.

Food allergies

It's natural to worry about allergies when starting solids—knowing what the symptoms are, and where to turn, means you're prepared.

Food allergies are on the increase, but they are still relatively uncommon in babies, and are very often outgrown in childhood. Your baby is more likely to develop allergies if there's a family history of eczema, asthma, hay fever, or food allergies. If this is the case, discuss with your baby's doctor the best time to introduce the most common allergenic foods: cow milk products, eggs, peanuts, wheat, soy, fish, and shellfish. They should be introduced one at a time, so you can watch for any reaction.

Some food allergies are easy to spot, particularly if a reaction occurs soon after the food is eaten. See your pediatrician if your baby displays any of the following symptoms : flushed face, or a red and itchy rash around the mouth, tongue, or eyes, which can spread across the body; mild swelling,

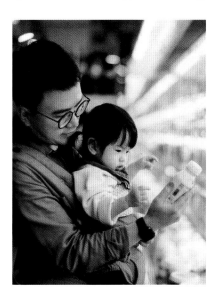

particularly of the lips, eyes, and face; runny or blocked nose, sneezing; nausea, vomiting, stomach cramps, and diarrhea. Very rarely, foods can cause a severe allergic reaction called anaphylactic shock (see p.372).

In some cases, reactions to certain foods are not so easily identified because the symptoms are less obvious and may not appear for hours to days after the food has been eaten. These are known as "delayed food allergies" as they involve the immune system. However, they do not cause anaphylaxis. Common culprits are milk, soy, egg, and wheat, and symptoms can include eczema, colic, reflux, diarrhea, and constipation.

If an allergy is suspected, your pediatrician may refer your baby for a skin prick test and/or a blood test for a definite diagnosis. Sometimes you may be advised to eliminate the suspected food or foods for at least two weeks to see if the symptoms subside. It may then be possible to reintroduce foods slowly, or you may need to adapt your baby's diet to include alternative foods.

Don't be tempted to cut out food groups from your baby's diet without professional guidance. (See p.241 for further information.)

Food labels It is important to develop the habit of reading food labels to check the suitability of the ingredients for your baby.

ASK A NUTRITIONIST

I'm worried that my baby might be allergic to peanuts. Should I avoid them? There's no reason to avoid offering foods containing peanuts, or any other nuts or seeds from 6 months of age, but introduce them in small portions. Advice suggests that your baby may be at a higher risk of developing a food allergy if they have early-onset or moderate-severe eczema or already have a food allergy. In these cases, your baby has a higher risk of developing a nut allergy, and you should talk to your pediatrician before giving your child food containing nuts (such as peanut butter) for the first time.

Can I arrange for my baby to be tested privately to diagnose a food allergy? It's very important to see your pediatrician in the first instance to rule out any other possible cause for any symptoms your baby is experiencing. Your pediatrician will likely refer you to a pediatric allergist, who will be best equipped to decide how to test your baby for allergies. To find a local certified allergist, visit acaai.org. Seeing an allergist for a definitive diagnosis is best. Commercial allergy-testing kits are not recommended by pediatricians. They're also costly and are not covered by insurance.

Less vital statistics

If you are still struggling to return to your prepregnancy weight and fitness levels, cut yourself a bit of slack.

Most pregnant people put on weight steadily over the nine months, so it makes sense that it may take time to lose any extra pounds after the birth. While exclusive breastfeeding can encourage continual weight loss, some say that any extra pounds refused to shift until they stopped breastfeeding. Losing weight can depend on your individual build and metabolism. Most pregnant bodies change completely and never return to their prepregnancy shape. You may find, for example, that while you've lost the weight, your waist is thicker, your breasts may be smaller or heavier, and your hips may be broader or rounder. Change doesn't have to be viewed as a bad thing. Focus on what amazing things your body has done and continues to do for both you and your baby.

If you are a healthy weight, try to reframe your thoughts from negative to positive, or just neutral. If your health-care practitioner does advise weight loss, take a look at your diet to see if there are areas where you can make healthier choices. Reducing the size of your portions can help, as can cutting back on foods high in fat or sugar. Avoid highly-processed foods, opting instead for whole foods, filling up on vegetables and whole grains. Switch to low-fat versions of milk and cheese. Don't forget to stay well-hydrated: try adding a squeeze of orange or cucumber slices to water.

Exercise helps weight control, as well as firming muscle and skin tone, all of which can help you feel better.

Sound combinations

Speaking is a complex process that requires lots of nerve and muscle control, which is one reason why speech comes slowly.

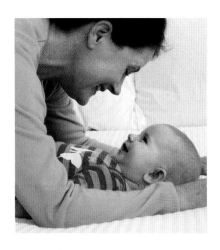

When we speak, we must coordinate many muscles, including the larynx, which contains the vocal cords; the teeth, lips, tongue, and mouth; and the respiratory system.

By now, your baby has established some of the groundwork for speech acquisition. At the moment, they are using a combination of vowels and consonants: lip consonants with vowels that are generated in the center of the mouth, with the tongue flat ("mama," for example); tongue-front consonants in front of vowels that come at the front of the mouth ("dada"); and tongue-back consonants in front of vowels that are created in the back of the mouth ("gaga").

Your baby is starting, therefore, to create some interesting sounds that sound more like adult speech. At this stage, though, it's still baby babble. Always respond to their babbling and be very interactive and positive.

Words of praise Encourage your baby with praise when they try to communicate with you and uses their "words."

Not so silent nights ...

Your baby's sleep may not be quiet. You may hear the baby snort, breathe irregularly, bang their head, and rock themself to and fro as they sleep.

Not all babies sleep in tranquility—many snore and sniffle, have irregular breathing patterns, or even rock or bang their heads to soothe themselves. Most of the time, this is nothing to worry about and babies grow out of whatever peculiar sleep habit they happen to adopt, but occasionally you may need to take action.

Snoring and sniffling

Babies often snore, snort, or sniffle when they have a cold or a blocked nose. Try using a vaporizer in the bedroom to add moisture to the air, which can ease breathing. You can also raise the head of the crib a little to help mucus clear from the nose. Talk to your pediatrician if you see a change in your baby's habits, for example, sniffling more than usual, difficulty breathing, a fever, or difficulty feeding due to congestion.

Irregular breathing

Lots of babies experience changes in their breathing patterns while they sleep. For example, your baby might breathe rapidly, then slow down, and even pause for several seconds before breathing again. Breathing may also change as they become excited or frightened by dreams. These pauses in breathing should start to happen less frequently now, but if they continue and you are concerned, consult your pediatrician. If your baby seems clammy or blue, get emergency medical attention. Very occasionally, a pause in breathing may be caused by sleep apnea, although this is more common in babies who are one year or older. Your pediatrician will need to diagnose sleep apnea and recommend treatment.

Head-banging and rocking

After the age of six months, some babies adopt rhythmic activities, such as head-banging and rocking, to soothe themselves. From their time in the womb, they are used to rocking as well as being in a head-down position, so may feel comforted by rhythmic pressure on the top of the head. If your baby isn't harming themselves, leave them to it. Most children outgrow this by the age of three, and many stop long before that.

There is no indication that rocking or head-banging is a sign of an emotional disorder. Sometimes babies bang their heads to distract themselves from a sore throat, teething, or an ear infection.

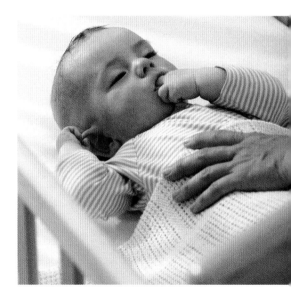

Comfort habit Your baby can find it soothing to suck their thumb or fingers, which can help them settle and fall asleep.

ASK A PEDIATRICIAN

I've heard of something called ALTE. What is this? Rarely, babies stop breathing for a longer period than a few seconds, which causes oxygen levels in the blood to drop. This can give the skin a white or blue appearance, and the baby can also choke or gag, and/or become floppy or stiff. Such an episode is called an Apparent Life-Threatening Event (ALTE), which used to be called a "near miss crib death." This should be treated as an emergency, and the baby may need resuscitation. Even if a baby recovers fairly rapidly on their own, an ambulance should be called and they should be assessed in hospital, and their condition prior to the episode assessed. Monitoring over the weeks following ALTE is important to ensure that the baby has recovered fully.

Separation anxiety

Your baby is approaching the age at which separation anxiety sets in, which can be difficult not just for them, but also for you.

Suddenly, your happy, independent baby may cry each time you leave the room or put them down. They may hate to be alone, and spend more time looking for you than engaging in the activities they usually enjoy. This is completely normal, even if it is a little frustrating. Your baby doesn't want to be without you, and will do what they can to prevent your departure.

At this age, your baby is learning to develop trust, so to support this it is important that you recognize their fears and emotions, and do whatever you can to help them feel secure.

Go to them whenever they call you. Do what you can to help them feel more confident. Talk to them when you are out of sight, so they know you are there, and return to them frequently so they understand that you will always return.

While frequently stopping whatever you are doing to reassure your baby can be time-consuming at the outset, they need to learn to feel safe and to anchor an understanding of the fact that you will always be there for them, even when they can't see you. When you leave, they must learn that you will always come back. These feelings are the foundation of trust and emotional well-being, so constant reassurance at this stage will go a long way toward encouraging confidence and independence later on.

Hands together

Your baby is now aware that both hands are theirs, and is beginning to learn that they can operate them simultaneously.

Your baby may reach for a toy with one hand and peruse it. Suddenly, their attention is captured by another toy. They know that one hand is busy, so they'll put the other to work to grasp what they see. They may look at both toys with interest, or perhaps drop one as they focus on the other. They may see something else and the process will begin again. They can use both hands, but they haven't quite figured out how best to use them together for even better results! They may pass a toy from hand to hand, and bang toys together, but their actions are likely to be uncoordinated and slightly clumsy as they are probably not intentional at this stage. They may manage to place two hands on the same object, pick it up, and turn it over, but when their attention is caught by something else, they'll forget that they're holding something at all, and drop it.

If you guide them, your baby may be able to hold a cup with both hands, but they're likely to let go unexpectedly and may find it difficult to pick it up and guide it to their lips.

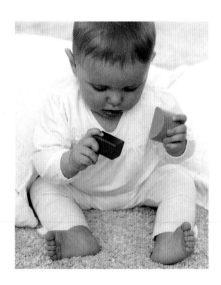

Better grasp Babies develop hand skills by touching, reaching, exploring, and grasping, so give lots of opportunity to do just that.

Your baby's drinks

Are follow-up formulas beneficial for your baby, and what else should they be drinking—or not—in the second half of the first year?

If you're breastfeeding, breast milk is the ideal drink for your baby for the first six months and, together with an increasingly varied diet, can form the basis of their nutrition up until one year.

If your baby is formula-fed, you are mixing breast and formula, or thinking of weaning off breast milk, you may wonder which type of formula is suitable after six months, and whether you should switch to one marketed for older babies.

Formulas contain two types of protein: whey and casein. First formulas, suitable from birth, are whey-based, which is easy for your baby to digest. Follow-up and "hungry baby" formulas marketed at babies over six months, are casein-based, which takes longer to digest and is thought therefore to keep babies satisfied longer. However, there is no significant nutritional difference between these formulas, and first formula is suitable for your baby for the whole of their first year.

Soy formula is not suitable before six months. After this, some choose soy if they wish to exclude animal proteins from their baby's diet. Soy is also promoted as an option for babies allergic to cow's milk formula. However, these babies can also be allergic to soy milk, and there are more suitable formulas, known as fully hydrolyzed formulas, that pediatricians prescribe for babies with an allergy. Soy also contains glucose, which can damage your baby's teeth. Talk to your pediatrician before giving soy formula milk.

Goat's and sheep's milk and oat drinks are also promoted as an alternative for babies with cow's milk allergy. However, these are not suitable under one year as they contain insufficient iron and other nutrients. Goat's milk also contains lactose so isn't a good low-allergenic alternative. Full-fat cow's milk should not be given until one year.

Quenching thirst

Once your baby is on solids, you can supplement feedings with another drink. Tap water is best, and there's no need to boil it unless you have well water or you know of issues with the water in your town's supply. Bottled water is also suitable for babies. Fruit juice contains vitamin C and it's fine after six months, but to protect your baby's teeth, give it only at mealtimes, in a lidded cup, and diluted to a ratio

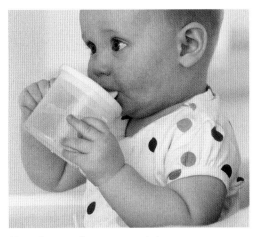

Mastering a cup Encourage your baby to start drinking from a cup after six months.

of 1:10. Fruit drinks and flavored milks should be avoided under one year, and limited or avoided after this; and carbonated drinks, and other caffeine-containing drinks, shouldn't form any part of a young child's diet.

ASK A MOM

My baby cries and spits out all the solid food I give them. What can I do? Offer some breast milk on a spoon to get them used to the idea of the spoon itself. Mix vegetable puree with breast milk to make it seem more familiar, then slowly reduce the amount of milk you add. Give them their own spoon with a chunky handle and a little puree in a bowl. Let them use their hands and spoon to play with the food; most will probably end up in their hair, but their instinct will be to put some into their mouth. This may be an easier way for them to make the transition to new tastes and textures. If they still resist, rather than force the issue, leave it a while. You can try again later when you know they're hungry and in a more receptive mood.

Using the right words

Your baby is too young to understand instructions, but it's valuable to begin using the words "yes" and "no" to introduce these concepts.

While your baby will not yet understand the concepts of "yes" and "no," do use them to start conveying the meaning of these important words. It is helpful to use "no" paired with a firm tone and a shake of the head or finger if your baby is in danger, for example, if they reach out to a hot stove or pull at a fireplace screen. When you say "no" like this, you will also need to act quickly because they won't stop on your say so at this age. As your baby grows, it is most helpful to tell them what you want them to do: for example, "Hold the teddy bear," rather than "No, don't drop it." Children respond more quickly when they know what you want.

When you want your baby to stop doing something, try to distract them by entertaining them with a new toy, making funny faces, or waiting while they calm down. It's not appropriate to introduce discipline now, as scolding at this age is more likely to distress them.

Equally, don't hesitate to say "yes" when they do things correctly. Praise, a big smile, and a positive, cheerful "yes," while you nod, will encourage them to continue in the same vein.

Enjoying music

The best way to teach your baby musical appreciation is to fill life with all kinds of music and enjoy it with them.

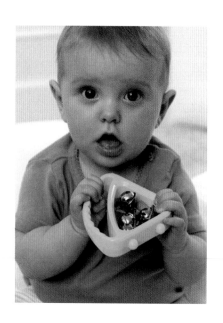

Your baby may display a preference for certain types of music. There may be a calm song that always soothes them if they are frustrated or helps them fall asleep, and some favorite playtime music that makes them giggle and has the power to entertain even when they are unsettled.

Music encourages the development of speech, and research suggests that babies exposed to lots of music are better able to understand the patterns of speech and grammar, and language development is enhanced. Also,

Making music Take out the baby musical instruments and create music together. Dance along to the shakes and rattles.

studies show that soothing music can reduce the stress hormone cortisol, while lively music will engage your baby, but may overstimulate them if they're tired. One study on the effect of music on young children found that soft music (in this case, lullabies) relaxed restless children.

Whatever the long-term effects, there is no doubt that your baby will enjoy listening to and making music. Sing along and hold them in your arms or on your lap as you move to music. Bear in mind that they can learn from all types of musical genres. It isn't only classical music that works on their brain's neural pathways— any music will do the same.

Practical baby clothes

Now that your baby is bigger and more mobile, you may need a few more items of clothing that allow them to move about comfortably.

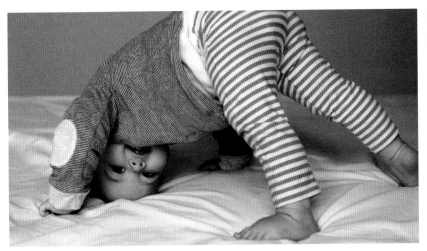

Loose clothing Choose garments that do not restrict your baby's movements. Stretchy baby leggings are ideal and are very versatile.

Choose garments that are a little on the large size to give your baby space to maneuver. They'll be on their hands and knees a lot, so patches, reinforcements, or padding on the knees will help keep your baby comfortable (and the pants intact). Long-sleeve shirts can protect little forearms and elbows. Find fabrics that will wash well, not require ironing, and that will be kind to your baby's skin (there will be a lot of chafing as they learn to crawl and walk).

T-shirts and onesies with easy-to-fasten snaps at the crotch will keep them cozy and clothes with snaps and elasticized waists are excellent for quick changes as your baby inevitably tries to wiggle away.

All change!

Weaning is a messy business and you can expect several changes of clothes a day. Go for tops and bottoms that can be mixed and matched. Don't spend a lot of money—clothing will be stained (and then outgrown)!

Feet first

Your baby may be trying to move, so they'll need to get a grip on the floor. Socks with little grip pads on the soles are ideal. If the weather doesn't call for socks, let them go barefoot—the best grip of all. Babies need socks and bootees only for warmth; they don't need shoes to learn to walk and should not, in fact, be fitted for their first pair until they are cruising or walking confidently.

ASK A PEDIATRICIAN

I always put my baby to sleep on their back to lower the risk of SIDS. But now, they've started to flip over and sleep on their stomach. Should I turn them back? There isn't much point in turning them over again once they've learned to roll over. If your baby prefers sleeping on their stomach, that's where they'll end up. While you keep putting your baby to bed on their back until they're one year old, the high-risk period for SIDS is generally passed by the time a baby can turn over. Just make sure your baby's crib is safe and continue to follow the guidelines for preventing SIDS, such as avoiding pillows and duvets (see p.31). But try not to worry if their position changes during the night.

My baby's hands and feet are very cool at night, but they're sleeping well. Do they need more layers? Hands and feet will always be cooler than the rest of your baby's body. A better gauge is to put your hand under their neck and feel their face. If these are warm, they're probably dressed appropriately; if they feel cool, try a baby sleep sack or pop on a pair of bed socks. Sweating around the face, head, or neck is a sign that they're overheating—it is very important to avoid this. Provided your baby's room is kept at a temperature of around 61–68°F (16–20°C), ideally 65°F (18°C), they shouldn't become too cold or too hot.

Talking with gestures

Your baby is beginning to understand how words and gestures go together. Activity rhymes can encourage this development.

Your baby may begin to make gestures, such as raising a hand toward something they want, which will rapidly develop into pointing over the next couple of months. Encourage your baby to pat or touch things in books by saying, "Where's the cow?" or "Where is the dog?" and then point to them to help your baby make the connection. When they look at and gestures to their favorite soft toy, bring it to them so they know their signal is understood. They may direct you to what they want with their gaze, and babble, or wave their hand.

Until they learn to point, your baby may gesture with a fist rather than a finger: they may ball up their hand and stretch out their arm. At about nine months (and, in some cases, a bit earlier),

they will learn instrumental pointing, which involves an outstretched arm and an extended index finger.

Imitating gestures

Around this time, your baby may be able to imitate some of the hand movements in their activity rhymes, and copy you when you stroke a soft toy. Say, "Pat-pat" when you stroke the toy, so your baby may learn that actions and gestures are associated with words, too. Two US studies have revealed that babies who are encouraged to gesture in advance of, and then in conjunction with, speech, learn to speak more quickly and experience faster cognitive development.

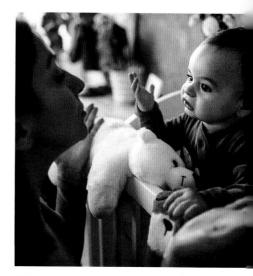

Giving clues Help your baby learn simple concepts such as "hungry" or "tired" by pairing hand gestures with your words.

USING A CUP

Once your baby can hold onto things and starts to eat finger foods, you can introduce a cup for drinking water. Choose one with a spout, preferably soft, and a large handle they can easily get ahold of. It will be dropped, so look for one that will bounce without the lid falling off! Learning to drink from a lidded cup is important, because by now your baby should be giving up bottles with slow-flowing nipples. Avoid giving fruit juice, even if diluted, so emerging teeth are not bathed in sugars (see also p.229).

ASK A PEDIATRICIAN

My baby is constantly teary-eyed. Will this clear up? Newborn babies have tiny tear ducts in the corner of each eye. When tears start being produced, at around one month, they drain away through these ducts. Occasionally, the ducts in newborns are blocked. However, this is not great cause for concern, and most blocked tear ducts resolve themselves by the end of the first year. Your pediatrician may show you how to massage them to help unblock them. If the eye becomes crusty, use cotton pads dampened with water to clean it. If you notice any redness in the eye or a yellow discharge, consult your pediatrician as your baby may need antibiotic drops.

Should my baby be vaccinated against the flu? Yes. The Centers for Disease Control and Prevention (CDC) recommend that all children aged six months and older receive an annual flu shot, so if your baby is old enough, you should have them vaccinated.

Is it normal for my baby to pull up their legs and grimace when they have a bowel movement? This just helps their bowels move. Drawing up the legs gets them into a squatting position and makes it easier—they're not in pain. As long as their movements are regular and there's no blood in the stools, they'll be fine.

Building awareness

Your baby's grasp of the concept of object permanence is maturing. They will delight in games of hide-and-seek and may hide from you!

Your baby's cognitive development is continuing steadily, and they will now show that they're beginning to gain the concept of object permanence—that an object exists even when they can't see it. This means they may continue to look for a toy if it is covered with a cloth or has fallen out of sight, and will delight in games that involve the disappearance and reappearance of an object, face, or toy.

They will apply this understanding to other parts of life, too, for example, pulling the covers away from your head when you are sleeping to check that you are still there, and moving toys to find something underneath.

Emotional implications

Your baby is approaching the age when separation anxiety starts to set in (see p.263). This development, coupled with the increased understanding of object permanence, may make your baby much clingier than usual. While once they may have played happily on their own, oblivious to your presence even when you popped in and out of the room doing chores, they will now start to wonder where you are when they can't see or hear you. After all, you are not in sight, so you must be there somewhere. It's no longer "out of sight, out of mind," and they may shout and cry to bring you back. Reassure them by responding when they cry out so they begin to feel confident that you are nearby even when they can't see you, and that you are still there to answer their needs when they call out.

DEVELOPMENT ACTIVITY: PEEKABOO

Your baby will be a big fan of peekaboo games now and will love to play them with you—and they can join in, too! They may think they're invisible when they can't see you, and find it great fun to "reappear," even though they've been there all along.

Playing peekaboo at this age can reinforce understanding of the concept of object permanence. With lots of chances to rediscover that "missing" things are not gone forever and will eventually reappear, your baby will eventually learn to cope more effectively with feelings of anxiety when you are not able to be with them.

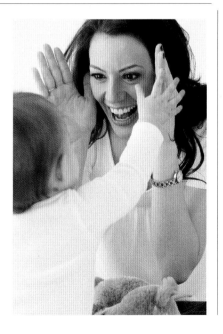

Surprise! As your baby gets used to this game, you can make them enjoy it even more by using a range of silly expressions.

ASK A PEDIATRICIAN

How can I reduce the risk of my baby getting asthma? If one of you, or another one of your children, has asthma, breastfeeding your baby for as long as possible will reduce the risk of developing it. You can also reduce the risk by both you and your partner avoiding smoking during and after pregnancy. Replacing old carpets and rugs with laminate, wood, or linoleum flooring, and replacing old bedding and cushions reduces your baby's exposure to dust, which in turn reduces the risk of getting asthma. Some children experience increased symptoms with certain pets, so research this before introducing a pet into the home.

Emotional awareness

Your baby's emotional antennae are sensitive. They'll pick up on stress in their immediate environment and will be affected by it.

We know that if they are hungry and not fed, or not given physical comfort when distressed, they experience symptoms of stress. Because babies are still developing their sense of security, and are not equipped physically or emotionally to deal with high levels of stress, this can have a profound effect on their physical and emotional well-being. Your baby needs you to reduce their experience of stress by meeting their needs for food, warmth, and love, and by soothing them when emotions overwhelm them. When you respond rapidly to calm and contain their emotions, they learn that feelings need not be overpowering. They will learn to self-soothe efficiently when they experience stress.

Studies have shown that babies have sensitive social barometers and pick up on parental stress and emotional upheaval, causing them to feel unsafe, afraid, and even unwell. If an argument becomes heated, even if raised voices aren't directed at them, they'll be startled and upset. Work to ensure discussions are calm; agree that if they get heated, you both take a break. Your baby doesn't understand the context of your disagreements, but calm resolution helps them learn that disagreements are healthy when respectfully handled.

Gentle guidance

Your baby certainly knows their own mind, so if they're veering in an unsuitable direction, you'll need to steer them gently elsewhere.

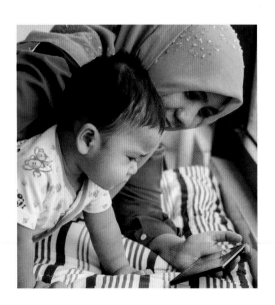

Guiding your baby toward appropriate objects, activities, and behaviors is a technique all parents will need to adopt. Babies may be single-minded, but they are also easy to distract as their memories are still fairly short and their interest in new things is limitless.

When your baby wiggles while being changed, heads for the potted plant for the twenty-fifth time in a row, or tries to eat an outraged siblings' snacks, it's time to employ some diversion tactics.

Look at this! If your baby is doing something unwanted, divert their attention by grabbing a toy you know will distract them.

Keep toy stashes dotted around the house so you can grab a toy when you need to capture their attention. Change the toys frequently so they always seem new. Choose a song or activity rhyme and launch into it when your baby is heading for trouble. Pick them up and move them to a different room, tickle their toes, or point out a bird in the sky.

Your baby is too young to reason with, so instead of facing a battle with them, quickly divert them. Over time, your baby may begin to realize that they won't be allowed to wiggle away from you while they're being changed—but it still probably won't stop them from trying!

Toys for seven months and up

At seven months, your baby will be ready for new toys that stimulate their reasoning, coordination, and gross and fine motor skills.

Toys don't have to be expensive to entertain your baby and promote their development. In fact, many household items can keep them occupied. There are, however, some great toys for this age.

Balls and toys on wheels encourage mobility and promote hand–eye coordination. Rolling a ball back and forth encourages motor skills and coordination. Also, go for a toy on a sturdy string that you can pull just out of reach, or that they can pull toward themself.

Toys that make your baby think will sharpen reasoning skills. Look for toys with features that hide behind or inside part of the toy. Very basic puzzles with chunky handles for lifting and moving will stimulate your baby. Ensure they are not too difficult or they will become frustrated and give up.

Toys that help your baby explore different shapes and sounds as well as cause and effect, nurture thinking and motor skills. Shape-sorters; noisy blocks; toys that ring, rattle, and crinkle when you squeeze or touch different parts of them; and stackable toys that fit inside one another will all entertain them. Musical instruments designed for their age, such as a baby rainmaker, can intrigue them with the sounds they make.

An activity board attached to their crib or the back of a chair will help them practice their coordination, and they'll love learning they can open doors, twist, squeeze, shake, and pull things to get a good reaction. Blocks that can be piled, knocked down, banged together, and dropped in and out of containers are a good investment, as they'll be put to different uses over the coming years.

Finally, don't forget books! If books form a regular part of playtime, your baby will develop an avid interest in stories and reading, and their vocabulary and speech will continue to improve. A love of books will help promote lifelong learning.

ASK A CHILD PSYCHOLOGIST

Is there such a thing as a toy for a boy or a toy for a girl? Toys are toys and are genderless. Focus on the quality, design, and purpose of the toys you give your baby—aiming for those that are designed to stimulate development (which includes emotional and physical development) as well as to entertain. Until they are three or four years old, children will have no real understanding of gender differentiations in either themselves or anything else in the world, so encourage them to play with anything and everything that captures their attention.

DEVELOPMENT ACTIVITY: TREASURE BOX

Fill a basket or box with a selection of baby-friendly objects, and encourage your baby to investigate the contents one by one. The box doesn't have to contain toys—household items such as a comb, and clean kitchen utensils such as a whisk or spatula are ideal. Your baby can rummage through the box and touch, bang, chew, smell, and study the items. This type of game encourages hand–eye coordination, imagination, speech development, and, above all, a sense of fun!

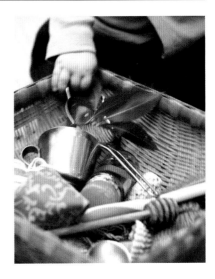

Box of fun Place an assortment of child-safe items in a box for your baby to investigate.

Stage two solids—lumpier foods

As soon as your baby is enjoying a variety of pureed foods, they're ready to move on to the second stage of solids. Now you should introduce a greater range of foods as well as new textures and some finger foods.

A TYPICAL DAY'S DIET

To give you an idea of what your baby should be eating at this stage, below is an example of a day's food intake for a 6- to 7-month-old baby. Your baby should still be having around 24 fl oz (720 ml) of milk each day. At first, some parents prefer to feed their baby at breakfast and lunch to give them time to digest their meal before sleeping at night. A simple, easily digestible meal can then be introduced in the evening.

- **Breakfast** Breast milk or formula, cereal, and mashed fruit. You can offer a variety of fresh or canned fruits or applesauce, and toast can be plain or served with a spread that is sweetened with fruit juice (not artificial sweeteners or sugar).
- **Lunch** Meat, poultry, or lentils with vegetables and mashed potato or baby pasta shapes or sweet potato; soft pieces of fruit; water to drink.
- **Mid-afternoon** Breast milk or formula.
- **Dinner** Vegetables and starchy foods like mashed baked potato. Also, fresh fruit, vegetables, and cereals/grains, including mixtures of these products (such as peaches and oatmeal); water to drink.
- **Bedtime** Breast milk or formula.

As your baby starts this next stage, they will begin to cope with soft lumps in foods, as well as mashed foods rather than runny purees. They don't need to have teeth to deal with lumps, but they do need to learn to chew rather than just suck and swallow.

They will start to learn to move foods around in their mouth, and this will be a different sensation. So it's important to vary the textures of your baby's food to get them used to chewing and moving food around, which will also help develop the muscles used for speaking.

Moving on from purees

Your baby will be familiar now with the taste and consistency of the usual purees, so it's important to alter the texture of foods, doing so fairly quickly if you have waited until the recommended six months to start solids. You can adjust the texture of these familiar foods as well as adding new foods to them. For example, you can add finely chopped, mashed, grated, or ground "new" foods to the purees. This will provide a different texture and flavor as well as improve their nutritional value.

Start by adding very tiny, soft lumps to familiar foods. Don't be surprised if the lumps reappear—simply scoop them back up again and spoon them back in. Try well-cooked, baby-size pasta shapes, mashed potato, or some soft cooked vegetables, which you can gently mash with a fork.

Introduce some finger foods—a little bowl of bite-and-dissolve foods such as baby bread sticks; soft cooked carrots; eggplant and potato cut into fingers; slices of banana; pear; and cubes of melon, papaya, or avocado. They will investigate these foods and over time will learn to chew or "gum" them, and then swallow. Make sure you stay there in case they choke.

Larger lumps

After this, it's time to introduce some slightly bigger lumps and textures, and different new foods. For example, coarsely blend cooked chicken breast so it is not a smooth puree and stir into mashed potato with pureed peas. Offer a cauliflower puree; and mash banana into baby rice.

If you are bringing up your baby as a vegetarian, try lentils or chickpeas ground up with pureed carrots or apples, or add to sweet potato or carrot puree to thicken the texture.

The idea is to introduce a much wider variety of foods over the next few weeks, mixing them with their favorite fruits and vegetables, while increasing the number and size of the lumps until they are able to move toward eating a similar texture of food to the whole family.

The atmosphere around mealtimes is really important, so give your baby plenty of encouragement and praise and don't press them to eat if they obviously don't want to. If they're really reluctant, check how much milk they are having and avoid giving a milk feeding in the hour or two before mealtime to see if this helps.

How much?

Most babies won't eat much more than a tablespoon or two of a puree at the beginning of this stage, but this can dramatically increase as their milk feedings start to decrease a bit. Your baby needs a diet that contains protein, carbohydrates, and fat as well as a range of vitamins and minerals. To achieve this, they need to have foods from the four food groups (see p.193). You'll be able to work all these foods into two or three small meals per day.

Checking for reactions

If your baby has not reacted to foods up until now, you may prefer to jot down what they like and keep on trying the foods they seem to dislike. However, if your baby has reacted to foods, it is likely you'll have discussed this with your pediatrician, who can advise you on how to introduce other potentially allergenic foods.

IDEAL FINGER FOODS

• Vegetables steamed or cooked in the microwave until soft, then cooled: carrots, sweet potato, baby corn, green beans, broccoli, or cauliflower florets.
• Plain cooked potatoes cut into wedges, steamed new potatoes, slices of eggplant.

• A few pieces of chicken, with a vegetable puree for "dipping."
• Toast fingers or puffed baby snacks, sold at baby stores nationwide.
• Miniature, unsalted, and unflavored rice cakes.
• Pureed fruit, vegetables, or beans spread on pita bread fingers, or baby crackers.
• Small cubes of ripe avocado.
• Soft ripe fruit, such as sliced pear, melon, banana, peach, nectarine, and berries.
• Cooked pasta shapes served plain or with a small amount of sauce or a little olive oil drizzled over.
• Resist the urge now to start giving your baby highly processed food. Stick with whole foods, or packaged foods that have ingredients you would have in your own kitchen.

NEW FLAVORS AND TEXTURES

• **Meat, poultry, eggs, and pulses** Once thicker purees are going down well, add small chunks or ground pieces of cooked poultry or meat to get your baby used to lumps. A casserole with vegetables can be pulse-blended to keep some texture. Add to mashed potato, couscous, or baby pasta shapes.
• **Fruit and vegetables** Introduce a wider variety of fruits, including berries and dried fruits, and offer green vegetables such as spinach and broccoli.
• **Carbohydrates** Provide a range of cereals: unsweetened breakfast cereals can be softened in milk and used as finger foods. Try pasta, couscous, sweet potato, rice, and potatoes, as well as baby crackers, toast, or pita bread.
• **Temperature** There's no reason why your baby can't eat food warm, chilled, or at room temperature. However, it's important to be sure that whatever you're serving isn't too hot.
• **Consistency** Mashed foods at first with tiny lumps and progressing to larger soft lumps.
• **How often?** 2–3 meals a day.
• **How much?** 4–6 tsp (more if they are hungry) of 2–3 different foods at each meal, with at least 2–3 vegetables and one fruit each day, plus some foods from the other food groups.
• **Flavors** Add spices and herbs you use in your regular cooking, avoiding salt. Your baby will learn to enjoy all the flavors of the foods that you love, too.

Happy meals Babies love to grab food and some may be happier if allowed to feed themselves. Learning to feed herself is a huge step in your baby's physical and intellectual development, so encourage all her efforts and don't worry about the mess.

Growing up fast

The way your baby looks is changing as they grow, and you may also find that their little rolls of fat are starting to disperse.

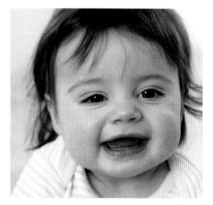

Million-dollar smile Your baby may now have four to eight teeth, just two, or even none, but that cute smile is still irresistible!

Some babies look a little leaner as they become more mobile—all the activity burns off fat stores so they begin to lose some of their chubby rolls of dimpled flesh.

Your baby's fontanels are closing over, and, as your baby begins to bear weight and walk, their feet will begin to flatten. Although they will continue to bounce up and down when held upright, they'll straighten their legs at the knees for longer periods. Their head is becoming more rounded as they spend far less time on their back, and, as the body grows, it looks more in proportion to the rest of the body than it did previously. They may have a full head of hair by now or a just few delicate wisps.

Your baby will continue to grow at a tremendous rate in the lead-up to their first birthday, but that rate will now slow down a little. They will probably put on about 1–1¼ lb (450–600 g) per month, and grow about 2½ in (6 cm) before turning one. Your baby's base eye color will have reached its final color by now, although very subtle changes may continue into adulthood.

Kitchen hygiene

Preparing your baby's food requires scrupulous hygiene; their immune system is still immature so they're susceptible to food-borne illnesses.

Use one cutting board and set of knives for meat and another for vegetables and fruits. Keep raw and cooked foods separate. Cook meat and poultry until it is well done, and wash fruits and vegetables or peel them before pureeing.

Use your baby's food immediately or freeze it for future use. If you store leftover food in the fridge, keep it in there for only two or three days, then discard it. Pour some into a bowl for serving, and refrigerate the remainder for later.

Wash all your baby's spoons, bowls, and food containers in hot, soapy water or in the dishwasher to kill any germs. You don't need to sterilize them. After all, your baby always seems to have something in their mouth, even when it's nowhere near feeding time. A few more germs won't make a difference. Also, wash your hands (and your baby's), clean surfaces frequently, and change dish towels fairly regularly.

YOUR BABY'S FEEDING AREA

Clean your baby's high chair after every meal with hot, soapy water. Pay particular attention to crevices around the tray and seat, where they may have dropped bits of food. Mop the floor around the chair and look for food that they may have thrown across the room; they'll undoubtedly spend time on the kitchen floor and put anything that looks interesting straight into their mouth, even if it is a week-old meatball.

Coping with chaos

Babies are messy! You may find that your once-tidy kitchen is in shambles, and your living room looks like a cyclone has hit it!

Try not to let the mess get to you. You may have to lower your standards and expect things to look less tidy than usual. Time with your baby is precious, and it's much more important to spend it interacting than it is to follow along behind them cleaning up.

Having said that, you can put into place a few routines to help keep things a little more organized. Put away the toys at the end of every play session. Make this easier by keeping them in baskets or boxes placed on open shelves, or screening off an area of your living room in which toys are piled out of sight.

Create baby areas in several rooms in your home, each with a large basket or a shelving unit in which to keep all your baby's things together. At the end of the day, do a pick-up, gathering the single socks, dropped toys, bibs, wet towels, and books, and put them back into their homes, or wash them. Take a few minutes to refill your diaper bag, so you are ready to go out on impulse. It may seem like one extra thing to fit in, but you'll be able to relax more if things are ready for the next day.

When you're loading the dishwasher, give your baby some toy pans and cutlery to organize, too—just like you. If you're washing up by hand, a little bowl of warm water with bubbles from a spot of baby shampoo is the perfect plaything (even better if the bowl has suction pads to prevent it going on the floor!). Protect the floor around the high chair with a mat—which is as useful at mealtimes as it is when pretending to do dishes.

If you can afford help with cleaning, don't hesitate to organize it—if some of the heavier cleaning is done regularly, it's easier to stay on top of the general tidying. If a cleaner isn't right for you, spend some dedicated time each weekend cleaning with the help of your partner while your baby sleeps; or pick one room a day—it may feel like your home is never completely clean and tidy at once, but it means you can stay on top of things.

DEVELOPMENT ACTIVITY: CLEAN-UP TIME

Encouraging your baby to become involved in cleaning up the toys at the end of a play session will help establish good habits, and they'll soon accept it as part of the routine. Show them how to pile toys back into the basket and put books on the lowest shelf of the bookcase. Demonstrate how to neatly line up soft toys and put everything in its place. Explain what you are doing, and repeat the fact that you are making things "nice and neat" to establish a positive association with the activity rather than making it sound like a chore! Praise them when they manage to put a toy in the basket. Your baby will enjoy this activity because it's with you, and as they notice your pleasure, they'll be more likely to join in next time, too.

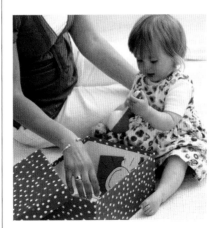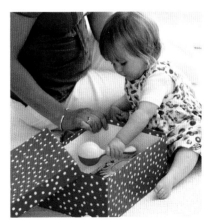

The clean-up game Make a game out of putting away toys so your baby learns what to do after playing with them. This is a great way to introduce the idea of cleaning up.

Is baby a bottom shuffler?

Not all babies like to crawl, so don't be surprised if your baby seems determined to stay on their bottom and move in their own sweet way...

Learning to move around can be frustrating for babies, which is probably one reason they all have different approaches. Some crawl before they walk, some don't crawl until after they walk, and others don't crawl at all. Instead, they shuffle on their bottoms, sometimes using a hand behind and a foot in front to propel themselves. Because bottom shuffling involves being able to sit and wiggle forward on their buttocks, it typically develops two to three months after a baby is able to sit unsupported.

Around nine percent of babies are bottom shufflers and it is thought to run in families, so if you or your partner were shufflers, there's a chance your baby will be one, too. Many bottom shufflers walk a bit later than usual, often because they are so successful at scooting around on their bottoms that there's less incentive to stand up. As long as your baby can get around, it doesn't matter how they do it.

Taking turns

From time to time, your baby may express a strong preference for one parent, and even cry or hide their face from the other. What's going on?

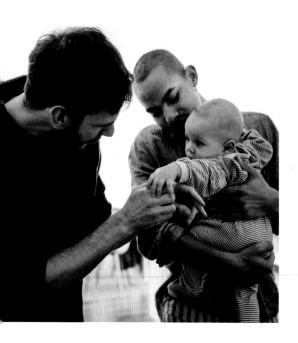

As your baby develops, they may at times show a preference for one of you over the other. Try not to be disheartened by this favoritism—it will swing around to you again at some point, and is not because you have made a mistake, or because they haven't bonded with you. Most often, your baby will show a degree of preference for the person most tuned into their needs and communication, and who knows all the best ways to soothe them. This is usually the parent who spends the most time with them, and who therefore has more opportunity to "read" their signals and gain confidence in responding.

The opposite can also be true on some occasions. For example, a fresh face may be what they want at the end of the day. So if you are returning from work, you may be the one getting the squeals of delight and a greeting of raised arms ready for a hug.

Balance these preferences by taking turns. Each establish your own special activities with them when you are together, and don't be disheartened when they show an unashamed preference for the other parent. They don't know it may feel hurtful, and they're definitely not doing it deliberately to upset you.

Showing favoritism Many babies go through phases of "preferring" one parent to another, so try not to take it personally.

Coping with a food allergy

Having a baby with an allergy can present a number of challenges.
Thankfully, many babies outgrow their allergies with proper care.

There is often confusion between allergies and food intolerances. A food intolerance is when your baby has difficulties digesting a specific food or group of foods. A reaction will often take several days to detect, and presents as mild symptoms such as diarrhea, skin rash, bloating, and flatulence. If you suspect your baby has a food intolerance, speak to your pediatrician and always check with them before removing any foods from your baby's diet.

On the other hand, a food allergy is when your baby has an abnormal immune reaction to a particular food or substance that will occur within just minutes of eating it. Symptoms of an allergy can include itchy skin and rash, swollen lips and throat, blocked and runny nose, sore and itchy eyes, a cough, vomiting, and diarrhea. If you suspect your baby has an allergy, speak to your pediatrician who can refer you to an allergy specialist. They will conduct a skin prick or blood test, so you know exactly which food or group of foods you should avoid.

Occasionally, an allergy can lead to a severe and life-threatening reaction, called anaphylaxis. This normally occurs within minutes and symptoms come on and worsen quickly. Symptoms include clammy skin, wheezing and difficulty breathing, rapid heartbeat, signs of confusion, collapsing, and losing consciousness. Call an ambulance immediately.

If your baby has an allergy, you

DEVELOPMENT ACTIVITY: WASHING-UP TIME!

Babies like nothing more than joining in with parents' activities, and a little help with the dishes can provide an opportunity for fun. Give your baby a bowl of warm, soapy water, set them up on a mat on the floor, and allow them to "wash" their own dishes using a big sponge and a clean dish towel. They'll love being involved and doing things they see you doing, and they'll also learn a helpful skill, develop hand–eye coordination, and enjoy the sensation of playing with water.

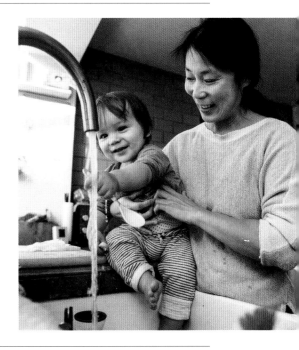

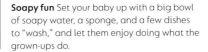
Soapy fun Set your baby up with a big bowl of soapy water, a sponge, and a few dishes to "wash," and let them enjoy doing what the grown-ups do.

should speak to your doctor about whether you need an antihistamine that's appropriate for babies. If your baby's allergy is severe, you may also need to carry an EpiPen Auto-Injector for emergency anaphylaxis. You should also ensure that anyone else who spends time with your baby knows about their allergies, and how to administer any medication.

Prepare food using implements that have been washed to avoid cross-contamination, and rigorously inspect labels on foods you buy.

Maintaining a food diary

Keep a food diary to help you identify a food or group of foods that cause a reaction in your baby. You may feel anxious about the possibility of an allergic reaction, but it's important that you don't pass these feelings on to your baby, which could make them nervous about eating, trying new foods, and relaxing during mealtimes. A food diary may prove a useful reference for a dietitian or allergy specialist should your baby be referred to a specialist.

Bed sharing

Your baby may be sharing your bed—perhaps it's time to encourage them to sleep in theirs.

Unless you plan to co-sleep with them for an indefinite period of time, you may need to get them used to their own bed again.

Try to resist the temptation to bring your baby into your bed when they wake up. Instead, stroke them, sing to them, and snuggle with them, then leave the room. Return whenever they call to reassure them that you will come whenever they really need you—if you leave them to cry, they'll simply become more insecure. Implement this new policy for the first time on a night when you don't have to wake up early the next morning. Be calm and patient and remind yourself that even if it takes an hour or so for your baby to fall back asleep, only to wake up again an hour or so later, it's worth the effort in the long run because you will all get more sleep.

Over the coming nights, they'll whine and complain for shorter and shorter periods of time about being on their own, until they understand that they aren't going to be invited into your bed.

If you need more advice about encouraging your baby to sleep on their own, ask your pediatrician. For more on sleep strategies, see pp.324–325, too.

Time-saving strategies

Most parents feel there are never enough hours in the day, but there are ways to save time and buy a little more freedom for you.

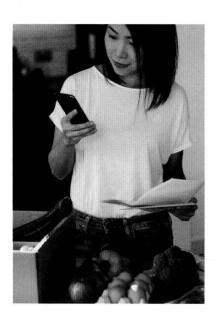

Now that life has settled into some sort of routine, you may really want a little spare time in which to pursue an interest or hobby. To gain yourself a bit more freedom, start by taking an objective look at how you prioritize your day and how much time each activity takes up. This can be a really good way of taking control of your time and assessing where too much is devoted to unimportant things, and too little to what really matters, such as your relationship, friendships, and health. Then try to find ways of reducing time spent on what you least enjoy, such as household tasks. If you iron regularly, for example, think about hanging up your laundry as soon as it's done to prevent creasing. If you're cooking a family meal, double the recipe and freeze the leftovers. Shop online for food and other staples, if you find it quicker and have them delivered or do a curbside pickup.

Speedy shopping Save staples in your online grocery basket to save time having to find and add them week after week.

Pulling up to standing

Your baby may start to pull up and stand with support, but probably won't find it so easy to sit back down again.

Over the next few weeks or months, your baby will start to pull up into a standing position. At first, they may need your help, but eventually, they'll realize that by putting one hand above the other, they can haul themself upward. From this fascinating new vantage point, they'll be able to see lots of exciting new places, and increase their motivation to get moving.

Unfortunately, at first, what goes up doesn't always come down easily: your baby might well find that they're stuck! They haven't figured out how to move their hands and feet to inch along the edge of a piece of furniture. They don't know how to walk. Nor do they know how to lower back down to the floor. You may need to help them sit back down gently and reassure them many times before they feel confident enough to plop down safely on their own, but eventually they'll understand that they won't hurt themself. They may even begin to have as much fun dropping down with a thump on the floor as they did pulling up in the first place.

While they're standing, leaning on furniture for support, they'll be practicing maintaining their balance, supporting weight on their legs, and shifting their weight to enable them to lift one foot or the other. Once they've mastered the art of standing and balancing, they will at some point take a step while holding onto whatever they used to pull themself up. This development is called cruising and is a precursor to walking (see p.249).

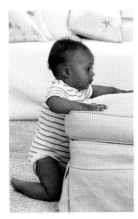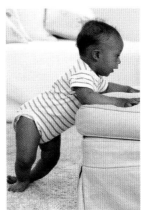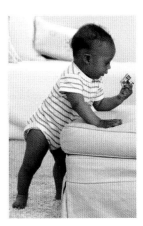

Pulling up A favorite toy positioned on an armchair provides your baby with an incentive to pull themself up. From there, they can cruise around, using the chair as support.

Update your babyproofing

Once your baby starts to pull up to standing, consider what they can now reach. Also, is there any furniture that might topple over if used as a support, or might they climb on something and fall off? Is your bookcase securely fastened to the wall? What is reachable from on top of the sofa? Your baby is intrepid and curious, and will be out of sight in no time, so make sure you are prepared and have done everything you can to keep them safe.

ASK A PEDIATRICIAN

My baby's feet are curving inward. Is this normal? When your baby is born, their feet turn inward and their legs bow slightly, which is a result of living in the small confines of your womb for many months. As they grow and develop, their legs become straighter and their feet flatter, to aid their ability to walk. Later on, as they approach the age of three, their flat feet will probably develop arches.

At about 7 months, the feet should sit quite flat on the floor when your baby is held upright. Your baby may balance on the outsides of their feet from time to time to establish balance, and then adjust position. Sometimes a baby's feet, or even lower legs, may be slightly misaligned, and turn or even twist inward (known as intoeing). Your doctor will be able to check if there is a problem. Be reassured that in virtually all cases, intoeing will correct itself naturally, and will not hinder your baby's ability to walk.

8 months

TOYS THAT ENCOURAGE EXPLORATION OF DIFFERENT SHAPES STIMULATE A BABY'S MIND.
Shape-sorting and stacking toys test motor and cognitive skills and encourage problem solving.
Help your baby to learn about sequences and sizes by demonstrating how these toys work. Your
baby's speech is more complex now, and they're getting better at imitating the pitch of speech.

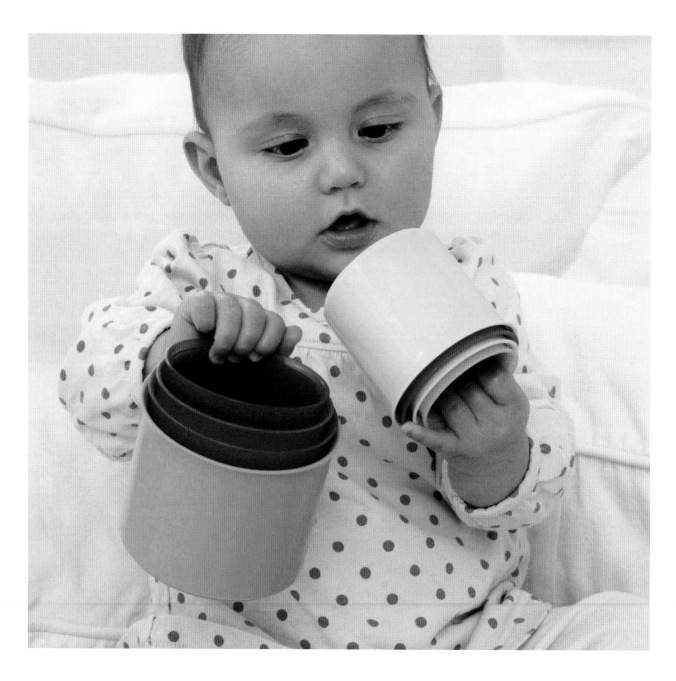

Babies and antibiotics

Antibiotics are not a cure-all for every illness or infection—you may like to know why they may or may not be prescribed.

Should your baby become sick, their illness is likely to have been caused by one of two main types of germs: bacteria or viruses. Bacteria are organisms that can be found inside and on the body (such as on the skin) and can cause infections including tonsillitis or strep throat and ear infections. However, not all bacteria are bad—some help keep your baby's body in balance, such as the beneficial bacteria in the intestines that help your baby use the nutrients in milk and food.

Viruses are organisms that cause disease by invading healthy host cells in the body. Viruses can cause chickenpox, measles, flu, and many other diseases.

Antibiotics are used to treat bacterial infections, or infections that are very likely to be bacterial. They have no effect on viruses, so will not work for coughs, colds or flu, sore throats (not strep throat), or runny noses.

Frequent and inappropriate use of antibiotics encourages strains of bacteria that can resist treatment. This is called bacterial resistance. These resistant bacteria require higher doses of medicine or stronger antibiotics to treat. Doctors have even found bacteria that are resistant to some of the most powerful antibiotics available today.

More complex chatter

Your baby's chatter is changing all the time, and they now have a greater variety of sounds than they did in the first six months.

Moving on to solid foods helps your baby develop lip control as they learn to keep their lips sealed when chewing and swallowing. Chewing takes on a circular motion, which in turn helps with tongue control. These changes allow your baby to start to create more complex vocalizations.

Your baby's babble now contains more syllables and different consonants and vowels. They're moving beyond repeating a syllable, such as "mamama," to combining them: "digabu," "apaba," or "babamado." They're also becoming more accomplished at imitating the pitch and intonation of the speech around them, and maybe even imitating individual sounds. So at a lively gathering, they may babble more loudly and in a higher-pitched voice, and when you read at bedtime, they may murmur and use a softer tone of voice, just as you do. This is known as echo talk: instead of simply imitating the tone and vowel sounds of your speech, as they have been doing over the past few months, they start to pay much more attention to pitch.

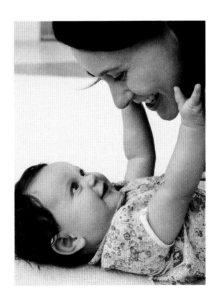

Early speech Your baby's communication skills are more consistent and understandable now. It won't be long before their first word!

Positive relationships

Grandparents are a wonderful part of your child's life, as they will often lavish them with their love, attention, and gifts.

It is very normal for grandparents to want to "spoil" their grandchildren, and it can give them great joy to provide your baby with things that you may not be able to afford yourself. While it can be a godsend to have some of the more expensive items provided by your baby's grandparents, you may feel it conflicts with your desire to be independent. There may also be an inequality between what different sets of grandparents are able to offer, which can lead to resentment.

Material possessions aside, you may find that grandparents are more relaxed about behavior and household rules than you are, which can be confusing for a baby or young child.

Talk to your baby's grandparents about your concerns. Explain that, while you appreciate their generosity, you would prefer that expensive gifts were agreed with you first, and that, as your baby grows up, you want them to realize that sometimes we have to wait for what we want, and to value love and care above gifts.

Share with them the values you want to teach your child. Whether these are about positive relationships, working for what they want, or a cultural ethos. Open dialogue will help you understand each other.

Taking turns

This is a good stage to begin teaching your baby about cooperation by taking turns when you do things together.

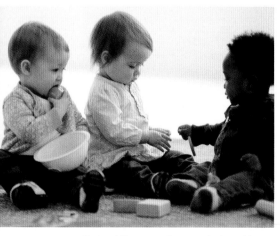

My turn When you take turns playing with toys, your baby learns the give and take of communication and social interaction.

Roll a ball to your baby and encourage them to push it back to you. Push the button on the toy telephone (my turn), then ask them to do it (your turn). Opportunities to teach taking turns are virtually limitless: your baby can lift the flaps or turn the pages of a book, then you can; they can "wash their face" with the wash cloth in the tub, then you can, or they can hold a teddy bear and hug him, then you can, too.

Your baby will begin to experience satisfaction when they have an opportunity to experiment and become involved in activities, which over time will build self-confidence and help introduce the notion of sharing and even (way down the line) that it's okay for other people to do things for us, too. However, they won't begin to understand the concept of sharing for a while yet, even when taking turns playing with toys. In fact, it won't be until around three to five years old that they'll begin to understand how to put sharing into practice..

With twins, while it's a good idea to set up both babies with their own toys and important to remember that they are individuals as well, and will behave as such, you can also start to encourage them to play "together," taking turns with toys—although you'll need to supervise.

Healthy food on the go

As well as your baby's regular meals, it's a good idea to also have a supply of healthy snacks and drinks on hand.

Get into a pattern of giving your baby a healthy morning and afternoon snack, including a drink, in addition to the three main meals. This helps prevent grazing throughout the day, which can lead to being too full to eat a proper meal, increase the exposure of teeth to food, and can override their innate capacity for appetite control.

Watch how much your baby drinks, too. If you are using formula milk, make sure you don't let them drink more than the recommended amount, and use a fast-flowing nipple or cup so they can

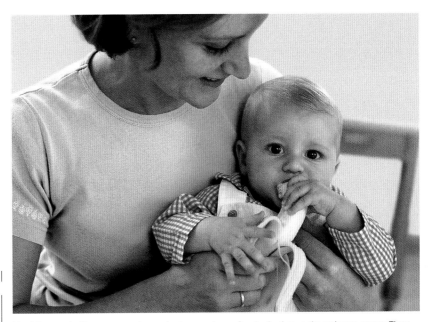

Healthy snacks Bananas are the perfect convenience food, whether you're at home or out. They don't need preparation, are easy to digest, and contain important nutrients, including vitamin C.

ASK A NUTRITIONIST

Won't regular snacking make my baby overweight? Nutritious snacks are part of your baby's healthy diet, helping to ensure they get the nutrients they need throughout the day. It's important to look at snacks as part of their overall diet, rather than as treats, to help you choose nutritious foods. Try to avoid feeding snacks to distract them when they are bored or unhappy. While it may seem like a good quick-fix solution, they may learn to use food to alleviate boredom, and to associate food with comfort. This may increase long-term risks of becoming overweight. Offer regular snacks when they seem hungry, and at regular intervals, leaving a good break between snack and mealtimes, to ensure they develop an appetite. Water is the best drink at snack time as an alternative to milk (see "Your baby's drinks," p.229).

finish quickly. If they constantly have a bottle of milk in hand, their appetite may be poor for other foods.

A snack can add important nutrients to your baby's diet. Opt for mashed beans and a few peeled, cut-up grapes, which supply essential calcium and vitamin C, as well as calories, sugar, and fat. Dried foods such as mini rice cakes, raisins, and dried apricots are good for keeping in your diaper bag. A banana, hard-boiled egg, cheese, tomatoes, and peppers make a good baby picnic. Try to avoid processed food. If you do buy prepared food, be sure to check labels for real food ingredients.

Meals on the run

If you're going to be out at a mealtime, pack a suitable puree for your baby in an insulated bag. Find out if you can heat up your baby's meal, making sure it is piping hot throughout, then let it cool. Alternatively, keep it hot in a wide-necked thermos. You can also carry some foods that can be pureed, mashed, or cut into chunks on the spot, such as bananas, melon, papaya, avocado, carrots, and ripe pears or peaches. Chunks of soft chicken, turkey, and fingers of pita, baby crackers, or bread can all be eaten cold.

Fidgety baby

Your mobile baby is less content to sit and watch the world go by—so you may need to adapt your routine to give them a bit more action.

Now that your baby is older and more mobile, you may find that they're less content to be confined to the stroller or car seat for even short periods of time. Generally, they are now more restless and likely to become fractious if expected to remain still for too long.

This is all part of growing up, so your best bet is to adapt your routine a little to suit you both. For instance, you might want to arrange to meet friends at a soft play area where you can grab a coffee and chat while you watch your babies crawl, climb, and explore. You could take turns with other moms to host get-togethers in each other's homes (your babies will love to discover an entirely new range of toys) or, in the summer, arrange picnics in the park. If you dread shopping with a wailing baby, go alone when your partner is at home and can take care of the baby. Just a few small changes can make a difference.

ASK A NUTRITIONIST

I'm trying to move my baby on to solid foods but they gag. What can I do?
Rather than backtrack to familiar purees, offer soft finger foods or a spoon so they feel in control. On their high chair tray, place small pieces of food so they can explore with their fingers. If all else fails, have a couple of days on familiar purees then try small spoonfuls of lumpier foods, such as mashed potato.

Nighttime acrobatics

Your baby isn't only active during the day; they may turn in their sleep and roll over onto their tummy.

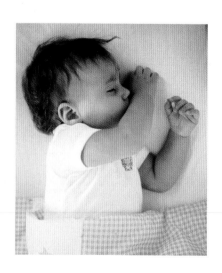

If your baby is strong enough to roll onto their tummy on their own, don't worry if they flip over off of their back during the night. At this age, the risk of SIDS (see p.31) is greatly reduced, as some 90 percent of cases occur before a baby is six months old. It's important that you don't restrict your baby's movements or try to force them to sleep on their back. It is also suggested that you avoid swaddling at this point. Confining your baby will disrupt their sleep and possibly encourage them to develop negative sleep associations.

A wiggly sleeper may kick off their blankets. Firmly tuck in the blankets at the base of the crib at bedtime to prevent them from covering your baby's face as they move around in their sleep. Alternatively, invest in a baby sleeping bag appropriate for their age. Start them off on their back at night (the position they will probably find most familiar) and continue to avoid pillows and duvets, and placing soft toys in the crib.

Roly-poly Although they may roll over in their sleep, still place your baby on their back when you first put them in their crib.

Learning to walk

From standing and balancing to cruising around the living room holding on to the furniture, your baby's progression toward walking may occur any time from now on, so make sure you are prepared!

All babies learn to walk at different ages, from as early as 9 months, right up to 18 months, so if your baby is in no hurry to walk, there is no rush. Follow their lead. Help them develop strength in their legs by holding their hands and bouncing them up and down. Continue to give tummy time to strengthen the back and neck muscles and improve coordination and balance, and offer them a good, sturdy push toy that will tempt them to get up onto their feet and push it along when they are ready.

Before your baby can walk, they'll need to master getting up into a standing position while holding a support, then bending their knees and sitting down. It can take many months for them to develop these techniques. When they can stand for short periods without support, they may be ready to take their first steps.

First steps

Your baby's first steps represent an enormously important milestone in their physical development as they put together balance, gross-motor skills, control, coordination, and especially courage! In advance of walking unaided, they will spread out their feet to increase their balance, giving them a waddling gait. They may launch in the direction of something stable, such as a table or even you, and probably throw out their arms to cushion a fall.

Over the coming weeks, your baby will learn to take a single step at a time, stopping to regain their balance before continuing. One thing they won't be able to control for a while is speed—at first they tend to hurl themselves forward, then lean too far back in an effort to regain balance, resulting in a series of stumbles and falls. Brush them off and help them back onto their feet. They'll learn through their mistakes and realize soon enough that they really must learn to walk before they can run.

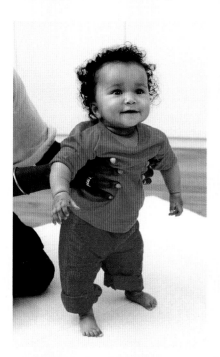

Twinkle toes Your baby should practice walking barefoot, as this encourages good balance, coordination, and grip.

WALKING SAFETY

Check that your baby's environment is safe when they are learning to walk. Although they'll take many tumbles, you can help to cushion their falls.

• Tape down loose rugs or carpets, so they don't become a trip hazard.
• Watch out for obstacles around the room that may hamper your baby.
• Keep out of reach small objects that could be swallowed and cause choking.
• Tidy away loose or tangled cords that could cause entanglement.
• Erect baby gates at the top and bottom of the stairs.
• Install guards or locks on windows.
• Secure or remove any furniture that is unsteady and could tip over when your baby grabs it to help them balance.
• Consider padding sharp corners or edges on furniture (such as tables), or remove the piece of furniture.
• If you have a glass-topped coffee table, consider temporarily replacing the top with Lucite or acrylic.
• Keep drawers shut—your baby may use open drawers to climb up onto uneven or slippery surfaces.
• Cover heated surfaces, and install a fire screen if you have an open fire.
• Ensure the toilet seat is kept down; get a clip to lock it into place.
• Position pan handles facing inward on the stove.
• Keep dangling electrical appliance cords out of your baby's reach.

Strong emotions

Your baby will be unable to control their emotions, and may end up in tears of frustration or become sad when you need to leave the room.

A young baby has highly changeable emotions, one minute squealing with delight, the next upset or frustrated. While these changes may be difficult to predict at times, each is an important communication from your baby to you, telling you about their needs and wants. Try to remember that what they are doing is communicating with you, and that this is a good sign.

In the first year, your baby will experience strong emotions as physical feelings in their body—their task is to separate out these emotions gradually, and, eventually, with your help and guidance, to label each one.

At first, strong feelings can be frightening for your baby, and they will need your help to tolerate the sensations and return to a calm, regulated emotional state. According to "attachment" experts (who study the deep relationship between a child and their main caregiver during the first few years of life, and the profound influence this has on a baby), your role is to show your baby you accept their feelings, that the feelings don't scare or overwhelm you, and that baby doesn't need to feel out of control or afraid of the feelings.

One way to do this is through "mirroring," which involves reflecting your child's emotions, but in a milder, version. You may naturally tilt your head during mirroring to signal your understanding. Holding them while a feeling grips them can also reassure that they are safe. You can mirror your child's emotions no matter how young

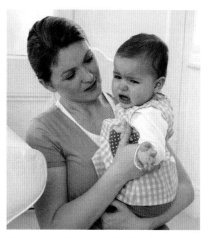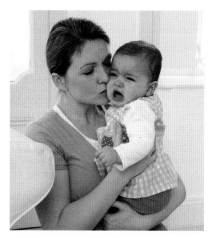

Reassure, comfort, and calm Your baby can't handle their emotions and will look to you to calm them down when they're feeling angry or frustrated.

they are. Your steady reaction will give them confidence that feelings need not overpower them. Help your baby put a name to their feelings by talking about what is going on. For example, when you say "You look angry" or "Is that a sad face?"

Good role model

Be a positive role model for your baby by showing them how you are able to manage your own strong feelings and recover from them. If you find yourself struggling to cope with a prolonged period of distress from your baby, seek help from your partner, or a trusted friend or relative, while you take a break. It's important to be realistic about your own limitations and needs, and to recognize when you need time out yourself.

ASK A PEDIATRICIAN

Why has my baby suddenly developed regular bouts of diarrhea, even though they don't seem ill? A change in your baby's diet may cause diarrhea and/or constipation, as their digestive system makes the transition to solid foods. Sometimes, new foods can appear undigested in the runny stools as they're introduced in the diet, a phenomenon known as "toddler" diarrhea (although this is more common after one year). If this is the reason, your baby will be otherwise well, and the diarrhea should settle down as the bowels get better at digesting new foods. Make sure your baby drinks plenty of fluids—give cool water on top of their usual milk feedings—and avoid fruit juices, as these are the most common cause.

Is fresh always best?

Using a mixture of homemade and store-bought baby food increases the range of flavors your baby experiences and gives you more time.

Many parents feel they should feed their baby exclusively homemade food, and feel guilty about using commercially produced baby foods. Nutritious and wholesome homemade food is ideal, but jarred baby food is getting better by leaps and bounds, and there are now nutritious and appetizing foods available that are salt-, sugar-, and additive-free. In fact, combining homemade and quality store-bought foods may introduce your baby to a wider variety of flavors, colors, and textures. Also, a pouch or jar of ready-made baby food is a convenient option to use when you're out and about.

When shopping for baby foods, it's important to compare ingredient labels closely, because some brands add sugar, water, and fillers to their foods. Whenever possible, it's best to serve your baby food that contains no extraneous ingredients—nothing but peas, for example, if the label says "peas." You may also want to factor in whether foods are grown organically when making your decision. Even the size of the jar or container may matter, since some babies eat less at each sitting, and you may prefer to serve your baby right out of the jar, rather than pouring half into a bowl.

In addition to store-bought meals, make sure that other commercially produced food you give your baby is suitable. For example, your baby needs "baby" cereals since these are fortified with vitamins and minerals and don't have added salt or sugar; and baby yogurts are made with whole milk and contain no artificial sweeteners, colorings, or other additives found in regular yogurts. They also come in baby-size containers so there's less danger of overfeeding your baby.

Measuring nutrients

Some baby foods are sold at room temperature, which means they have been treated at high temperatures to ensure they keep safely on the supermarket shelf. This can destroy some of the vitamins, but these are often added back in. On the other hand, some baby foods are frozen at high speed, which ensures that a high proportion of vitamins is kept.

When making your baby's food, look for the freshest ingredients and steam or lightly boil vegetables to make sure that your baby's purees have the optimum nutritional content.

Ultimately, home-cooked food tastes different than store-bought, and it's important that commercial foods do not become the mainstay of your baby's diet.

ASK A NUTRITIONIST

Which is more cost-effective—store-bought or homemade baby food?
Commercially produced baby food is a relatively expensive way to feed your baby. Making meals at home gives you complete transparency on what ingredients make up a dish, plus you can make a dish in bulk and freeze batches. Also, it's easy to give your baby some of your own meal by putting their portion aside before seasoning and then pureeing it to the desired consistency.

USING STORE-BOUGHT BABY FOODS

• If you are out, a jar or pouch of baby food that doesn't need to be kept cool can be extremely helpful, and wait staff should not object to you bringing your own baby food into a restaurant (See p.247 for more ideas on healthy food on the go.)
• When buying commercially produced baby foods, make sure that your baby doesn't stay on thin purees for too long. Make sure the progression of textures and tastes you make for them at home is reflected in the store-bought foods that supplement their diet.
• If your own diet is restricted in any way through choice or intolerance, commercial baby foods are a convenient way to give your baby flavors you don't tend to eat. However, try to make sure you also cook foods at home specially for your baby, so they don't develop an aversion to homemade foods.

Mini parent?

Your baby's personality is beginning to unfold, and you might notice certain traits that seem very familiar—and a few that are unique.

Your baby is their own little person, with their own likes, dislikes, and foibles. If these don't match yours, it's important to accept this and allow them the space to grow in their own way. It can be easy to regard your baby as a "mini-me," but don't be surprised or frustrated if they don't behave as you expect. If they are an extrovert who loves attention and being around others, but both you and your partner are shy, try to give your baby lots of opportunities to socialize. (This may change in the coming months as they experience separation anxiety—see p.263.) Equally, if your baby is shy and from a family of extroverts, don't force them into situations that cause anxiety. Let them play on your lap while you talk; they will probably get bored and, in time, choose to investigate what else is going on at their own pace.

Likewise, if you are fairly laid-back and tend to go with the flow, it doesn't mean that your baby will enjoy this; on the contrary, they may crave routine. As the parent, you need to try to structure the day so your baby feels comfortable and secure, even if you are not the sort of person who relishes routine.

Caring for your baby's hair

As your baby gets more active and makes more of a mess at feeding times, you will find regular hair care becomes essential!

If your baby was born with a full head of hair, by now they may need their first hair cut. Be gentle and—if you are doing this at home—very careful, combing the hair first, and making sure that cut hair doesn't go into your baby's eyes or ears.

Baby hair doesn't need to be washed every day: twice a week is usually enough. However, you will inevitably find bits of food in their hair as they get more involved at mealtimes, so you may need to wet sponge it after they've eaten. Before you wash their hair, gently tease out any tangles with your fingers or a fine-toothed comb. Start at the tips and work your way up to the roots to avoid tugging the roots. Use a baby shampoo that doesn't contain harsh chemicals (such as parabens and sulfates) or perfume that could sting their eyes, and has a balanced pH of between 4.5 and 6. If your baby has very curly hair, you might want to comb conditioner through to help keep it soft and loose. Sponge it off with water.

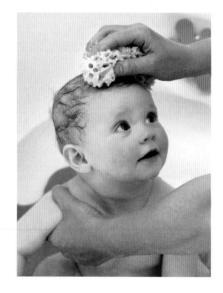

Hair care Using a sponge or wet washcloth to rinse the shampoo from your baby's hair will stop soapy water from trickling into their eyes.

All sorts of sounds

As your baby hears words repeated regularly, many will start to sound familiar and they will be stimulated to babble even more.

Although babbling seems nonsensical, studies show that the way babies babble is modeled on how we talk, in that they use the right-hand side of their mouths slightly more in the same way that adults talk (watch yourself in the mirror!). Research shows that the left brain, which controls the right side of the body and is responsible for understanding and language, is therefore also instigating babbling, confirming that babbling is important in language development. Psychologists believe that babies begin meaningful talk long before we realize (as early as between 8 and 10 months)—we just don't recognize the words!

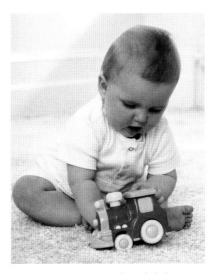

Choo-choo! Toys with sounds can help language development. "What noise does a train make?"

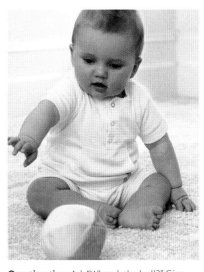

Question time Ask "Where's the ball?" Give a running commentary as they play.

Speech development

While most babies won't utter their first comprehensible word until close to a year, or older, babies are like sponges, soaking up sounds, so keep talking. Your baby will watch your mouth intently as you talk, so face-to-face talk helps speech development, as do games that involve distinctive sounds. Point to animals in books with phrases such as "What does a cow say? A cow says moo!" Even if your baby doesn't make the sound, they might copy the shape of your mouth. Use every chance you find to play sound games, for example, talking about their toys ("an airplane goes whoosh!"), and talk to them constantly during everyday tasks such as dressing and bathing.

Naming people and objects all the time, including using your baby's name, helps their word recognition. Although a baby's recognition of their own name is usually around nine months, there are clear indications that before this, babies grasp that words have associations.

If your baby isn't babbling by now, or doesn't respond to loud noises or you calling their name out of their range of vision, speak with your pediatrician who may suggest a hearing test for your baby.

DEVELOPMENT ACTIVITY: SONG AND SPEECH

Studies suggest that babies who are sung to a lot learn to speak more quickly than those who are not. Singing separates out syllables in words, breaking them down so they are easier to pronounce, and listening to songs helps improve attention spans in young babies. There are lots of musical and singing activity groups for parents and babies, but simply singing to your baby at home is enough. Don't worry if you think you're tone deaf; your baby won't mind and will enjoy being held by you as you sway and move to a song. Sing nursery rhymes and introduce your baby to songs with actions to help them get involved.

Stopping breastfeeding

Many babies are breastfed throughout the first year—and beyond. However, if the time is right for you and your baby to stop, take things slowly and drop one feeding at a time to make it a painless experience for you both.

ASK A NUTRITIONIST

Our family has a history of allergies. Should I wean my baby onto soy or goat's milk formula instead of cow's milk formula? If you are concerned that your baby has a higher risk of being allergic to cow's milk formula, it's essential to talk to your pediatrician before deciding how to wean your baby off breast milk; they will be able to give you unbiased advice on the pros and cons of different types of formula. They may also advise you not to make any assumptions before you have started weaning.

Goat's milk also contains proteins that your baby may react to, so is not a good alternative. Most importantly, though, goat's milk isn't advised for babies because the level of proteins are too concentrated.

Soy is sometimes promoted as an alternative for babies allergic to cow's milk. However, a significant proportion of babies who are allergic to cow's milk also react to soy milk formula. If, while weaning your baby, you notice that they develop a rash or are experiencing stomach upsets, for example, talk to your pediatrician, who can prescribe a special type of formula called fully hydrolyzed formula (see p.229), in which the proteins are broken down so they are easier to tolerate.

Some babies naturally lose interest in breastfeeding, preferring instead to drink their milk from a bottle or a cup because it's easier for them. If they enjoy formula, this allows you to wind down breastfeeding fairly easily. Other babies enjoy the comfort of nursing and breast milk long past the point at which you have had enough, and it can be a hard task to wean them.

The length of time you breastfeed is a personal decision. Common reasons to reduce, or stop, breastfeeding are that you want to allow other caregivers a chance to feed your baby, or, that you are going back to work (you can still express milk, mix breast milk and formula, or you may want to stop entirely). Whatever the reason, it is gentlest to your baby emotionally, and better for you physically, to drop feedings gradually, one at a time.

A successful transition means planning ahead and carefully timing the dropping of feedings. Try to avoid times when your baby feels unsettled, for example, if they've just moved to their own room, or are feeling sick.

Milk, whether breast milk or formula, remains the most important

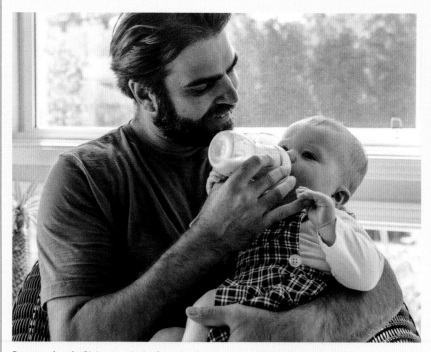

Breast to bottle Giving your baby formula allows your partner and other relatives to get involved in their care, helping them strengthen their bond with your baby.

source of nutrition for the first year of your baby's life. When your baby starts on solids, milk still forms the bulk of the calories, while the baby gets used to new textures and tastes. Weaning from breast milk in the first year therefore involves substituting formula (not cow's milk) for breastfeedings.

You can begin to substitute one breastfeeding at a time for formula in a cup or bottle. While there is no set timetable, it's recommended that you drop just one feeding a week to start with—or allow a minimum of four to five days in between dropping feedings, to give your baby and your breasts time to adjust. Make the first feeding you switch one where they aren't ravenously hungry, like mid-afternoon.

You might like to continue the evening feeding for as long as possible, since it's a relaxing way to unwind before bed and often a cherished part of the bedtime routine. Your baby may also be more resistant to losing this feeding, especially if you've been at work. There's no reason why you can't continue to give your baby one or two breastfeedings a day for as long as you both want.

When your baby resists

If your baby is finding it hard to give up breastfeeding, ask your partner or a friend to give a formula feeding in a bottle or cup. Change your routine slightly so your baby isn't as aware that the bedtime breastfeeding hasn't materialized. Distract with a book away from the place that you usually feed them, and offer a cup of formula before the story instead of after, or the reverse. Try to keep your baby away from your breasts, and avoid changing in front of them. Sight and smell can remind your baby of what they're missing. You could try enticing them onto a bottle or cup by offering expressed milk at first so it's a familiar taste.

Dealing with discomfort

A slow approach helps prevent your breasts from becoming engorged or leaky. If they feel full, a cold washcloth can be soothing, and make sure to wear a supportive bra. If your breasts are very full and the excess milk does not leak naturally, try expressing a tiny bit extra, at feeding times only, to relieve the fullness without stimulating them to make more. Taking off small amounts of milk can decrease the milk you make so your body adjusts. If it doesn't and you become feverish or suspect mastitis (see p.59), see your doctor.

Weaning can be difficult for you both; rest assured your baby won't starve themself, and will be happy if they otherwise get the comfort and affection they are used to.

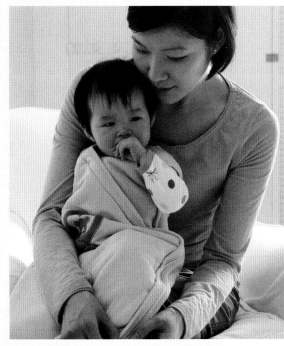

Bedtime hugs Make sure you still have a lot of cuddling before bed so you continue to feel physically close to each other.

ASK A BREASTFEEDING EXPERT

My friends are stopping breastfeeding, but I want to keep going. Is it a good idea to continue? There is absolutely no reason you can't continue to breastfeed for as long as both you and your baby enjoy it. This could be for their first year, or much longer. Plenty of research suggests that breast milk continues to offer antibodies well into toddlerhood, which can help your little one resist infection. It also contains protein, essential fatty acids, vitamins, and minerals, complementing a healthy, varied diet. There are also health benefits for you: breastfeeding beyond infancy has been shown to lower the risk of developing certain forms of cancer, for example.

Breastfeeding offers emotional nourishment and comfort, and can play a strong role in a healthy relationship with your baby. If you are worried that returning to work means an end to breastfeeding, it may reassure you to know that you can keep it up with a little organization (see p.185). You can express and freeze milk so your baby can be fed in your absence. This can be a comfort for them and means you keep up your supply of milk. Of course, you can also keep just the evening feeding to enjoy that reassuring bond at the end of the day.

It's important to focus on what's best for you and your baby, and try not to be swayed by the actions or opinions of others. In retrospect, the time you spend feeding your baby can seem all too fleeting, so follow your instincts and enjoy this special bond with your baby for as long as you want. (For more on extended breastfeeding, see p.331.)

Encouraging good behavior

Your baby is now establishing patterns of good behavior that will help them grow into a kind and helpful child.

Your baby is highly inquisitive, which sometimes means they do things you would prefer they didn't do. While she doesn't understand "good" and "bad," you can start to set boundaries, which in turn forms the foundations of good behavior later. Make lots of positive noises when your baby does something you approve of, and make little fuss if they do something you would prefer they didn't! If they hand you a toy or offer some of their food, praise them. Likewise, if they let you wash or dress them without making a fuss, tell them

"Good job!" and give a great big hug! Gently patting animals is also worthy of praise.

Babies of this age don't intend to be naughty, so respond appropriately to unwelcome behavior. For example, it is perfectly normal for them to grab toys from another child. Gentle admonishment—holding their hands, making eye contact, and saying "No, you shouldn't grab" is adequate to establish boundaries. If they repeatedly grab, gently move them away so they sense their actions are not welcome.

YOUR FRUSTRATED BABY

As your baby grows, they become more aware of their needs, yet have a limited ability to convey them—and no patience! Pay attention when they're frustrated, and help them cope by communicating all the time. Even if you can't get to them immediately, respond to babbles and cries, talking to them and vocalizing what you think might be wrong: "Are you hungry/tired?" Knowing you're paying attention will be the first step to calming them.

Regular "me-time"

Now that you and your baby have a more predictable routine, you might want to schedule "appointments" to pursue your own interests.

Taking care of your baby and making sure they're entertained, stimulated, and content leaves very little time for relaxation. However, by now, you and your baby have probably settled into some sort of routine. Rather than feel overly anxious about how your baby will manage if you're not there, reassure yourself that regular "me-time" will recharge your batteries and help you maintain a balance between self and family that will allow you to tackle parenthood with a clear head and a sense of calm. Take the pressure off yourself and trust

your partner or a grandparent to take care of your baby for an hour or so. Ideally, join a weekly class so you make a commitment to the time off. Alternatively, reading the newspaper in a local café for half an hour, going for a swim, or just settling down with a book, will all give you rewarding and rejuvenating time off. Your baby will be in good hands and you will be a more relaxed, happy parent.

Time for you Give yourself a little space—read a book, go for a run, or just indulge in a long soak in the bath. You deserve it!

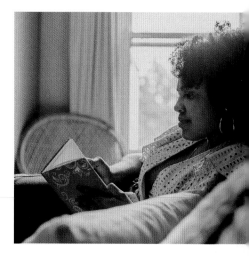

The monthly cycle

If you've recently stopped breastfeeding your baby, you may find that your periods have returned and you are fully fertile again.

All the hormonal changes that your body experiences during pregnancy and breastfeeding can affect your body in a number of ways.

You may find that problems such as PMS are no longer as debilitating as they were before you became pregnant, or that you now experience stronger symptoms. Your previously regular cycle may be all over the place now, or the opposite may be true—some find that everything goes like clockwork once they've had a baby, even if they've never had a reliable cycle before.

If you do find that having a baby has brought on some uncomfortable symptoms, such as heavier and more painful periods, talk to your doctor. They can discuss ways to relieve pain or discomfort and check your hormone levels if necessary.

Still breastfeeding

If your periods have returned and you are still breastfeeding while your baby moves toward solids and therefore starts to drink a little less milk, you may find that your cycle becomes a little unreliable. You may skip periods for a month or two, and sometimes experience only spotting at the time when your period would usually appear.

If it's usual for you to experience some breast tenderness just before your period, it can make breastfeeding uncomfortable. Although easier said than done, try

THINKING AHEAD

Even if you have not started having periods, once you are not fully breastfeeding, you are likely to be fertile. You may decide to try to have another baby right away, for example if it took a long time to become pregnant, but keep in mind that having two babies under two years old can be exhausting. Also, caring for a baby while pregnant is no easy task. You won't get to catch up on your sleep this time, and may find it hard to juggle your pregnancy needs with those of a young baby. You may have an exhausting third trimester just as your toddler is into running and climbing! If you are struggling to cope now, it might be a good idea to take a break and wait until

your baby is a bit older and more independent.

Having said that, extending a family is a joyous experience and your baby will no doubt benefit from having a loving relationship with their sibling. If they are close in age, they are likely to be doing fairly similar activities as they get older, and you and your partner will experience the wonderful, but tiring, early years all at the same time, rather than have to readjust to diaper-changing mode a few years down the line.

to relax during feeding, since any tension will increase the discomfort. To help ease the pain, hold a warm cloth on the side of the breast from which your baby is feeding, and massage the milk downward. If all else fails, try a mild analgesic, such as acetaminophen, to ease discomfort.

Return of fertility

Breastfeeding stops being a reliable form of contraception once your baby is more than six months old, or you begin to reduce breastfeeding. In fact, ovulation may occur at any time, so it's possible to become pregnant again before your period returns.

You may want to discuss contraceptive options with your doctor. If you are still breastfeeding, the combined oral contraceptive pill is not recommended since it can interfere with your milk supply. Your doctor may suggest the progesterone-only mini-pill, or talk to you about other forms of contraception, such as an IUD.

Scaling new heights

When your baby starts to negotiate their way around, it's time to make some changes to your rooms. Everything moves upward!

As soon as your baby can pull up to standing, from around eight months, they will realize they can use their new-found technique to climb. The first step is often the stairs! Negotiating the stairs requires a great deal of both brain and brawn, so it marks an important stage in your baby's development. The hands, legs, and feet move in synchronicity to keep weight stable with each upward movement. The hoist needed to push up comes from the coordinated efforts of one arm and the opposite leg, which alternates with the opposite arm and leg at each step. Climbing therefore requires fairly sophisticated control of limbs, and considerable muscle strength.

Babies know danger only because we alert them to it, and although scaling stairs is potentially risky, it is an activity that, with constant, close supervision, helps develop a baby's confidence. Allow your baby their foray into the danger zone of the stairs, but stand right behind them; they will have a surge of self-confidence, especially with you there praising their every effort.

Safety considerations

Never leave your baby unattended on the stairs. Although going up is a fairly foolproof adventure, the slip of a hand or knee can make a tumble likely. Furthermore, coming down requires a completely different skill set and, at this age, it's important to teach your baby to descend in the least risky way possible. Feet first and on their tummy

| ASK A PEDIATRICIAN |

Our home isn't ideal for safe climbing. What can I do to help my baby climb safely? You can encourage your baby to climb in a completely safe environment by making regular visits to a local soft-play toddler gym. Most gyms have areas that are cordoned off for babies which are furnished with small, baby-friendly play equipment designed for their little limbs, and with soft, spongy mats to break their fall when they tumble. Your baby will learn from watching other children as they move themselves up and down the play equipment, and will enjoy the social nature of this kind of play. However, your child will still want to practice climbing at home, so if your home isn't safe, you will need to be extra vigilant.

is best, since this minimizes the risk of toppling forward.

Install gates at the top and bottom of the stairs and shut them when you are not there to help your baby. If you have large gaps in your banisters, consider investing in mesh to fill them for the time being. Now is also the time to take a fresh look at the rest of your home and make sure it's safe for your baby.

Mini mountains

It's not just stairs your baby will want to climb. Onto and over sofas or chairs, cribs, and low tables are other common options for infant explorers. Try to babyproof these mini mountains as much as you can. Keep sofa backs against walls so baby is less likely to try to climb over the top, and try gently to steer your baby away from unstable items of furniture that might topple as they climb them. If they are trying to climb out of the crib (they'll manage to get a leg over the side with increasing

agility), adjust the base of the crib so it's at the lowest height and remove anything inside the crib that might give your baby a leg up.

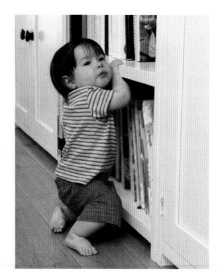

Getting up It's very tempting for your baby to use any furniture they can pull up on just like a jungle gym.

Post-pregnancy fitness

Usually it takes at least six months to lose any weight gained during pregnancy, but the more important focus is health and fitness.

Feeling good about yourself helps you give the most to your baby. Try to focus on feeling healthy and more energized—rather than on the goal of fitting back into an old pair of jeans. Opt for a nutritious whole food diet rich in vitamins and minerals, especially if planning another baby in the future. Also, if you're breastfeeding, you need a slightly higher caloric intake so shouldn't actively diet unless advised to. Keeping fit also helps you stay trim, as well as enabling you to keep up with the physical and emotional demands of parenthood.

Getting active

The key to reaching your health goal lies in motivating yourself to get active. You may already feel that your baby never lets you sit down, and this constant activity is definitely beneficial. There are other simple changes you can make to bring fitness into your routine. Whenever possible, walk your baby in the stroller to places, rather than drive. If you walk at a fast pace (enough to raise your heart rate a little), a mile takes 15 minutes—there and back is 30 minutes good exercise.

Resisting temptation

Try to resist picking at your baby's finger foods. Eat your lunch when your baby eats, introducing the notion of sociable eating to your baby and reducing the temptation to your picking at their food.

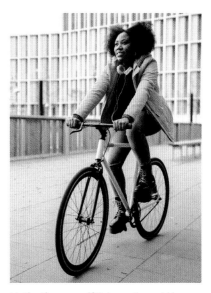

Motivating yourself Being active quickly becomes a habit, but to get started requires a little bit of self-motivation.

HEALTHY EATING

While you may be eager to shed the extra pounds gained during pregnancy as soon as possible, it's judicious to avoid trendy diets and quick-fix solutions. Instead, concentrate on maintaining a nutritious diet and moderating your portions. This will help you lose weight steadily and instill healthy eating habits that will enable you to maintain a constant healthy weight, rather than yo-yoing up and down. The following tips can help keep you on track.

• **Eat regular meals** Eat three meals a day and ensure that each meal contains at least one vegetable portion, as well as fruit.

• **Choose foods that give a sustained release of energy** This will help you feel full longer and resist snacking between meals. Try oatmeal and whole-wheat toast for breakfast along with some fresh fruit. Lunches and dinners should contain whole grains, lean meat or fish, and, ideally, two portions of vegetables.

• **Opt for low-fat dairy products** Fat contains twice the amount of energy as carbohydrates and proteins, so choose reduced-fat milk, dairy spreads, yogurts, and cheese, and measure out oils, mayonnaise, and salad dressings with a spoon. It's important, though, not to eliminate dairy entirely since it plays an important role in your diet. There's also evidence that calcium has a part to play in weight loss.

• **Include protein** All meals should include some protein, which helps keep hunger at bay.

• **Maintain your fluid intake** Drink water regularly; this helps keep you hydrated and can stop you from mistaking thirst for hunger. Try adding in a squeeze of lemon for a zesty, fresh flavor.

• **Eat healthy snacks** Keep cut-up carrots, celery, and cucumbers in the fridge for quick, healthy snacks.

A flexible routine

Planning a day out or a short trip can play havoc with your baby's routines, but by using familiar cues you can help them adjust.

A certain amount of predictability can make a baby feel secure, and most respond well to having a routine to their day. However, it's not a timetable; your baby notices and understands a series of events, not the hands of a clock.

So if occasionally it is better for you to shift your baby's nap time up by half an hour, this is fine, as long as they aren't fussy. They are unlikely to expect to have a nap until you take out the sleepy-time story and settle them into the crib. With these on hand, they will probably offer up no more or less resistance than they would have done had they been put down for their nap at the usual time.

Thinking of the routine as a sequence of events allows you to be flexible, for instance when you go on vacation or want a spontaneous day out. Implementing a familiar routine on trips and visits can help calm your baby. As much as possible, do the same things, so if it is a quiet game, bath, book, then lullaby, do it in the same order as usual and keep it up while you're away. They'll recognize the cues and realize what's coming, whatever the time or place.

Question time

Your baby is beginning to understand that objects (and people) have names. Have fun with simple questions that reinforce this learning.

The more you read to your baby, sing songs to them, and talk to them, the quicker they will learn everything has a name. Brightly colored board books with clear pictures can help you teach the names of objects. Ask "Where's the ball?" and guide their hand toward it. One of the best ways to teach your baby names is through song—try "Head, shoulders, knees, and toes," putting your hand on the different parts of the, then follow up with a game. Ask "Where is [their name]'s nose?" Then touch it yourself, saying "Here it is," and move their hand to touch it. Use the third person, because their language skills are not developed enough to understand possessive pronouns and adjectives (such as her, his, your, my).

They'll want to please you, so if you ask them something simple like "Bring me the book" while pointing to it, they'll enjoy getting it for you.

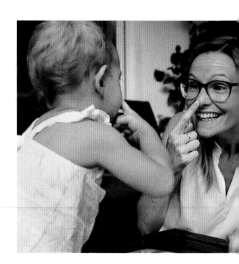

Where's my nose? Asking simple questions as you point to your nose is a game they'll enjoy. Soon they may point to it themself!

Using a babysitter

You and your partner may want to go out and leave your baby with a sitter, but how do you find someone you feel confident in?

BABYSITTING CHECKLIST

• Leave a list of emergency contacts—your cell numbers, the phone number of where you will be, and details of a trusted neighbor and your baby's doctor.

• Very importantly, make sure the babysitter knows if your baby is allergic or intolerant to any particular foods or medicines.

• Tell your babysitter about your baby's health or state of mind that day. For example, whether your baby is teething, was grumpy, or refused food, so the sitter is prepared.

• Tell your babysitter how to settle down your baby if they wake up, or explain the bedtime routine if the sitter will be the one doing it.

• Show your sitter any bottles, or meals, your baby is allowed to have during your absence, and how to heat them appropriately.

• Leave clear instructions on whether or not the babysitter should answer the door or phone, for example if you are expecting a delivery.

• Make sure your baby has all the necessary comfort toys, and let the babysitter know what they are and how they are used.

• Be prepared to return in a hurry if necessary—make sure the babysitter knows they can call you at any time.

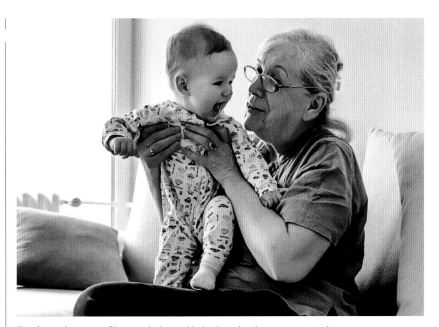

Getting to know you Give your baby and babysitter the chance to get used to each other before you leave them alone for the first time.

Family and friends who have spent time with your baby are an obvious choice for babysitting, but that is not always an option. If you are back at work, you might consider asking someone from your baby's daycare center. Or perhaps friends can recommend a babysitter.

A professional babysitting agency that specializes in finding caregivers, and who will check their credentials, is a good option. Or if there is a parents' babysitting circle in your area, your local library or pediatrician will have details. If not, perhaps you could set up your own babysitting circle with parents from your childbirth class or other families you know well.

Teenage children of neighbors are a traditional option. You may want to gauge whether you think they are mature enough to care for a baby.

You should always feel confident in your choice of babysitter. Talk to them and find out how they would calm your baby and how they would handle an emergency. Find out if they have any references from parents you know. Ask a new babysitter to arrive at least half an hour before you put your baby to bed, so they aren't a total stranger if your baby wakes up.

Getting creative

It's time to get artsy! Your baby will enjoy trying a new activity and might even create something to treasure.

Simple painting activities that don't involve holding brushes or creating neat lines are easy to arrange with your baby. An ideal place on a warm day is outside on grass; otherwise, clear a space on the floor, or a low table, and put newspapers or old towels down to soak up spills. Have water and washcloths ready.

Nontoxic paints are available at toy stores, stationers, or even big supermarkets. Check that the ones you buy will not stain your baby's skin or clothes. You'll need large sheets or a roll of blank paper. Spread the paper flat on the floor, pour some paint into an old dish or saucer. Daub your baby's hand in paint or let them put

their hand in it, then help them press onto the paper and make prints. You can use their feet, too. Their first attempts will probably be splotches, but you should at least get one lovely hand print to frame or put in a book. Remember to date them! It's a great way to see your baby's growth and reactions to painting each time.

Fussing at bedtime

Resistance at bedtime needs careful handling to prevent bad habits from forming. What should you do when your baby wants to stay up?

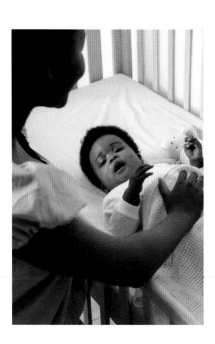

It can be unsettling for everyone if your baby suddenly starts to create a fuss about going to bed, especially if previously they easily settled down. Many babies go through a phase of resisting bedtime at about this age. Your baby has realized that events in life follow a predictable sequence, and they will begin to know what's coming next. They are increasingly aware that sleep time means separation from you. Separation anxiety (see p.228 and opposite) is a normal developmental stage, and can lead to tears when you try to leave at

Resisting bedtime Being firm about sticking to the bedtime routine will encourage a reluctant baby to settle down for the night.

bedtime, or when they wake up and you're not near. How you react now can affect the future routine, so do your best to get them back on track.

Make sure they've had an active day so they are physically tired. There's no need to cut back on naps, but stimulate with trips to the park or a soft play area. Stick to the bedtime routine, making sure it's an enjoyable experience that they want to take part in: say goodnight to the pictures on the wall or soft toys, read a story, or sing a song. Finally, be firm that this is bedtime; don't be tempted to let them play a bit longer. Be reassuring when you settle them, and return if they call, but try not to pick them up. Eventually, they'll settle down again.

Separation anxiety

Your baby's growing independence reminds them that they are separate from you, and they may become anxious about you leaving.

From around eight months, your baby is very likely to experience separation anxiety. This milestone signals their deep attachment to you and their recognition that you are their main source of care and protection. At the same time, they are gaining the concept of object permanence, becoming aware that when not in sight, you have gone away. The source of their safety and care has left them and they're unable to understand that you'll be back. They'll show how they feel through genuine distress, tears, and tantrums.

Reassuring your baby

When you leave the room, keep your voice calm and positive, and tell them you'll be back in a moment. If this phase coincides with your return to work, try to leave them for short periods only to begin with, getting them used to the fact that you always return. When you leave them with a caregiver, talk about what you're doing, "Mommy is going to put you in the car and strap you in." Avoid sounding anxious, and don't be impatient—they are more likely to be calm if you are calm, even if you have to be firm. Leaving a transition object, such as a comfort toy, blanket, or piece of clothing smelling of you, will help soothe them while you're apart.

When you drop them off, don't prolong the agony by spending too long cuddling, or telling them you wish you didn't have to leave—at this age, this sends a mixed message because the outcome will be the same. Talk to your baby while you hand them to the caregiver, tell your baby that you love them and will see them soon (or after lunch/nap/at dinnertime); give them a big kiss, a wave, a smile, and leave. Wait until you are out of sight and earshot before you burst into tears, if you need to!

Like most things in a baby's life, this is a passing phase (although one that often lasts, albeit in a milder form, up until three years old). If, however, you think your baby is genuinely unhappy with a caregiver, you may want to consider other childcare options. Keep in mind, though, that a change may not make a difference. You may just have to ride out the storm and build their self-confidence so they learn to separate more willingly. Visit play areas so your baby gets used to being around other babies, and grows in confidence while in your company.

DEVELOPMENT ACTIVITY: TICKLING GAMES

Now that your baby has a greater sense of anticipation, they will squirm and giggle with excitement and expectation long before the moment at which a tickling rhyme actually becomes a tickle! Among the traditional favorite tickling rhymes is "This Little Piggy" (in which you say the rhyme while wiggling each of the toes on your baby's foot in succession, then, at the last "piggy," tickle their feet and run your fingers all the way up their leg to their armpit for "wee, wee, wee, all the way home!"). There are a host of other tickling rhymes they'll enjoy and they will learn to anticipate the part when they're tickled.

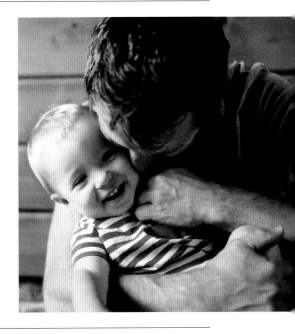

Tummy tickling You can tickle your baby on the tummy to squeals of delight. Their reaction will probably make you giggle, too!

Learning to focus

Your baby's brain is not yet mature enough to stream sounds, which means that they cannot select what they hear by focusing on it.

Adults can filter out background noise, but babies are less able to do this which is one reason babies startle so easily at loud noises—everything is heard at full-blast and in conjunction with the other sounds in the environment. Try to keep things quiet from time to time to allow your baby to concentrate on their activities and focus on your voice. They are learning all the time, but this learning can be hampered if they are subjected to constant background noise. This doesn't mean your household has to be completely silent, but many sounds will distract them from their activities. Turn off the television when you are reading or playing together, and turn off or turn down the volume of any music during playtime. Tone down the noise level at baby's bedtime, but don't try for total, or almost total, silence because falling asleep with a little background noise means your baby is less likely to wake at normal evening sounds.

If your baby is struggling to reach some of their developmental milestones, give some peace and space in which to try again.

Problem solving

While learning through play, your baby develops skills that enable them to look at a problem and find solutions on their own.

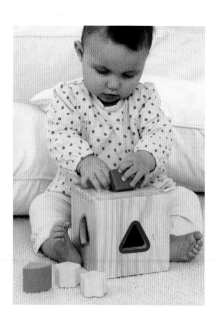

Studies show that, once they reach eight months, babies' cognitive awareness has developed enough to enable them to understand cause and effect ("If I want to drink from my cup, I need to tip it"), and that one problem might have several solutions.

To encourage these important skills, you don't need to do anything more complex than allow your baby to play with toys that require them to move objects around or press a button and see what happens. Sorting cups (which you can stack, and they can enjoy knocking over), shape sorters of different kinds, and toys with lids that need replacing or removing (ideally to discover something hidden inside) are all fantastic toys for encouraging their problem-solving skills.

Watch as your baby uses their ingenuity to solve problems such as reaching a toy that isn't in hands' reach—they might crawl to it, or protest until you get it for them, and by nine months, they may start to point at it! These are all signs of developing cognitive skills. As always, offer your baby encouragement and praise their efforts.

Think and play Shape-sorting toys help improve your baby's problem-solving skills as they try to fit the pieces into the right slots.

Your baby and screen time

Is it okay for your baby to watch television briefly, or is any screen time bad for their development? There are arguments for and against.

Many of us will have an abundance of technology in our homes—smartphones, tablets, TVs, laptops, and game consoles to name a few. Handing over your smartphone or tablet to your baby, or turning on the TV may seem like a blessing, providing a little distraction for a fussy baby, or keeping them temporarily amused while you get on with other tasks or catch up with friends. However, after decades of research on screen time and child development, there remains mixed evidence revealing both positive and negative developmental outcomes.

Who's right?

The information available can be confusing and contradictory. Some research suggests that high-quality TV programs and apps designed for babies can help with their language development, shape, and color recognition, as well as promote problem solving and visual thinking. Other studies link babies who are overstimulated by screen time to physical health concerns such as obesity, diabetes, and poor sleep patterns, as well as negative impacts on their mental health later on including issues with anxiety and low self-esteem. Also, research has shown increased links between excess screen time and attention deficit disorders (ADHD). Although more conclusive research is needed, there's little doubt that watching a screen eats into your

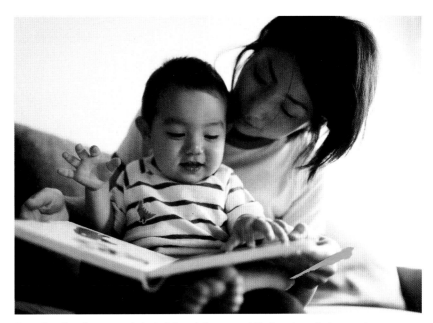

Story time Reading to your baby builds early language skills, introduces first concepts, and nurtures a bond between you and your baby.

baby's time to play, observe, and explore the real world, and to be stimulated by physical games, reading, and creative play.

Research has shown that screen time cannot match the educational value of time spent with you, family, or friends. For example, studies show that language is acquired most effectively through face-to-face interaction rather than from passive observation of TV shows, however, child-centered. Rather than ban screen time, the best solution is probably to use technology mindfully and for limited periods only.

Keeping it interactive

Make sure that your baby is not in front of a screen for long; encourage your baby to engage with a book or enjoy some playtime. Interact with your baby while they watch a show or program to bring any learning to life. Point out objects and name them as they appear, and repeat any rhymes featured on the program to reinforce the rhythm. Try acting out the roles of their favorite characters using different facial expressions and voices. This level of interaction will make the experience together more fun and memorable.

Testing your reactions

When your baby does something repeatedly, you may notice that they're watching you carefully to see how you will react.

This will usually work to your advantage because they'll repeat sounds, actions, and behaviors that make you smile, or give them praise, attention, or a hug. But babies will also repeat behaviors and actions that get a reaction from you—including a negative one!

No baby is willfully naughty, they just want your attention. You can begin to teach that things such as hair pulling or grabbing are not okay simply by calmly saying, "Stop, that hurts" and showing in your expression (a frown, say) that it's painful or unwanted. You can go on to demonstrate gentle, for example moving your baby's hand to stroke your arm, saying, "Let's touch gently." Ignoring negative behavior is not a recommended strategy at this age because you need to stop the baby if they are doing something potentially harmful to themself or others. If your baby receives the best reactions from you for the positive things they do, they will repeat those actions. So if they stroke the cat gently, eat their food without throwing the bowl, and copy you by putting a toy in a box after playtime, praise them, clap your hands, and give them plenty of attention. In this way, you will begin to teach them the boundaries of acceptable behavior.

Great communication

Your eight-month-old baby is open to learning, so explain things and respond to their communications to support their development.

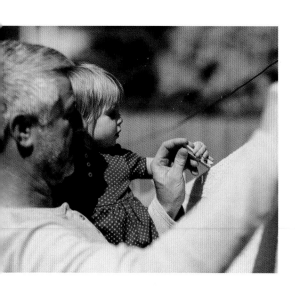

Talk to your baby to describe your activities throughout the day so they develop an understanding of the world. Everything is new and exciting to a baby, so stop and look at the cracks in the sidewalk and the butterfly perching on a pretty flower. Lie on your backs in the grass and look up at the clouds and show them the leaves on the trees.

Also, listen and respond to your baby's communications as if you are having a conversation. Show an interest when they babble to you, repeat their sounds and intonation, and allow them to respond. Pay attention when they shout, laugh, gurgle, or gesture toward something they want. While it can be frustrating to figure out what they want, responding to their needs and efforts to communicate will help them become confident about expressing themself. They'll also get an early grasp of the subtleties of sociability and manners. Everything you help them understand in these formative months forms the basis of their curiosity, self-belief, memory, vocabulary, imagination, and much, much more.

Running commentary Explain to your baby what you are doing around the house, and what comes next in the daily routine.

Going swimming

Swimming with your baby is fun and relaxing. It also promotes
a healthy respect for water and encourages their development, too.

Water supports your baby's weight,
which means that they're able to move
around freely in a swimming pool even
if they're not yet particularly mobile
on dry land. This gives them a feeling
of freedom and independence, and
allows them to work their muscles
while kicking and splashing around.
It also helps them build their
confidence in the water so they don't
feel afraid of it.

Before you go

To avoid unwanted accidents in the
water, you'll need to buy swim diapers
for your baby (ordinary disposables
will disintegrate in a pool). You can
choose between disposable or
reusable diapers—just make sure
whichever you choose fits snugly.
You may also want to invest in some
inflatable baby arm bands or a
swimsuit with buoyancy inserts, to
help keep your baby afloat.

If you're using a public pool for the
first time, check the water temperature
beforehand. If it's below 86°F/30°C,
your baby may find it too chilly. Plan
your visit for when the pool is not too
busy or noisy. Make sure you feed your
baby at least an hour beforehand—
don't go swimming just after a meal—
and take a drink and snack
for afterward.

Getting started

Take things slowly. Introduce your
baby to the water gradually, holding
them close to you and giving them

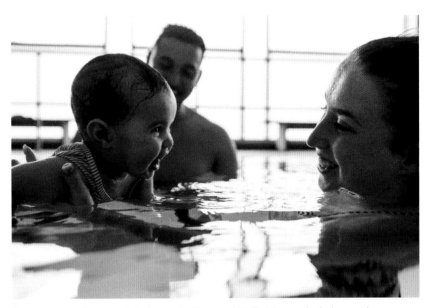

Free movement Once your baby learns that they can kick their legs and splash around
in the water, they'll love the freedom of movement that being in the pool gives them.

time to get used to the sensation of
the water before you start to play.
Once they are comfortable, splash
gently, sing, and kick their legs for
them so they realize the range of
movement they can achieve in the
water. Show them how to blow
bubbles, which helps teach them to
avoid inhaling water.

Keep your first session reasonably
short—20 minutes or so to start
with—supervise your baby at all times.
If, at any point, your baby seems cold,
or if their skin or eyes are irritated by
the chlorine, it's time to get out. Give
them a warm shower afterward and
dress them before you dress yourself.

ASK A PEDIATRICIAN

**My baby has eczema. Is it okay to take
them swimming?** While chlorine can be a
potential irritant to children with eczema,
taking a couple of precautions can help
make it an enjoyable and stress-free
activity. You can apply a barrier cream
first to protect their skin from the chlorine.
Since this can make them slippery in the
water, you might want to put them in a UV
swimsuit or baby wet suit after applying
the cream so you can hold them securely
during the swim. After swimming, make
sure you shower them to wash off the
chlorine, then pat them dry, and apply
their usual emollient cream.

9 months

ABOUT 12 PERCENT OF BABIES ARE WALKING BY THE AGE OF NINE MONTHS. Now that your baby is increasingly active and alert throughout the day, they may be tired enough at night to sleep through until morning. This shift in their sleep pattern may also affect their daytime naps. What remains the same is that when awake, they'll be eager to play and learn.

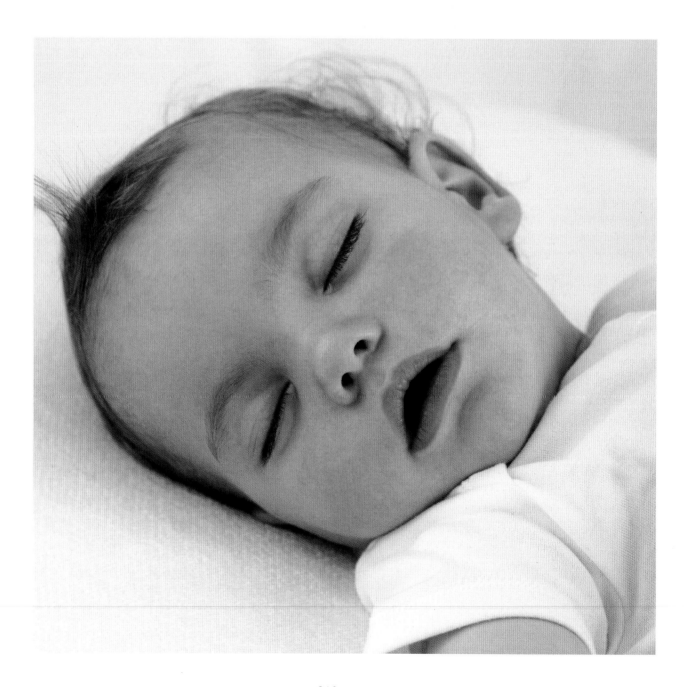

Going cruising

Once your baby pulls up to standing, the next step is to start edging their way around the furniture—it's time for cruising.

Over the next few weeks, or months, as your baby experiments with their new ability to stand upright and step, they will be cruising from one piece of furniture to the next. Try to arrange your furniture so they always have something to hold on to. As they become more confident, you can create small spaces to encourage a few tentative, free steps. Just make sure the furniture is sturdy and never leave them alone to explore. Cruising is a developmental milestone of its own, but one that some babies never go through, preferring instead to bottom-shuffle (see p.240) to get around before going straight to unsupported walking.

There are several defined stages of cruising. A first-time cruiser uses both hands to hold onto their support and will keep their body close to it. Later, they'll stand a little farther back from the support, holding on with one hand only, and then—at some point—they will try letting go. Your baby may also develop an interest in climbing—over cushions, up the stairs, and even up onto the sofa. Keep an eye on your babyproofing and make sure they can't get into danger when doing this. Once they're feeling confident about their balance and control, they will enjoy walking while holding your hands and may even attempt a step or two on their own. Take off their socks so their toes can grip the floor and help them balance more effectively.

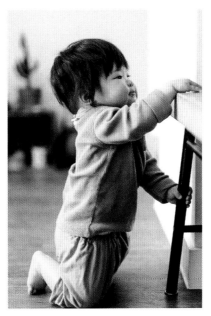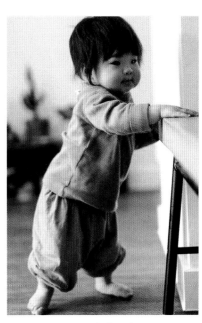

Baby steps Your baby may spend weeks pulling up to a standing position before they are willing to step out and cruise between items of furniture

ASK A PEDIATRICIAN

How many milk feedings does my baby need at this age? At nine months, most babies need 2–3 milk feedings a day, along with 2–3 meals of solid foods. It's recommended that they have approximately 20 fl oz (600 ml) of breast milk or formula each day alongside a varied diet until they are one year old, at which point they can drink cow's milk. If in doubt, be guided by your pediatrician who will be able to advise on the correct amount.

My baby is cruising on their tiptoes—is this normal? Don't worry—quite a few babies do this and before long they should start to use their whole foot to support themself while moving around. If it continues, mention it to your pediatrician.

Tiny tears

At this age, your baby is sensitive to other people's distress. Their cries in reaction to your tears are a forerunner to their later empathy.

By now, you have noticed that your baby is mimicking some of your facial expressions and tone of voice, and engaging in exchanges of babbles and sounds. They have also been noticing others' emotional reactions and reacting with distress if someone else is upset. This is known as "reflexive" crying. You may have noticed this when, for example, your baby is calmly settling in at day care, but then starts to cry when another baby cries.

This gesture of comfort is probably copied from you and, although it is not truly empathic, such gestures will gain genuine meaning in time—it won't be until their toddler years onward that they will really start to identify emotions. Over the coming years, they will gradually gain an understanding of others' perspectives and recognize the effects of their behavior. To help them develop an understanding of emotions,

it's important not to hide your own feelings; but you also need to make sure that if you are showing strong feelings, they see you manage them rather than seeing you become overwhelmed.

When you soothe your baby, you are teaching them how to comfort. This is an invaluable life lesson, and they will use methods such as stroking or hugging to show their empathy for others.

Changing sleep patterns

If your baby is sleeping through the night, they may be ready to drop their morning nap and make it through the morning in a good mood.

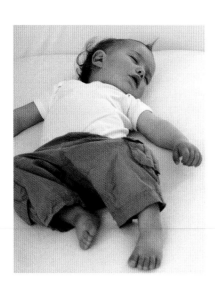

Some babies will need two naps a day well into their second year of life, but if your baby is happy in the mornings, and resists attempts to settle down, they may be ready to switch to one nap. Settle them for their morning nap. If they play quietly instead of sleeping, they'll still get a little respite from their busy day and will benefit from the quiet time. There will, however, come a point when they resist being put down.

Siesta time Your baby's afternoon nap may last longer when you drop the morning nap.

For a smooth transition from two naps to one, alter your routine a little to give your baby their lunch and midday feed a little earlier and put them down for their afternoon nap an hour or so earlier than usual. Watch for signs that they are becoming overstimulated. Without a morning nap, they may sleep longer in the afternoon, so if they don't stir, wake them after a couple of hours, or they won't be tired enough to sleep at bedtime. If they seem tired the next day, they may need two naps again, then just one longer one the day after. Let them be your guide.

Keeping love alive

Parenting a baby is tiring, so while being intimate together may seem like too much effort, it will help keep your relationship strong.

Falling into bed (straight to sleep) well before your partner; feeling a little resentful that you've been at home with your baby all day; being too busy to make time for each other—these are all reasons sex can end up on the back burner in early parenthood. The physical closeness you share with your baby, and the affection you lavish on them, can also leave you feeling as if you need space rather than touch. If you're breastfeeding you may feel that your body isn't your own.

A healthy relationship can cope when there is a period without regular sex, but it is a powerful way of expressing feelings, and it can also lift your mood and help you relax. For now, being more affectionate with one another will help to revive your physical relationship over time.

Romantic moments

Try booking a few "date nights" to spend time together. Curl up in front of the TV or, better still, switch it off, light some candles, and give each other a massage. Share a bath or just snuggle up in bed and chat. Simply savoring the warmth of each other's bodies and becoming familiar with them again is a good stepping stone toward regaining a sex life.

Respond positively to each other's suggestions. Even if you aren't in the mood for sex, a positive response to gestures of tenderness will reassure both of you that you are still lovable

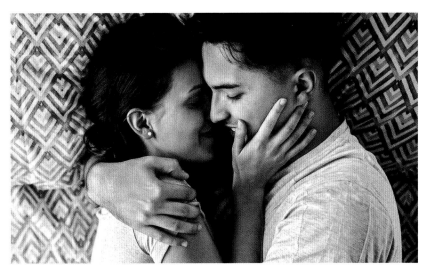

Staying close Make time to be physically close with your partner. Even if it doesn't lead to sex, the intimacy will help you both to feel more connected and in tune with each other.

and attractive. A little foreplay or even some passionate kissing can help you feel more in the mood and rekindle a little sexual excitement.

Equally, however, sex may not be a priority at the moment, and if you are both happy with the situation, it's absolutely fine to show your love in other ways. If you and your partner's sexual desires do not match at the moment, and one or both of you is feeling pressured—or lonely, frustrated, and isolated—try to come to a compromise. Expressing your love is an important part of your relationship, whether you do this sexually or through words and actions.

ASK A DOCTOR

Sex is still painful after my baby's birth. Is this normal? If you had a difficult birth, your body may still be recovering, and you may feel emotionally bruised, too. The anticipation of pain may be making you tense, which will increase discomfort. Using a lubricant can help, especially if you are not becoming aroused due to fear of discomfort. Take things slowly and experiment with positions. Practice Kegel exercises (see p.65) to improve muscle tone and encourage circulation, which may help. Occasionally, episiotomies or tears cause long-term discomfort. A yeast infection may also cause discomfort or pain. If you continue to feel pain, consult your gynecologist or obstetrician right away.

New tastes

Although it can be tempting to feed your baby exactly what they like, it is important to expand their menu to include new foods.

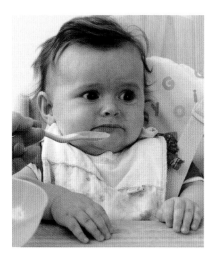

Picky eater Some babies actively resist trying new foods. It's worth persevering, but you may need to try some new tactics.

Keep offering a new food, using different accompaniments to alter the flavor, texture, and appearance of the meal to help them accept it.

If you've gotten into the habit of batch cooking, use these as a base for many new meals. So if your baby loves mashed sweet potato, you could stir in some ground chicken and some peas—you'll have an instant casserole, packed with nutrients. If they're a fan of potatoes, mix mashed potatoes with finely chopped chicken or beef and chopped spinach for a "chicken pot pie." If they like mashed carrots, blend them with equally sweet foods such as sweet potato, parsnips, and butternut squash.

Dippers are a good option, too. Show your baby how to dip healthy finger foods, such as carrots, cucumber, or toast fingers, into their favorite mashed foods. Try chopped spinach in with mashed carrot with buttered pasta pieces and cucumber sticks to dip.

Getting dressed

Your baby may be far too busy for anything as trivial as getting dressed! Distraction tactics will help get clothes on them.

When you want to dress them, catch your baby off guard! If they dress at the same time or stage of their routine each day, you can alter things occasionally so they don't begin to resist as soon as they anticipate what's coming next. Alternatively, if your baby thrives on routine and always likes to know what's coming next, make sure you dress them at the same point each day, since this type of personality will probably resist less if they know what's coming.

You may find it easier to dress your baby on your knee, so you can hold them firmly to stop them wiggling away. This change in routine might also surprise them into cooperation. Or, as long as they will be warm enough, dress them in stages, letting them play between layers.

Do your best to make dressing fun for your baby. Give a commentary to distract them—for example, "Here are your red leggings and we'll pull them up over your legs and around your tummy! Now it's time for your striped T-shirt. Arms up, over the head, good job!" Tickle your baby when you pull down their T-shirt, encourage them to help you put on their socks, play "This little piggy," or sing one of their favorite songs. If they're engaged and having fun, they'll forget that they don't like getting dressed. Whatever you do, practice speed and efficiency, and it will be over before they know it!

Successful child care

Whether you leave your child with a family member or paid caregiver, it's important to build a good relationship with them.

Whoever takes care of your baby, trust, understanding, and mutual respect are key, along with good two-way communication, which will help childcare run more smoothly.

Paid-for care

If you have a nanny, keep your relationship friendly and formal. You don't need to be best friends, but you do need to be a good boss. Listen to their concerns, pay them on time, keep to the agreed hours, and be willing to oblige if they need you to be flexible from time to time. You'll need the same from them, too.

Remember that they aren't just an employee. You may be paying them, but they are the most important "other" person in your child's life, so make time to get to know them, remember birthdays, and ask about things that are important to them.

Communicate as fully as possible. Pass on salient information—teething, attachment to comfort objects, particular clinginess. Similarly, your baby's caregiver should report on all developments, no matter how minor, at the end of each day.

Share your philosophy on childcare and take time to explain why you want your baby to eat the food they eat, or why you'd rather they didn't watch television, and how you are maintaining their routine at home. If your caregiver feels involved, they're more likely to follow your lead. Show respect for their

experience, though, and open your mind to new ideas—you may well learn some important tips from them.

Set up regular reviews to air any concerns (from either of you) and give a sense of being a team. Show sensitivity to their needs and they're likely to do the same in return.

Family help

If a family member is caring for your baby, show them your appreciation regularly. It is not easy caring for

a young child all day, and if no (or little) money is changing hands, the situation can become resentful. Talk through any problems as soon as they arise, and show willingness to shoulder extra responsibilities if they are finding it difficult to cope. Understand that anyone caring for small children needs a break from time to time, as well as some adult company. Show that you do not take them for granted.

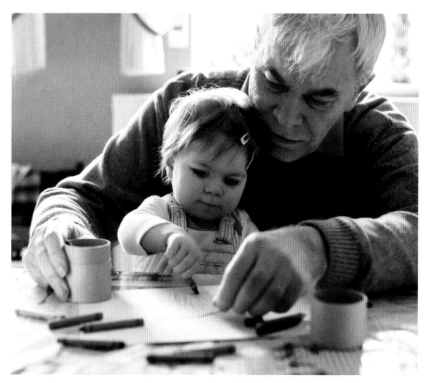

A harmonious arrangement Grandparents are often caregivers; make sure your baby's grandparent feels valued and respected, even if they feel it's a privilege to help out.

Self-chatter

Your baby will happily babble away whether you are listening
or not, and they'll start to experiment by turning up the volume.

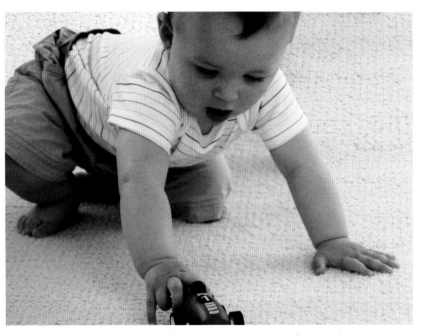

Range and volume As your baby goes about the important business of playing, they may
hum, blow raspberries, squeal, make burring noises, and laugh as they entertains themself.

DEVELOPMENT ACTIVITY: BYE-BYE!

Waving goodbye as someone leaves is one of our most common gestures, and one that babies love to watch and copy. Most babies give their first meaningful wave between 10 and 12 months. Some do so earlier; especially if you have held their arm to wave from an early age. If your baby isn't waving on their own, you can show them how as you say "Bye-bye." After plenty of repetition, they'll start to respond. Soon they will automatically raise their hand and wave unprompted when leaving friends or in stores!

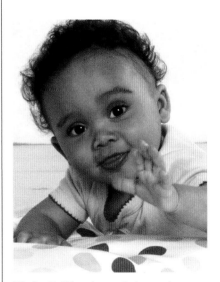

Waving By 37 weeks, your baby may be linking the action of waving to hearing the words "bye-bye."

At 37 weeks, your baby will be practicing speech patterns and inflections by talking, singing, and even shouting to themself. This is an important step in the development of language skills. Don't be surprised if they practice a single sound for a long time, before confidently combining it with another. They'll also be eager to experiment with volume, and emit some amazingly loud, high-pitched shouts that may make them laugh at their own capabilities. Listen for them blowing raspberries and making other funny noises as they practice their vocal range!

As your baby hits the nine-month mark, they continue to respond to you by mimicking the sounds you make, including the pitch and inflection. This copying helps cement the rhythm and cadence of language. You may notice that they end some of their "sentences" with a higher-pitched sound like a question, or even an exclamation. Repeating what they say helps this process. Your baby will watch your mouth closely, but their understanding comes from association, so keep pointing to things and explaining what you are doing.

Growing up fast

Your baby has now evolved from a helpless newborn to an active, curious infant, trying out sounds ready for their first word.

Your baby may be two or three times the size they were at birth, and the dramatic developments in physical and cognitive skills are increasingly evident. Their milk-only diet has made way for a variety of foods. They are increasingly independent and happy to play on their own at times, and learn from their experiments and explorations on a constant basis. They're a willing communicator and like nothing better than a good "chat." While crying was once the only way for your baby to express their needs, signals, gestures, increasingly sophisticated sound combinations, and even an occasional "real" word make up their new repertoire of communication skills. What's more, their ability to interact and respond to people shows a huge leap in their social competence, which has been fostered by their sensory awareness.

Your baby's gross motor skills have developed to the extent that they can hold up their head and sit unassisted, and also roll over, possibly crawl, and perhaps pull up to standing. Their fine motor skills continue to mature, so they can manipulate objects with both hands, and may be able to use their fingers efficiently.

If your baby seems slow to reach milestones, you may wonder if they're developing at the right rate. If they haven't yet achieved the same social, language, cognitive, and gross and fine motor skills as peers—or your other children—don't panic. All babies develop at different rates. However, if you are concerned, do speak with your pediatrician for reassurance or help.

If your baby was born prematurely, you can expect them to lag behind on some developmental tasks. This is entirely normal. Use your premature baby's adjusted age when you assess their development, and as with any developmental issues, seek advice if you're concerned.

DEVELOPMENT ACTIVITY: PUPPET TIME

Your baby will love to watch a puppet show, and probably want to take part themself! Make a sock puppet using a felt-tipped marker to make eyes, or purchase an animal hand puppet. Make the puppet play hide and seek behind a cushion, and laugh, cry, and even tickle your baby! Pop your baby's hand in the puppet and show them how it works. Finger puppets are ideal for playtime, and can easily slip onto your baby's little hands. Make your finger puppet dance, whisper, giggle, shout, and jump up and down, and ask your baby if their puppet can do these things, too. Puppets encourage creativity and imaginative play and help concentration and visual skills.

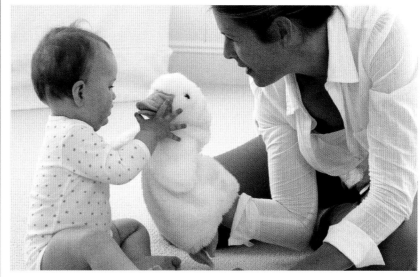

Was that a quack? Puppet games are great fun for your baby, and they won't even notice if your skills as a ventriloquist aren't up to snuff.

Slowed weight gain

Although your baby is more hungry these days, they may gain weight more slowly at this age because being mobile burns lots of calories.

It's normal to be worried about your baby's weight, but if it continues to follow the same percentile line on the growth chart, they'll be doing just fine. Continue to have them weighed regularly, around once every 2-3 months, to keep tabs on their progress and to reassure yourself.

Your baby's growth rate rapidly slows down during the first year of life, reaching a near plateau by 12 months. Breast milk and formula are more caloric than the foods your baby will be tasting and eating now, and it can take time for them to be able to eat enough to make up the difference in calories. Don't panic if they don't seem that interested in solid food at first; many babies take a while to show an interest. Be reassured that milk still provides the basis of their nutrition at the moment, and that your baby needs time to get used to and accept new tastes and textures.

ASK A PEDIATRICIAN

My baby's fontanels are still soft—is this normal? It can take up to 18 months for a baby's skull bones to fuse together. By 11 months, the smaller gap (the posterior fontanel, toward the back of the head) has usually closed, leaving only the larger gap (the anterior fontanel, at the top of the head) still soft. So there's no need to worry for seven months or so, but if your baby's fontanels are sunken or bulging, see your pediatrician immediately.

Mouthing toys

Now that your baby is able to hold on to toys without dropping them, they can move them around their mouth to explore all of their surfaces.

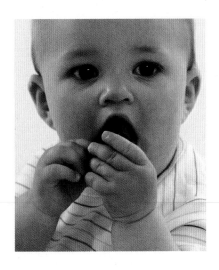

Your baby's jaw and tongue movements are quite coordinated, and their "mouthing" skills are sophisticated, allowing them to extract sensory information from whatever enters their mouth. Using their tongue, lips, and jaw, your baby will explore toys and other objects to find out about their size, shape, texture, and weight. They will use this skill to find out about the food they eat, assessing every mouthful.

Tool for discovery Your baby's mouth is often the first port of call when investigating objects.

Your baby will begin to gnaw on toys to ease the discomfort of teething. Chewing helps soothe gums. You can help by offering cold non-PVC teething rings to chew. Mouthing prepares your baby for chewing and swallowing solid food, and for speech, working the muscles of the jaw and tongue.

Now that your baby is more mobile and is in the throes of mastering their pincer grip (see p.311), be very careful not to leave potential choking hazards within reach.

Crib safety

Once your baby is able to pull up to stand in the crib, you'll need to take some steps to make sure they remain safe in there.

ASK A CHILD PSYCHOLOGIST

My baby wants to be picked up all the time. When I put them down, even for a couple of minutes, they cry. It makes life very difficult—what can I do? Some babies feel more insecure than others (perhaps as a result of separation anxiety, see pp.228, 263). Your baby feels safe in your arms and that's where they want to stay. However, carrying your baby around the clock not only prevents you from getting things done, it also stops your baby from practicing new skills such as creeping and crawling, that will eventually enable them to get around without being carried. Nor does it allow them to learn how to entertain themself for short periods.

Babies also cry to be picked up because they want comfort and attention, or because they need something. So ask yourself whether you are spending enough one-on-one time with your baby. Is their diaper dirty or is it time for lunch? If their needs are being met, then try to lengthen the time between pick-ups. Give enough toys to keep them entertained and leave them to their own devices for a short time. If they start fussing, play for a few minutes, and then move away. If they cry to be picked up, try distracting them by engaging them in an activity. Be realistic—all babies need lots of cuddling and carrying around. Once they start crawling and gains a sense of independence, they're less likely to want to be held all the time (and you'll probably miss it!).

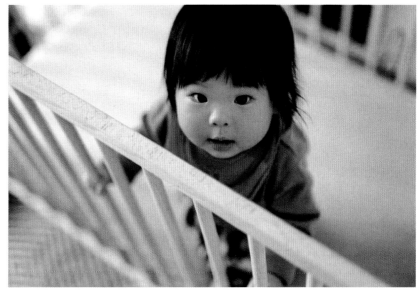

Safe height By now, the base of your baby's crib should be set at its lowest height. Ideally, they will be completely behind bars, even when they are standing up.

Ensure your baby's crib base is set at its lowest possible height now. Once they can stand up in their crib, your teething baby is likely to chew on the top rail. If the crib is painted, check that the paint doesn't contain lead. You may be able to purchase a plastic teething rail that sits over the top rail, to protect your baby from paint and splinters, and also keep your crib looking a little nicer, too!

Remove mobiles and adjacent wall shelves that your baby could reach and hold on to for balance as they maneuver themself up and out of the crib. Tie cords for lamps, blinds, or curtains up and out of reach.

Check that the mattress fits snugly. A moving baby can become trapped if their foot gets stuck in a gap between the crib and mattress. Cover cut-out designs or other spaces in which their arms or legs could get caught. Check that the spacing between the slats adheres to Consumer Product Safety Commission standards (especially if the crib isn't new). There should be no more than $2\frac{3}{8}$ inches between the bars, to prevent a baby's head from becoming lodged between them.

Finally, as a precaution, place a thick, soft rug on the floor by your baby's crib. With an intrepid baby, where there's a will, there's a way!

Brain power

Your baby's brain is developing faster than at any other time in life. What's going on in there?

Your baby's brain grows more during the first year of their life than at any other time. By 12 months, their brain will have doubled its volume and reached about 60 percent of its adult size. Your baby was born with their full complement of nerve cells (called neurons), but as they grow those used most frequently grow stronger and branch out to make more connections that enable your baby to think and learn new skills. By the end of the first year, your baby's brain will have made millions of new connections— and the more it makes, the more advanced their mental development will be. In addition, each of your baby's neurons has a coating called myelin, which insulates and protects it, and helps messages move faster.

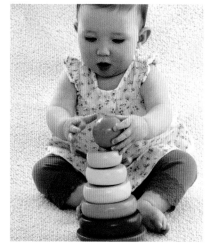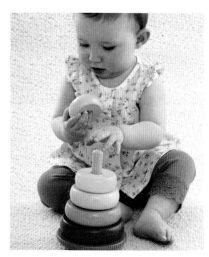

Stimulation and repetition While your baby's brain is developing, experiencing repeated stimuli will encourage the development of neural pathways, which is how information is stored.

Repetition

Neural pathways are formed as your baby's brain processes the experience of the world. Repetition in words, actions, and play cements these connections, and is much more beneficial to your baby's neural development than one-off actions.

Building skills

Your baby's development occurs in logical stages, with each milestone providing the building block for them to go on to reach a more complex or demanding milestone. For example, mastering the ability to lift their head and push up provides them with the skills for rolling, and enables them to practice the movements they will need for crawling. Once you add strength and balance, they will be able to combine all these separate skills and start to crawl in earnest.

Stimulating their senses

All of your baby's experiences—what they smell, taste, see; each voice, song, or noise they hear; and every texture they feel—will help develop their brain building a strong foundation. New neural pathways are made while others are reduced through a process called "pruning," which helps your baby's brain become more efficient. Give your baby plenty of stimulation, and keep repeating experiences so their brain grows strong.

SOFT PLAY AT HOME

Safe, soft play areas are not the province of toddlers only—babies love them, too. Set up a soft-play gated area in your living room— your baby will be fascinated by the transformation of the room, and playing in it will encourage the development of gross motor skills. Collect as many quilted or fleecy blankets and comforters as you can and cover the floor with them to give a soft landing whenever baby falls. Use cushions and upturned plastic boxes to create obstacles to climb over, and a cardboard box (open at both ends) to make a tunnel to crawl through. Don't leave your baby alone while they explore this fascinating play zone and, if needed, help them negotiate the ups and downs of your homemade adventure course.

Testing times

Your adventurous baby is pushing the limits of their ability, and sometimes they are going to get stuck!

Being endlessly curious, your baby may manage to pull up to a standing position, then feel unsure how to get back down. They may crawl up the stairs, then look back to see that they've gone a bit too far, and realize with dismay that they're not sure how to get back down. They may cry when they hear a dog barking or another loud noise, and even express a sudden dislike of their dark room at bedtime. These reactions are a form of self-protection. They may encourage your baby to be cautious, but this is often overpowered by curiosity and hunger to learn or practice emerging skills. There may come a time when your baby has really overreached and is afraid and in need of your support, reassurance, and comfort.

Show them how to climb and descend the stairs and sit down from standing. Encourage them to repeat the actions until they beam with new confidence. No matter what situation they've gotten into, stay calm. If you're frantic, they'll quickly grow alarmed. Help and reassure them, then let them try again with your help. Don't show them your fear of dogs or accidents, and be confident in unfamiliar situations. Set up opportunities for playtime success to boost their confidence and praise them when they do well.

Bumps and falls

It is inevitable that your baby will end up with bruises and bumps as they become more mobile and interested in doing things themself.

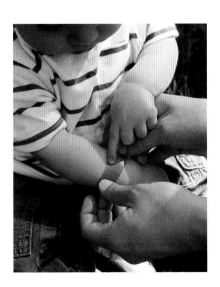

If you teach your baby that making mistakes, bumps, and tumbles are part of normal life, they'll take these minor setbacks in their stride and keep trying. Be careful not to overreact when your baby does take a tumble. They'll gauge your reaction before deciding how to respond, so if you panic, they'll do the same. If they become fearful of new experiences because they associate them with being hurt, they'll be much less likely to engage in healthy experimentation and exploration.

If your baby becomes distressed after an accident, comfort them, place a cold compress on any bumps, and check them carefully. Any bump to the head, awkward fall, or a cut that bleeds longer than a few minutes should be discussed with your pediatrician, particularly if your baby seems distressed. Consider contacting an organization such as the Red Cross to learn first aid, a useful skill for a parent.

Baby tumbles Take the sting out of falls and minor cuts with some fun bandages and lots of attention and cuddling.

Music and brain development

Listening to and making music supports the development of your baby's sensory coordination and memory. Singing nursery rhymes promotes their language skills and teaches them about rhythm.

Your independent baby will love to make music by themselves, so encourage this as much as possible. Their memory is improving, and they are making connections between sounds and objects. Toy musical instruments help develop your baby's fine motor skills.

Music can have a significant impact on your baby. Soothing music can calm them, while lively music can lift their spirits, proving an excellent distraction when they're tired or fractious.

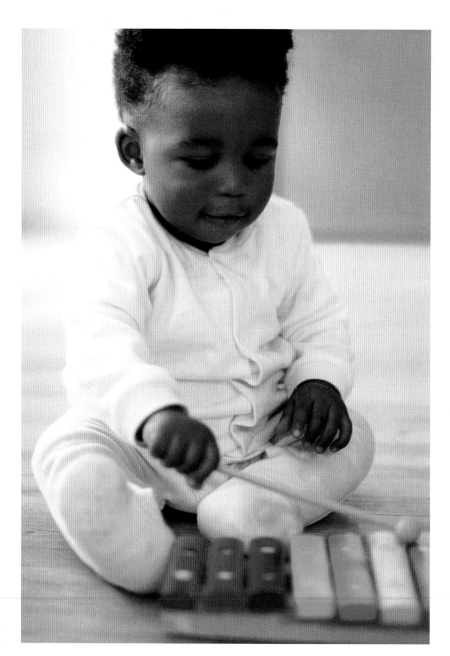

Xylophone Encourage your baby to explore music by making up their own tunes.

Music and movement

Stimulate your baby's natural sense of rhythm and encourage their enjoyment of listening to music and moving their body in rhythm.

Encouraging your baby to move in time to music will help them develop a sense of rhythm, improve their coordination and body awareness, and express themself creatively. Put on a tune you know they like, and they'll instinctively move their arms and legs when they're little, and bounce and sway as they get older.

Sing, clap and make music together. Share your favorite tunes, dance to the rhythms, and sing out loud. Hold your baby's hands to support them and "dance" with them, lifting them up for a twirl. Or put on a waltz or a tango and glide around your living room—ballroom style—with your baby in your arms. They will love to be swayed and twirled across the floor!

Research suggests that babies are born with a predisposition to move rhythmically in response to music. In a study of 120 babies between five months and two years old, researchers played recordings of classical music, rhythmic beats, and speech to them, and videotaped the results. They found that the babies moved their arms, hands, legs, feet, torsos, and heads in response to the music much more than to speech. The study suggested that the reason for this was that dance and music-making were important to our ancestors for social cohesion.

Music and movement will help your baby express their feelings and emotions, building their self-confidence and creativity. Besides encouraging their self-expression and imagination, music and movement stimulates the development of physical skills including hand-eye coordination and balance. Learning how to play music and dance with others will teach your baby social skills such as taking turns and sharing a musical toy.

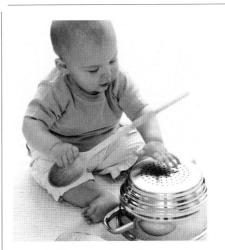

Musical life Make listening to music—and making it—a part of your baby's everyday life. It will stimulate them on every level.

DEVELOPMENT ACTIVITY: HOMEMADE BAND

Improvised instruments Anything can be a musical instrument, as long as your baby is able to make plenty of noise.

Your baby will enjoy making lots of noise with safe household objects. Make a shaker from a plastic bottle full of pasta or rice. But make sure that the top is securely sealed and taped so nothing can escape to create a choking hazard. Use pots and pans and plastic bowls and containers together with a spatula or a wood spoon to create a homemade drum kit. Use rattles as maracas. If you have a keyboard or piano, let them bang away on that, too. Make music together, but also leave room for them to make their own sounds. Play lively then quiet music and watch how your baby reacts to each; does their banging slow down when the tempo changes?

281

Comfort objects

If your baby has a comfort object, they've probably become very attached.
It may be difficult for them to settle down at night without it.

At this stage of babyhood, when separation anxiety sets in (see p.228 and p.263), a comfort toy can ease your baby into new situations by providing a link with the familiar. With their "comforter," they'll find it easier to sleep at Grandma's or sit on a stranger's knee. If you are going back to work, their comfort object can help them feel more at ease with their caregiver, and they can use it to soothe themself when distressed.

If your baby doesn't have a comfort object already, it's not too late to offer one. Choose a toy that they like with a soft, smooth texture they can rub or chew, or a blanket that's light enough for them to carry themself. Pick one that is easy to clean or machine wash, and safe for your baby to handle—and, ideally, something that's easy to replace if lost! Tuck it under your baby's arm when feeding, and make sure they have it with them when they go to sleep. Use it to soothe them when they're tired and grumpy, and they'll soon associate it with comfort.

Your social baby

Your baby is fascinated by other babies. They will chatter away to them,
imitate their actions, and enjoy playing alongside them.

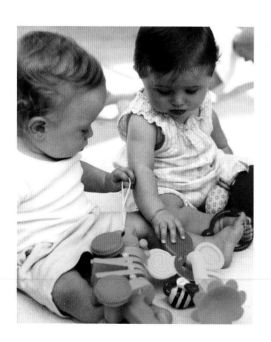

Parallel play Your baby will play alongside others but won't share for a couple of years yet.

Around now, your baby will engage in parallel play—alongside another baby, each doing their own thing. They may chatter to one another and look over to see what the other is doing. They may even tussle for the same toy or copy each other's activities, but they are largely playing independently. In fact, they may even forget the other is there.

However, they love to see others who are just their size and these early interactions allow them to become used to the company of other children. They'll learn things by watching other children, and make "friendships," which, at this age, means other babies become familiar and, therefore, favorites. They'll gravitate toward babies they know when you enter a playgroup or meet up with friends.

Don't be surprised if your baby wants to examine their companion and give their hair a good tug or poke at their face as they would with a new toy. They may enjoy getting a reaction when they bonk their friend on the head or climb on top of them. Be patient; this is experimentation, not aggression. Show them how to pat other people gently, then distract.

Repetition

You'll have to pick things up a lot over the coming weeks as your baby discovers the fun in dropping things, and does it over and over again.

So far, your baby hasn't had the motor coordination to be able to open their hands purposely to release an object they are holding. At around seven months of age, they begin to make the transition from involuntary release to intentional release. At first, this is almost forced—in passing an object from one hand to the other, the giving hand has to let go as the receiving hand pulls the object free. Also, when your baby feels the object they are holding pressing against another surface, they learn to let it go. Over time, they learn to extend their fingers and thumb to release an object deliberately. Although it seems obvious to us, for your baby this action is fascinating new skill that they want to practice.

At around the same time, your baby has an increasing understanding of the concept of object permanence (see p.233). They soon realize that if they drops something over the side of their high chair, it hasn't disappeared, but is now to be found on the floor. In addition, they are learning to point—so they can also tell you that the object is down there, and "request" that you pick it up, which, of course, you do.

Dropping objects also compounds lessons in cause and effect. When an object hits the floor, it makes a noise. Your baby will want to hear that noise repeatedly, reinforcing the connection between the drop and the thud as it hits a surface. The delay between the action and the noise teaches important lessons about timing and space.

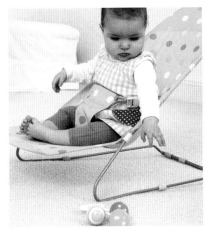 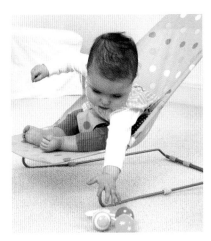

Pick and drop Your baby may decide that dropping objects is lots of fun, and will spend plenty of time playing this fascinating new game—if you'll help them!

Dropping objects is an important game, as irritating as it might be to repeatedly pick things up. Humor your baby for as long as you can bear to, reminding yourself that dropping something, looking for it, and pointing to it are all important developmental milestones. Once they get a little bit older, you can adopt the "rule of three"—once it's been thrown on the floor and you've picked it up three times, the fourth time means it stays on the floor! Your baby will soon understand and adapt.

DEVELOPMENT ACTIVITY: PLAY CATCH

Your baby is definitely interested in dropping their toys, and is about to find out about throwing. They're learning to let go of objects, so play catching games with them. Put them in the high chair and throw a soft beanbag toy onto the tray. They will pick it up and, with any luck, go to drop it from the chair. When they do, catch it and gently toss it back onto the tray. Before long, they will get the hang of the idea that they are to pick it up and drop it again, perhaps even copying your movement and giving the beginnings of a throw themself. You could follow the same principle when rolling a ball along the floor to them—now that they can let go purposefully, they'll eventually learn to bat or roll the ball back. These new experiences will help the development of cognitive and coordination skills.

Nap time

Your baby's naps, probably now down to one a day, continue to be important for their well-being, whether they think so or not!

Your baby may not want to miss out on any fun, but that doesn't mean they don't need to sleep. In fact, their rapid development and all the activities they enjoy will make them very tired, even if they don't admit it!

If you are having trouble settling them, try putting them down a little earlier. Set up a short pre-nap routine with a milk feeding, a wash, and a comforting lullaby. They may begin to anticipate these activities with pleasure and unwind sufficiently to sleep. Some babies will sleep in broad daylight, while others need silence and a good black-out blind. Figure out what works best for your baby.

If your baby is flagging but resisting a nap, have some quiet time. A nice, long walk in their stroller, or snuggling with a book on the sofa can be enough to keep them going.

Schedule play dates, shopping, or social visits for when your baby is alert. There will be times when they fall asleep in the car and you will have to transfer them to the crib, or they may doze off in their stroller, where you can leave them as long as they are strapped in and safe.

Developing recognition

As their memory improves, your baby may turn their head when you call them, and start to show they recognize familiar objects you name.

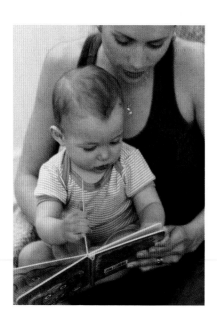

Your baby may be starting to point when they see something they want, and they show excitement and recognition of familiar places such as the park, even getting enthusiastic as they identify they are on their way there.

They will now recognize people they haven't seen for a few weeks, and will therefore be happier to be put down at night with a familiar babysitter. They will recognize the toys they enjoy, and maybe even vociferously request them with an urgent "uh-uh-uh" and a dramatically pointing finger.

I know that! Your baby may be able to gesture to things that you name in their favorite book.

Encourage these attempts to communicate by trying to figure out what they are saying and what they want. It may involve a lot of holding up objects and saying "This?" but they will appreciate your efforts to understand them, and when you get it right you will be rewarded with a very big grin.

If you generally keep to a daily routine, your baby will come to recognize the stages of the routine. They understand much more of what you say now, and will love to become involved in what is going on. They may even adopt a bold grin when you hold up your camera! They recognize what comes next, and they're game to do what is required.

284

Preventing tooth decay

The enamel on your baby's teeth is weaker than yours, and even a little sugar or inadequate oral hygiene can put them at risk of tooth decay.

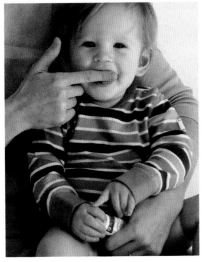

Applying toothpaste Rub your baby's teeth with a little children's toothpaste to prevent buildup of bacteria.

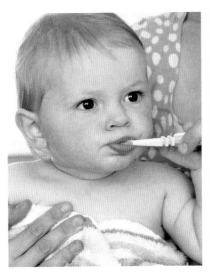

Brushing teeth Let your baby try brushing their teeth.

FLUORIDE AND BABIES

Fluoride is a natural mineral found in many foods and in drinking water. Fluoride promotes good dental health because it strengthens tooth enamel, making it more resistant to decay. It reduces the amount of acid that bacteria on your teeth produce. It can also prevent grooves from forming in teeth, reducing areas where plaque can collect. For these reasons, it's added to adult toothpaste to help make brushing more effective.

Since the 1940s, fluoride has been added to water in some areas in an effort to improve dental health. Water fluoridation has been proven to reduce decay by 40–60 percent. However, it is not added in every area, so you'll need to check with your local water authority if you want to find out whether your supply is fluoridated.

The American Dental Association recommends that caregivers should begin brushing children's teeth as soon as they appear. They should use no more than a smear of toothpaste the size of a single grain of rice. The teeth should be brushed twice a day.

Too much fluoride isn't good for children's teeth, so you want to make sure to use the correct amount of toothpaste.

Your baby doesn't yet have a full diet of solid food, and therefore they have less of the saliva that builds up when they eat (saliva helps protect the teeth and make them stronger). For this reason, it is important to take steps to guard against tooth decay, and to give their teeth every opportunity to become strong and healthy.

Encourage your baby to eat foods that contain lots of calcium, which will help both their baby teeth and the next set of teeth develop properly. Leafy green vegetables and soy are the best sources, so try to include these in their daily diet. Of course, they will be getting plenty of calcium from their regular milk feeding, but you're setting up good eating habits for later.

Brush your baby's teeth regularly and effectively (see p.200). Even if they don't have many teeth yet, rub or brush them with a tiny smear of children's toothpaste containing fluoride. This will prevent bacteria building up, and will encourage strong enamel.

Offer treats at mealtimes, when saliva is at its best. If you offer fruit juice—which contains natural sugars—do so only with meals. Snacks should be accompanied by water when at all possible, or milk, because the protein and calcium content of milk help keep teeth healthy.

Stage three solids—a varied diet

As soon as your baby is enjoying a variety of pureed foods, they're ready to move on to the third stage of solids. Now they'll be introduced to a greater range of foods as well as new textures and some finger foods.

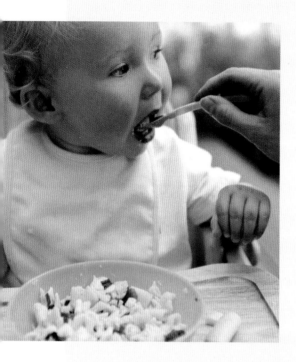

The third and final stage of introducing solids basically involves continuing with all the good work you've done so far, but adding more texture to your baby's meals—in the form of bigger lumps and foods they need to chew—as well as a wider range of flavors.

Your baby will now be familiar with a range of different tastes and should be able to eat some finger foods as well as enjoy mashed meals. They may also be able to drink water from a lidded cup.

In this third stage, which is generally from about nine months, you can introduce finely chopped or ground foods as well as finger foods since

Expand your baby's diet Once your baby is happy with solids, it's important to introduce a variety of textures and combined flavors.

they'll be able to bite and chew more confidently. Some babies will also be very happy trying to feed themselves at this stage even if the result is quite messy. Although they will be happy holding a spoon, the dexterity required to find their own mouth without spilling the contents comes later on in their second year, so don't expect success overnight. Some babies like to eat meals composed of finger foods, which they can hold more easily than a wobbly spoon that seems to have a mind of its own. However, it is good to let your baby experiment with a spoon since it's an important skill to master.

Your baby should now be eating three meals a day, plus snacks, and sampling a wide variety of different foods. If you're still mostly spoon-feeding, you shouldn't need to do much more than roughly mash the food with a fork first; by nine months, you should really only be chopping up or food processing the bigger lumps.

Whether you're spoon-feeding or taking the baby-led solids approach, you can also now take advantage of your baby's fast-developing pincer grip (the ability to bring thumb and first finger together to pick things up) to give smaller finger foods, such as peas, and halved cherry tomatoes or grapes. Or something altogether squishier.

Good eating habits for life

At this stage, it's important to introduce your baby to more complex recipes that combine different flavors, as well as

THREE MEALS A DAY

It's time to introduce more lumps, new textures, and a wider range of flavors and finger foods.
- **Protein** Your baby should have at least three servings of protein each day. One serving is approximately 1¾ oz (40 g). Sources include eggs, meat, fish (check for bones), tofu, legumes, and seeds.
- **Fats** About half their calories come from fat, some from their milk. Include healthy fats such as avocado and olive oil.
- **Fruit and vegetables** Aim for five servings per day.
- **Carbohydrates** Your baby should have approximately three servings a day.

Include cereals, bread, pasta, couscous, potatoes, rice, and pita.
- **Consistency** Mashed, chopped, and ground foods with larger lumps.
- **How often?** Three meals a day, plus a few snacks.
- **How much** Be guided by your baby; they may be hungrier on certain days. Start with a small amount so they aren't overwhelmed, and give them more if they want it. Keep in mind that they're not likely to be hungry if they're having more than two milk feedings a day (see p.291).

herbs and spices. Simply adding a sprinkle of mixed herbs to spaghetti marinara, for example, can turn a bland meal into something new and exciting for your baby. Hot spices may be difficult for babies to manage, but other fragrant options, such as coriander, cinnamon, lemongrass, thyme, and basil, are all good options. And broadening your baby's palate now can help make them less picky about their food in future.

Meals like chicken pot pie, tuna salad, and casseroles provide an appealing mix of flavors, as do mixed fruit desserts, and fruity breakfasts. Dishes that contain different combinations of ingredients add variety that educates the taste buds.

It's important your baby has a balanced diet that includes proteins, fats, carbohydrates, and vitamins and minerals. Offering your baby a wide variety of foods will ensure they get the nutrients and energy they need to grow and develop properly. It may take time for your baby to adjust to new foods, flavors, and textures. This is normal, don't worry. Be patient. (For more information on nutrition for babies, see p.193).

Following your lead

It's a good idea to sit down and eat as a family so you can lead by example and spend valuable time together. Your baby is much more likely to try a new food if they see you or a sibling eating it. They'll also learn something about table manners as well as enjoying the social aspects of mealtimes. Try to keep mealtimes fun and enjoyable, and don't push your baby to eat or try new foods if they really don't want to. Praise them for eating, even if they only manage to eat a small amount.

MEAL IDEAS FOR OLDER BABIES

Breakfast
• Oatmeal or unsweetened cereal with breast milk or formula and banana
• Toast, sliced into "fingers," with hard-boiled egg and slices of fruit, such as peach or pineapple
• Pureed apple, organic yogurt, and unsweetened cereal

Lunch
• Baked potato with yogurt and grated zucchini
• Small bites: for example, sliced cherry tomatoes, pita bread, cucumber sticks, and hummus

• Low salt-and-sugar baked beans and toast
• Mini sandwiches: for fillings, hard-boiled egg or chopped chicken and a little mayonnaise or yogurt
• Spaghetti with tomato and basil sauce
• Homemade tomato soup with soft bread sticks
• Pita with chopped cherry tomatoes and cucumber
• Fish (check for bones) or chicken fingers with carrots and tomato sauce mixed in or for dipping the chicken
• Bread sticks and vegetable crudités with fresh dips

Dinner
• Ground or chopped meat, mashed potatoes, and carrots
• Fish sticks, peas, and mashed potatoes
• Chicken casserole and rice and peas or broccoli
• Vegetable risotto or pasta
• Beef or lentil burgers, zucchini, sliced tomato, and boiled potatoes
• Baked chicken with cooked carrots and rice
• Meatballs with broccoli and carrots
• Poached salmon with rice and chopped up vegetables
• Chicken and vegetable kebabs

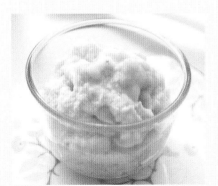

Breakfast Baby oatmeal with milk, yogurt, and mashed banana.

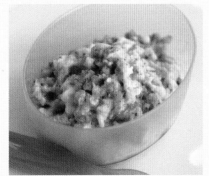

Lunch Fillet of whitefish and vegetable sauce, with a sprinkle of cheese.

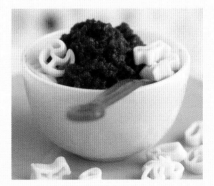

Dinner Baby pasta shapes with a simple tomato pasta sauce.

Feeling displaced

If you're back at work, you may be a little envious that your baby's caregiver is able to witness your baby's milestones before you do.

A professional caregiver will be aware that parents struggle with a sense of missing out, so do express how you are feeling. To help you feel close to your baby, ask your caregiver to keep you up-to-date with everything that occurs in the day, even if it means calling you while you're at work. Make it clear that you appreciate the efforts your baby's caregiver makes and comment positively on what they have taught your baby. If

you begin to feel a little left out, remind yourself that your baby is with you many more hours than with a caregiver.

Don't be surprised if your baby fusses or even cries sometimes when you come to pick them up. The transition can be stressful. You may be interrupting their play or a nap; they may be feeling comfortable where they are, and don't want to be wrapped up and moved. Take your time at the changeover, hold them

while you ask their caregiver how the day was, and get into the habit of waving goodbye to mark the end of your baby's time with their caregiver. Once you've picked them up, try to spend some one-on-one time together, even if there are other jobs to do. They'll appreciate some parent time now. Be reassured that most parents feel some degree of guilt about spending time away from their baby; you are not alone.

First words

You may find that your baby has their own words for familiar objects. For example, point to their comfort item to see what they call it.

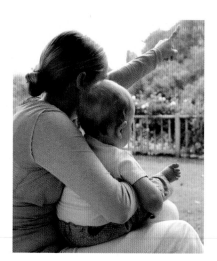

What's that up there? Ask your baby to tell you their words for everyday objects.

If your baby repeats a sound each time you show them an item, odds are they've developed their own word for it. It's common for babies to blend some sounds from the name for an object to create an identifiable "word." They may call their bottle a "baba"; they may say "mi-mi" for milk or "dob" for the dog. Encourage them to name things, and applaud their efforts. Listen carefully for patterns in their speech—do the same "words" crop up regularly? What might they mean?

Your baby may become frustrated when they try to communicate with you, pointing and repeating their words to try to get the message across.

To ease frustration, hold up familiar items such as their plate, blanket, or cuddly toy to hear what they call them. Repeat their words and give them the correct word as well. For example, say "Yes! Dob! This is the dog!"

Give your baby opportunities to practice their new words. Ask them to point to different objects in a picture book. Give the correct words and see how they respond. If you've been practicing your animal sounds together, they may actually use the noise an animal makes rather than attempt to say its name. Celebrate the fact that they are linking words and sounds with objects, and encourage them to continue.

Family vacations

Vacations with your older baby can be fun. As long as you are well prepared, they'll love having an adventure with their family.

Many babies feel unsettled in a new environment, so it is a good idea to take a few of your baby's familiar toys when you go on vacation, to comfort them and keep them occupied at your destination. Pack some toys and books into your carry-on luggage, too, to distract them while you are in transit. If you are staying in a hotel that provides a crib, or taking a travel crib with you, take your baby's usual sleep sack—they may find it easier to sleep in a different place if there is something familiar about it. Let them play in their new bed before you settle them down, so when they wake up at night they will know where they are.

USEFUL EXTRAS

On p.125, you'll find a list of items that you'll need to pack for your baby when traveling. Now that they are a little older, you may also want to consider bringing some of the following:

• A sunshade for the car, and a shade or umbrella for the beach
• A first-aid kit with some infant acetaminophen and teething gel
• A baby monitor or night-light
• A canopy for their stroller
• A baby backpack carrier
• Stroller books and stroller toys
• A universal bath plug that fits all plug holes so a shower can be run to become a bath
• Some laundry detergent to wash clothes after messy meals.

Milk and food

If your baby is bottle-fed and you are going abroad, take a supply of their regular formula in case you can't find the same brand at your destination. You might also worry about which solid foods they're going to be able to eat while on vacation. If they're used to jars or pouches of food, take a few with you so they still have some familiar meals as they adjust to a new place and different food. These also serve as a standby in case of emergencies. Individual containers of fruit puree appeal to most babies, and if there is a fridge at your destination, you can chill some of these treats for them.

Pack a few favorite snacks, too, such as baby bread sticks and rice cakes. Small boxes of baby breakfast cereal may also prove useful.

Between local supermarkets, markets, and your own plates, it's usually fairly easy to cobble together enough food for your baby to get by on. Fresh fruit and vegetables purchased in their country of origin are also particularly delicious—and you may be able to tempt a picky baby to expand their palate by offering them tastes of fresh local produce.

Sensible precautions

Wash the fruit and vegetables carefully, and peel fruit when possible. If you buy bottled water for your baby, make sure it's low in sodium. If you order a poultry or meat dish from a restaurant, always check that it is thoroughly cooked

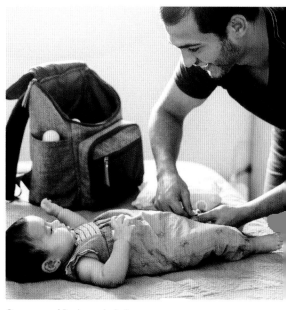

Go prepared Pack your baby's essentials in a diaper bag that you can carry with you.

before letting your baby try any. On arrival at your accommodation, check for potential hazards. If your baby is crawling, starting to stand, or even cruising, look to see if there are any steps they might fall down, wires or cords they might grab, accessible electrical outlets, unstable furniture, or anything else that could lead to an accident. If you are concerned about your baby's safety, speak to someone in charge to have it rectified. Finally, don't forget in all that to take your travel documents with you—including your baby's own passport, if you're leaving the country!

Shining locks

From a fine, downy covering to a mass of unruly tangles, babies' hair grows very differently and so needs caring for accordingly.

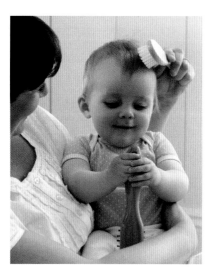

This is the way ... we brush our hair. Make routines more fun by involving your baby and making them an active participant.

During their first year, most babies lose their soft, downy hair as new, thicker hair grows. However, as with all things baby related, there's huge variation. Some babies might still have very little hair at 9, or even 12, months; others may have a mop of unruly curls, or hair down to their shoulders. If your baby is still lacking in the follicle department, don't worry—the hair will grow, and at least for the time being, it's easy to take care of. A wash with a gentle shampoo a couple of times a week and a brush with a soft-bristled brush is perfect.

For parents of babies with lots of hair, particularly if it's curly, use a small amount of conditioner after a shampoo and rinse, and then comb through with a fine-toothed comb to ease out tangles.

Thick, coarse, curly, or wavy hair requires special care because of its texture and curl pattern. Treat it gently, as the hair can be prone to breakage. Over-washing can also strip the hair of its oils, so it's best not to wash it more than once a week.

Hot and cold

Your baby's body is now better able to regulate its temperature, but you still need to make sure they don't overheat or become too cold.

Your baby may pull at their clothes or become fractious if they're too hot, or come to you for a cuddle if it's chilly.

In cold weather, dress your baby with the same number of layers you put on yourself. In the stroller, they'll be less active than you and will probably feel cold more easily, so pop a hat on their head and tuck a blanket around them. A double layer of socks will keep feet warm inside the stroller blanket. Mittens may be a challenge as they restrict hand skills, but if it is cold enough for you to need gloves, your baby should have some, too.

When it's hot, allow your baby to play outdoors in just a hat, t-shirt, and diaper; or dispense with the t-shirt, too (make sure they're wearing sunscreen). A red face, damp and clammy skin, or frequent tongue-poking may indicate the baby is too hot. Offer a drink and remove a layer of clothing.

KEY TEMPERATURES

The temperature of your baby's bedroom should be kept somewhere between 61°F (16°C) and 68°F (20°C). Your baby's bath water should be at a temperature of about 98.6°F (37°C). A "normal" temperature for a healthy baby is 98.6°F (37°C) when taken in the mouth. This can be up to one degree Fahrenheit lower when measured from the armpit.

Your baby's memory

Since birth, your baby's memory has come a long way. They remember many things and retain information for increasing amounts of time.

Your newborn baby operated mostly by reflex, and while your smell, touch, and voice would be familiar, out of sight was, quite literally, out of mind. From there, their memory has developed gradually.

One of the first things your baby remembered was your face, which allowed them to form a strong bond with you. Before they were six months old, they began to remember things that were significant to them on a short-term basis. This was evident in their ability to anticipate certain actions and events, indicating that they were drawing from their memory. For example, they would know what was about to happen next when their book was brought out or you sat them down in the high chair for a meal, and they may have shown excitement at seeing their comfort object or a favorite toy.

By the time your baby was six months old, they recognized you and your partner as the most important people in their life, and by now they turn if you call their name, indicating that they remember this sound refers to them. They will recognize familiar objects, too, and will remember where their toys are stored, or where their snacks are kept, and will recognize familiar faces and everyday routines.

There are, of course, some disadvantages to them developing a memory. For example, they may remember that they hate having their hair washed and begin to fuss and wiggle the moment they hear the bath water running.

Developing long-term memory

The development of your baby's memory is such that they have a steadily increasing ability to store and recall new information. The more they see and experience something, the more likely they'll be to recall it.

They are also gradually increasing the amount of time they can hold a memory. For example, if they see their grandparents infrequently, they may recognize them immediately if they see them again within a month, but will probably take a moment or two and/or need a reminder if it's been a longer break than this. How much your baby remembers can depend on various factors, such as familiarity and the reminders they receive about certain pieces of information.

DEVELOPMENT ACTIVITY: MESSY PLAY

Your baby is interested in textures, consistency, and generally getting their hands dirty. You'll already notice they want to put their fingers into their food, stirring it around, squeezing it, and patting it on the high-chair tray. They may also enjoy smearing it on their face and clothes. This playfulness with different consistencies is all part of understanding the properties of familiar items in their world so that, eventually, they'll be able to predict or anticipate how things feel. Give them some sloppy oatmeal, let them pull the leaves off Brussels sprouts, or push their hands into pliable pastry dough—it's all about learning how things look and feel.

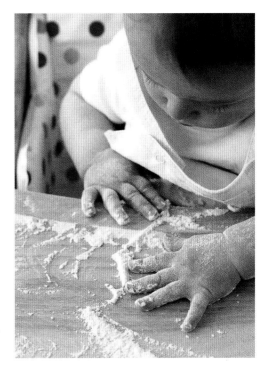

Flour power Making lots of mess with foodstuffs is not only fun but teaches your baby about texture and form.

Your baby from
10 to 12 months

10

MONTH 10: SAYS THEIR FIRST WORDS

There might be one or two words that your baby says regularly now—whatever the sound is, if they use it often, with meaning ("bah" for bottle, for example), it counts as a word. You might hear "dada" and "mama" said with meaning now, too.

11

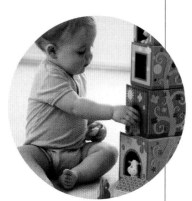

Your baby will start to enjoy complex play, such as **stacking and sorting**.

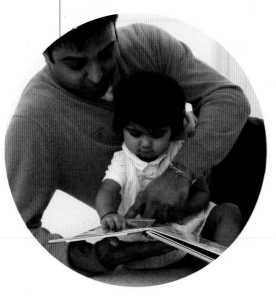

Your baby may be able to **turn the pages of a chunky board** book now and enjoy the pictures.

MONTH 11: LEARNS TO SAY THE WORD "NO"

Your baby is beginning to realize what "no" means but they won't always cooperate. They're more likely to think it's a game!

> " Your baby is now a sociable little person with a host of new skills and much greater control over their body. "

MONTH

12

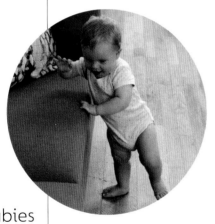

Your baby sees their **peers as objects** and wants to know how they look and feel.

A few babies will take their first independent **steps** during their first year.

MONTH 12: BECOMING A TODDLER

Your baby is becoming more independent, and will have their own ideas of what they want to do and when. With their improved speech, they will combine first words and gestures to try and communicate with you about what they want.

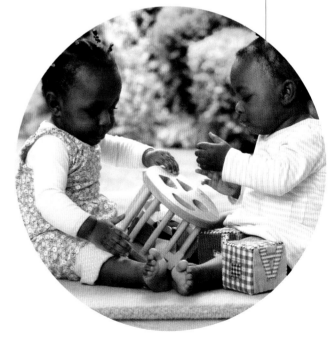

10 months

SEPARATION ANXIETY IS USUALLY STRONGEST BETWEEN THE AGES OF 10 AND 18 MONTHS.
Your baby can use both hands simultaneously with confidence, and is proud to show off their skills to you. Give them plenty of praise for their achievements. They will be more sociable now, and will enjoy and benefit from spending time with others.

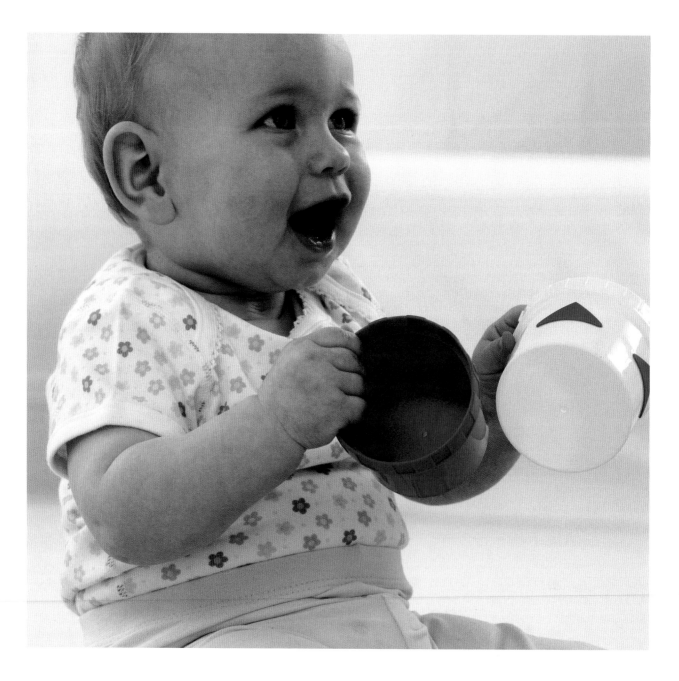

Expressing self-will

As your baby grows up, there are occasions when they might be less cooperative than you would like. Time for you to hone your skills in patience!

DEVELOPMENT ACTIVITY: PICK IT UP

As your baby approaches 10 months, their pincer grip is fully developed. You'll find they use their fingers to "rake" small items they want to hold until they've positioned them so they can pick them up between their thumb and forefinger. Mealtimes provide the perfect opportunity for practice—a small piece of soft fruit or lightly cooked vegetables put on their tray are tempting treats to pick up. Place two or three pieces at a time on the tray and let your baby pick them up and release them into their mouth by themselves. They'll enjoy dropping everything onto the floor from the high chair. This activity is also known as "casting," and to your baby it's great fun.

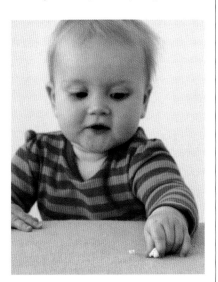

Motor skills Your baby will find many practical applications to practice their fine motor skills.

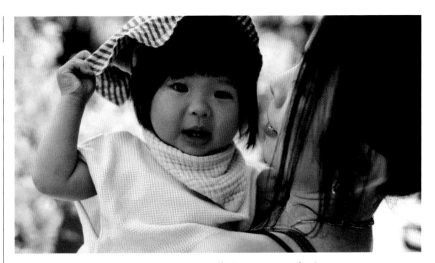

Hats off! You put the hat on. Your baby takes it off. It's a great game for them and a test of patience for you—especially if you're in a hurry to get out the door to enjoy a sunny day!

Although your baby won't be striving for independence just yet, they're certainly capable of objecting to or taking an instant dislike to something you are trying to do. What happened to your agreeable baby?

Perhaps you want their hat/socks/booties on and they keep taking them off, or they're objecting to having their diaper changed or their coat put on, or they empty their food bowl all over the floor. There may be days when you feel that your patience is being sorely tested. Keep a sense of perspective and remember that your baby—even though they seem to have developed quickly all of a sudden—is still very much a baby and doesn't mean to be difficult.

Time and compromise

Try to build some time into your routine so if your baby doesn't cooperate right away, you don't become flustered under time pressure.

Try to respect their wishes when you can—if they don't really need socks on and you can cover their feet with a blanket, let it go. If they prefer a cozy cardigan to being buttoned up in a coat, take the easy option. If they become frustrated, offer help; if they push you away, let them experiment and try to achieve whatever they're trying to do.

Above all, don't get angry. They won't understand and they'll be upset by it. Try to see the funny side and don't expect too much of your baby.

Consistent nap times

One of the keys to ensuring that your baby sleeps through the night is to give them a consistent nap time during the day.

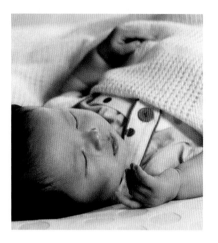

Good-quality naps Your 10-month-old needs one or two good naps every day.

Although at this age babies can manage with little shifts in their routine for the occasional day out, it's important that, by and large, nap times are consistent and your baby gets a good quality sleep when they nap. If they are overtired at bedtime, they'll be harder to settle and may be fretful at night.

Most babies at this age are down to one longer nap in the afternoon. If the nap is well scheduled (coinciding with your baby's signs of sleepiness) and of a good length (two to three hours), your baby should be able to make it through to bedtime without becoming overtired, then sleep well at night.

A consistent nap-time routine that is similar, but not identical, to your baby's bedtime routine is important. Keep to the same pattern each day so your baby learns to anticipate that nap time is coming and prepares for it, so they're more likely to settle in happily and fall asleep quickly.

Going naked

Our ancestors would be amazed at how we wrap up our babies. When cold isn't a factor, it can do a baby good to go naked at times.

Your baby will love some diaper-free time every day. For obvious reasons, summertime is best to do this, although just before bath time in the safety of a well-heated bathroom is good at any time of year. If you have carpet, invest in a waterproof mat, covering it with a couple of towels to quickly absorb accidents.

Giving your baby two or three short diaper-free periods each day will help prevent, or clear up, diaper rash. It will also enable your baby to become familiar with the sensations of urinating and a bowel movement, which means that, in time, they will learn what it feels like just before they need to go. In fact, some experts believe that diaper-free time every day hastens potty training. Although that might be a happy end-product of daily diaper-free time, don't make it the goal. Your baby is still very young, and their diaper-free hour should be nothing more than an opportunity for them to get a sense of freedom in their body, and for their bottom to get a good airing!

AS A MATTER OF FACT

The babies of our ancestors had very little in the way of clothing—in the Middle Ages, for example, cloth was considered a luxury. Babies were usually swaddled in linen strips until they were old enough to sit up on their own. Then they were often simply naked, or wrapped in blankets if it was cold. They may have been clad in simple gowns. It wasn't until the 18th century that baby boys were dressed in jumpsuits and girls in simple shift dresses.

Eating as a family

Your baby will benefit from regular family meals. This will encourage good eating habits and a willingness to try new foods.

It might not be practical to sit down as a family to eat all the time, but try to do it a few times during the week and also when you have more time on the weekend. Babies are social and they tend to be less picky in their eating habits when everyone is around the table together. If your baby sees their family eating foods they haven't tried, they'll be more willing to try them themself. Offer appropriate foods from your plate, and if you can, make meals you can all eat.

Your baby will see you using cutlery, drinking from cups or glasses, and perhaps using napkins. They'll notice that you don't throw your bowl across the room, and that family members ask to leave the table and help with the dishes. Although they won't develop these types of social skills for years, you are providing them with an excellent example of how people eat together and the kind of behavior and manners that are expected. Keep mealtimes cheerful. It's best if you don't use the time for heated debates.

Involve your baby in social or larger family meal gatherings—perhaps at Sunday lunch or festive occasions. Even though they may be naturally wary of strangers, the more opportunities they have to meet new people, with you at their side, the more confident they will become.

FAMILY MEALS

There are many family meals your baby can eat, too, remembering that they shouldn't have salt and sugar added to their portion. Make sure the texture is right for them by pureeing, mashing, or finely chopping. Ideas for baby-friendly family meals include:
- Chicken pot pie with vegetables and a crust on top.
- Thick vegetable or lentil-based soup with toast cut into strips.
- Baked chicken with spinach and potatoes.
- Homemade meatballs in tomato sauce with noodles or rice (if you blend the meat finely and make the meatballs small enough, they can be finger foods).
- Broccoli, carrots, or cauliflower and tofu with a pureed red pepper dipping sauce.
- Pasta with tomato sauce.
- Lamb burgers with avocado (form baby's patties into small, firm balls and mash avocado, or leave in slices).
- Meat and bean pie—be careful with stocks, which are high in salt.
- Mashed lentils with rice (avoid spice blends and pastes that contain salt).

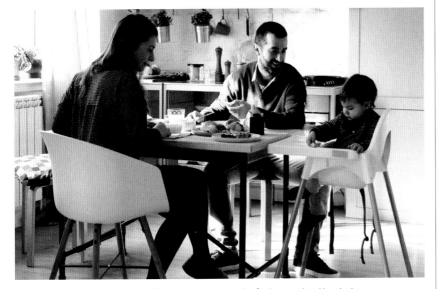

Social mealtimes Family meals offer a good opportunity for interaction. Your baby will observe your table manners, and when they see you eating something they're more likely to want to try it.

Learning to be sociable

It's common for even the most social of babies to become fearful and uncomfortable in the presence of strangers around this time.

Your baby's anxiety about strangers and separating from you may become more intense now. They understand that their relationship with you is special, and that other people need to be treated with caution. Instead of beaming with pleasure when they see the lady at the supermarket check-out, they may cry, cover their eyes, and cling to you.

This is a normal part of their development but can be tricky for close family and friends. Try not to be embarrassed if your baby fails to be always sociable. Some form of separation anxiety (see p.228 and p.263) can last until a child is three.

Introduce them to social situations slowly, and reassure them constantly, using a low, gentle voice. Give them time to warm up around strangers before you pass them to someone to be held. If they really don't want to go, don't force the issue. If you feel the need, explain to strangers that they're not comfortable with people they don't know right now, and not to take it personally. Show friends and family a few tricks that make your baby laugh, to relax them and make positive associations. Even if they want to be held by only you, let them get used to meeting new faces. As long as you are there, reassuring them, they will gain confidence. Above all, be positive and sociable in the company of others. If they see that you are relaxed and having fun, they'll soon realize that there's nothing to worry about.

Lots of laughing

Laughter is a developmental milestone—it shows your baby can respond positively to stimuli and is developing a sense of humor.

Your baby finding something funny is the clearest sign you have that they enjoy the company and actions of those around them. They have probably been able to let out at least a little giggle since they were about three months old but, by now, their giggles may well have turned into full-blown belly laughs.

All sorts of silly behavior will leave your baby in helpless laughter— blowing raspberries on them, tickling their thighs, or pretending that their feet are very smelly. Since they are now better able to read other people's expressions and feelings, they will love that their feet have made you make a face and groan in horror. They'll probably thrust them into your face for you to groan again! And when you find a thing that makes your baby giggle uncontrollably, you'll want to repeat it, too—because, for most parents, your baby's laughter is pure, feel-good parenting joy.

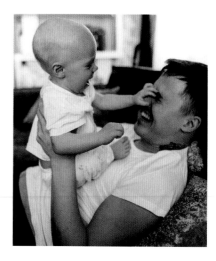

Cheesy! Try pretending that your baby's feet are really smelly—they may find it hilarious!

What's my baby eating?

Your baby can now eat food that is more like your meals. They may eat three meals a day with snacks, and can tolerate lumpier textures.

Now is the perfect time to introduce a wider range of finger foods into your baby's diet. Other than finger foods, the rest of their food will be mashed, and you can progress to giving them cut-up chunks of food (see Stage three solids, pp.288–289).

Your baby will likely have a few teeth by now, and their jaw and tongue have developed enough to allow them to "gum," chew, and swallow food efficiently. The more lumps, bumps, and different textures you give, the less likely they will become a picky eater.

Mashing together vegetables, rather than using a food processor, is a good way to provide plenty of texture. You can also mash well-cooked and raw fruits, or several vegetables and/or fruits together. Finely mincing foods such as meat also produces pieces that have a little bite, but are soft enough to be chewed and swallowed by your baby.

Once ground and mashed foods are acceptable, finely cut and chop your baby's food. As they become used to eating food in pieces, make the pieces gradually bigger. Some babies prefer large, identifiable chunks to smaller lumps that take them by surprise.

Variety of textures

Work toward giving your baby a dish made up of all sorts of different textures for them to enjoy. For example, you could mince chicken, mash potatoes and carrots, and give corn pieces as finger food. Or food process together some spinach with nutmeg, and serve this alongside baked or poached chicken, pasta shapes, and lightly steamed green beans or broccoli florets for your baby to pick up.

By the end of your baby's first year, they'll be eating three meals a day, although the amount of food they eat at each meal can vary considerably. If they find breakfast hard to manage, try giving them less milk in the morning so they have more room for a breakfast meal. If they still have a milk feeding during the day, give it after a meal, and not before.

Don't fret if your baby doesn't eat everything at each meal. As long as you offer three balanced meals and two healthy snacks over the course of the day, they will be getting the nutrition that they need.

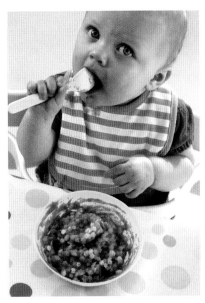

Changing diet Solid foods now become more important in your baby's diet, and the food they eat is much more like your own food.

ASK A PEDIATRICIAN

My baby won't breastfeed. What should I do? As they get older, they're likely to be more easily distracted from feeding by all the things going on around them, and may feel impatient with how long a feeding takes. Usually, the problem is temporary. Try the following tactics to get your baby interested in feeding: feed them away from the action, since they may settle down once the distractions are removed; feed them when they are sleepy and less likely to be distracted; offer a little skin-to-skin contact to encourage them to recall positive early bonding experiences; feed them when they are most relaxed and when they are in their favorite, familiar spot. Continue to give feedings around the usual times, working around mealtimes, and begin a session by rubbing a little breast milk on their lips. They may just need to be reminded about how nice it all is. If all else fails, offer them breast milk in a cup or bottle and express regularly to keep up your supply. Eventually, you'll be able to coax them back.

Shopping with your baby

Any parent knows that supermarket shopping with baby in tow can be a trial, so here are some ways to navigate the aisles without tears.

Write a shopping list before you go. If you know the supermarket layout, you can write your list in the order of the aisles you visit so you're super efficient when you get there!

Plan your shopping around meal and nap times so your baby isn't too hungry or too cranky. Try to avoid going at peak times, so you don't have to negotiate long lines at the checkout counter. Take a snack, such as some rice cakes or a bread stick, that your baby can munch on as you're walking around. If you're putting them in the baby seat of the shopping cart, make sure the harness is safely fastened. Bring a couple of their stroller toys, too, to keep them amused. Park as close as you can to the supermarket entrance and cart bay, so you only have to cover a short distance to return the shopping cart after loading the car. Last but not least, involve your baby in the shop. For example, pick up a pineapple, explain what it is, and let them touch it before you put it in the cart. Keep talking to them as you walk around the supermarket, and praise them, touch their hand, and make plenty of eye contact with them to let them know that you're pleased they're sitting calmly.

Standing tall

If your baby had already started to move around gingerly while holding onto furniture, they may begin to cruise more confidently now.

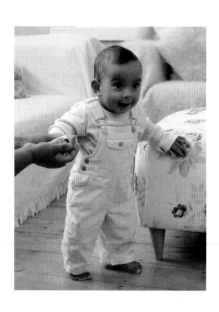

I'm almost off When your baby learns to walk, their feet will be set fairly far apart to provide stability, causing them, literally, to toddle.

The average age for babies taking their first steps is 13 months. Before then, your baby will be concentrating on spending lots of time pulling up to a stand, and becoming an increasingly confident cruiser. By now, they may be very happy working their way around the room holding onto furniture, and may stand more upright, leaving a larger gap between their body and the furniture as their confidence grows. At some point, they may even let go momentarily and stand with no support at all.

While you will want to wait until your baby is really walking to buy their first pair of sturdy outdoor shoes, there are plenty of soft shoes available that can be ideal for your baby around now, especially when they are outside (see p.302).

Try not to worry if your baby seems to prefer other methods of getting around, such as bottom shuffling. As long as they are showing an interest in being mobile, they're fine. Many bottom shufflers are so proficient that they are less interested in taking to their feet than other babies.

300

Home safety checks

With your increasingly mobile baby often on the prowl, it's a good idea to reassess your babyproofing to make sure they are safe from harm.

The best way to keep your home as safe as you can for your baby is to get down on your hands and knees and look at it from their height. If there are loose wires, tuck or tape them away; buy safety plugs to fill outlets; and look for any head-height edges and corners that might cause bumps or cuts. Babies often use the space between the door and the frame on the hinged side to hang on to, because their little fingers can fit in the gap—if the door swings closed, fingers get squashed. Invest in doorstops to hold doors open to prevent little fingers from getting trapped.

Leave floor spaces clear by removing rugs, if you have them, for the time being. It might also be a good idea to put away your coffee table temporarily. Not only will it have sharp corners and edges but, inevitably, drinks will be left on it, presenting spilling hazards and, in the case of hot drinks, the possibility of scalding.

Buy a cover for your oven door if your baby can reach it, and put child locks on cabinets that contain items such as knives and chemicals. Also, unplug hair dryers or straighteners and avoid leaving them lying around to cool.

Keep the washing machine, dryer, and dishwasher doors firmly closed so they can't open them and climb in. Internal glass doors should contain safety glass; if yours don't, you can arrange to have a special film put over them to make them safe. If you have pets, keep their food and water shut in a room that your baby can't get to, or put it out only when your baby is out of the room.

DEVELOPMENT ACTIVITY: MAKING FACES

Your baby was born with the ability and motivation to copy you, so if you make faces at them, they'll return them. Making faces to each other is important to their social development; they are mirroring your expression and you are reflecting this back to them. They are learning social turn-taking, and these facial movements will have meaning in later years as they connect the raised eyebrow to questions, or a frown to anger. Pairing an expression with a label such as "angry" or "happy" is the beginning of teaching your baby the labels for different emotions. They won't make the connection now, but it's good to start this emotional education early.

Making faces also helps develop your baby's facial muscles, which, in turn, helps develop their speech.

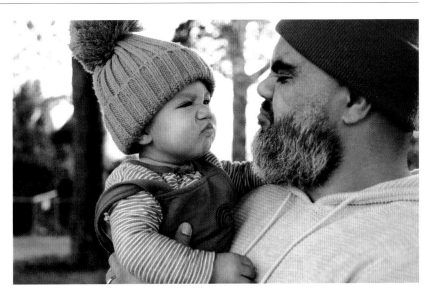

Copying faces Your baby can learn a lot from copying the faces you make to amuse them, and will have lots of fun with you at the same time.

301

Sweet tooth

Your baby may prefer sweet foods over savory, but avoid giving processed sugary foods that could harm emerging teeth.

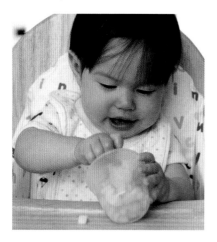

Natural sugar Fruit is full of sweetness and flavor, and will appeal to a baby's sweet tooth.

Many studies suggest that a sweet tooth is learned. Older babies can have their need for sweet foods satisfied easily with healthy foods.

Sugar is naturally present in many foods, including fruit, vegetables, and milk. Sugar in whole foods is less damaging to teeth than extracted sugar, such as that found in fruit juice, which acts on teeth in the same way as table sugar. As your baby's teeth are emerging, their sugar consumption needs to be monitored. Avoid giving refined sugar products such as cakes, cookies, candy, and chocolates. A treat in the form of grated apple or a mashed banana is sweet enough. Restrict dried fruit (pureed only) such as prunes to mealtimes since they can lead to tooth decay. For a drink, give primarily water. If you give juice, dilute it one part juice to nine parts water. While your baby is still fairly suggestible, though, offer savory foods as much as possible.

Shoes for cruising?

Once your baby starts cruising confidently, you may wonder whether their feet need support and protection.

Going without socks and shoes allows your baby to figure out how to use their toes to balance. As much as possible, let them practice walking in bare feet. Their feet are going through an important phase of development, and walking barefoot also helps build the arches and encourages the ankles to strengthen.

You may be concerned, though, about whether a standing baby's feet need more protection, especially when they are outdoors or moving around on slippery surfaces. Many outlets sell shoes specially designed for "cruising." While there is some debate as to whether or not these are a good thing for babies, proponents of cruising shoes state that they provide support for toes and heels, which gives a baby confidence on their feet.

Soft "cruising" shoes give complete flexibility, allowing your baby's feet to bend and ensuring they can still feel the floor. Choose a soft material and make sure you have them fitted at a store by a trained fitter used to working with babies.

ASK A MOM

Even "cruising" shoes are expensive. Can I buy a secondhand pair? It's not a good idea to buy cruising shoes secondhand because they mold to the shape of the previous owner's foot, which isn't advisable when your baby's feet are developing. If they'll be wearing them regularly, it's a good idea to buy a new pair. You could make an exception if you want an "occasional" pair for special events that won't see much action.

A real personality

Your baby's personality is increasingly evident now as they learn more ways to express themself and have distinct behavior patterns.

Many aspects of your baby's eventual personality have already emerged. They may be strong-willed or easy to please; they may be calm and quick to laugh or a little more highly strung and sensitive.

Whatever the case, avoid labeling them. Calling them "easy" or "difficult" can influence their personality. If your baby grows up thinking they are "the fussy one," they're more likely to act in this way. This is particularly important if you have twins or other multiples, which makes it easier to compare and label.

Celebrate your baby's individual characteristics, even when they are at odds with your own personality or, in the early years, somewhat frustrating. A nonstop, highly energetic baby may be exhausting for new parents, but keep in mind that these qualities will be admired when they are older.

Some characteristics may be a little extreme, and you can work to ease them a little during these formative months. For example, if your baby is relaxed to the point that they don't respond much to their surroundings, play lively music often and encourage them to be physically active. If they're easily frustrated when things don't go right, show them patiently how it's done, or distract them with another activity until they're calm. Their temperament may not change, but they'll develop the ability to tolerate frustration.

Keep in mind that it is possible to stifle your baby's natural characteristics by trying to impose your own. For instance, if you are quiet, you may find their noisy, ebullient personality exhausting. However, actively avoiding noisy play or situations in which these characteristics shine through could leave your baby slightly confused, without an outlet to express themself.

Try to celebrate your baby's unique characteristics, even those you find a little challenging, and look for ways in which to support your baby. With a gentle guiding hand, even the trickiest babies can become settled, well-behaved children and adults.

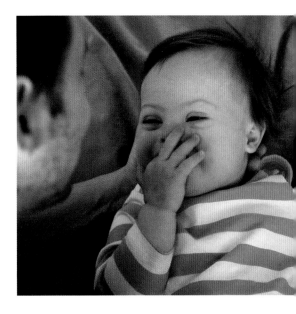

A real character Celebrate your baby's personality and find good ways to channel it.

DEVELOPMENT ACTIVITY: MAKING MOVES

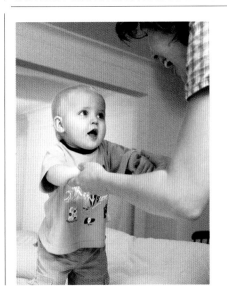

Wiggling, swaying, bouncing, clapping—these are all dance moves that your baby can achieve with very little effort. If they are comfortable with standing and holding on to something, you can put on some music, hold their hands or lightly grasp their waist to keep them steady on their feet, and dance with them. The bouncing in their knees will encourage them to bend and straighten, which is another step on the road to walking, and will also build strength in their legs.

Dancing together Get your baby moving to some music. Doing it on a bed allows for soft landings when things get rowdy!

Was that "dada"?

Studies suggest that babies are most likely to utter their first word at around 10 or 11 months. But what will it be?

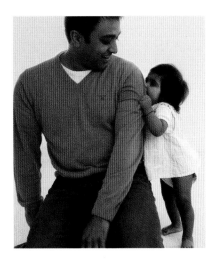

First words Most babies say "dada" before "mama," but that has more to do with how speech develops than relationships.

Your baby has now developed enough control over their vocal cords to be able to make sounds purposefully. Any friendly competition that vies for your name to be their first word can only help speech development as the adults in your baby's life concentrate on getting your baby to talk.

"Dada" is the most common first word, followed by "mama," most probably because the "d" sound is easier for babies to utter than the "m" sound. So don't be surprised if your baby says "dog" or "duck" before "mama." Other popular first words are "cat" (although it will probably come out as "tat") followed by "milk" ("mah") or "ball" ("bah"), while less popular but frequent contenders include "juice" (usually pronounced "juh"), "shoe," "dog," "bye," and "nana."

Words with easy consonant sounds (p, b, d, m, n, s or sh, g, and so on) tend to be the basis for first words, with words made up of trickier sounds (k, j, th, l, for example) coming later.

How your baby grows

It now seems inconceivable that your newborn baby was ever that small— just look at the size of them now!

Between now and 12 months, your baby should weigh somewhere between two and three times as much as when they were born. However, these are just guidelines and all babies gain weight at slightly different rates. They should also have grown about 10 in (25 cm) by the time they reach their first birthday.

If you notice slowed growth or a drop in weight, it could be due to illness—a couple days of not eating, especially if combined with vomiting or diarrhea, can lead to weight loss that your baby will regain when they recover. Or it could happen if your baby is crawling, cruising, or walking, as these all burn calories. If your baby is alert, happy, feeding well overall, and filling diapers normally, all is likely to be well. If there's any cause for concern, see your pediatrician.

If you are worried that your baby is too plump, discuss their weight with your pediatrician, who will tell you right away if there's a risk of your baby becoming overweight. Never withhold feedings, but pay attention to cues that the baby is full.

If your baby is a little overweight, make sure their calories come from nutritious sources—like fruits, vegetables, healthy fats, and grains— rather than sweets and processed food. Play with your baby to encourage physical activity, making sure they have a safe space in which to practice being more mobile.

Balancing work and baby

It's not easy to balance work and home life: add a baby to the mix and you'll need to put all your organizational skills into practice.

Nobody is perfect, so don't try to be superhuman. If the housework slides or your baby doesn't get their bath one night, the world won't end. Making things easy at home is the secret to survival. Babies are hugely resilient and their needs are actually very basic. As long as your baby is loved, cared for, and stimulated, they'll be fine. Sometimes they will be glad just to be in your presence, so relax with them, too.

Also, learn to say, "no." Your baby, family, and job are your priorities. Maintaining these will sometimes be all you can manage. Figure out the parts of and people in your life that you enjoy and say no to anything or anyone that doesn't add positivity.

Similarly, don't succumb to guilt. If staying at home with your baby is not an option financially, embrace your situation and find ways in which you can make it healthy and happy for all of you. In other words, be positive. How can you get the most from the time you have with your baby? Focus on the things you can do, rather than the things you can't.

Establish boundaries at work

You may once have been a 24/7 employee, but this will be hard now. It helps for your work colleagues to know your needs when you return to work. You may wish for more flexible or part-time working arrangements; don't be afraid to ask for these. Most workplaces value their employees

and are willing to try to accommodate the work-life balance you hope for. If you are in charge yourself, consider delegating some of your workload to give you more time.

Take care of yourself

An exhausted, underfed, emotionally drained parent isn't any good to anyone! You'll be able to keep more balls in the air if you eat well and sleep well. Time alone for yourself and your partner is also important for a healthy emotional life. Sometimes both home and work can feel tricky, but even if there isn't much time to spare, you both need to take time out without guilt and with support.

FOCUS ON TWINS: DIFFERENT INDIVIDUALS

Your twins' personalities will be emerging in earnest now, and no matter how alike in some ways, they will probably have different character traits, even if they are identical. You may find that one wants to crawl, and the other isn't interested, or one is relaxed and placid while the other is easily frustrated. The challenge with twins is to avoid comparing or labeling them. A label can stick, and one child being labeled the "shy one" and the other the "loud one" could put each child into a category that is difficult to change later on. As your babies grow, it's important that they feel valued as individuals as well as having a close relationship as twins.

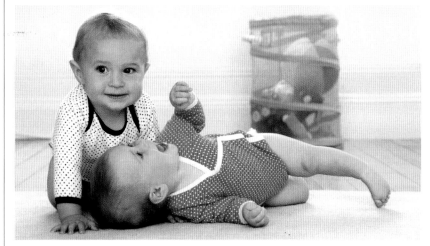

Same but different One twin may be more dominant or gregarious early on, but that doesn't mean it will always be so—the dynamics of the relationship will change as they grow.

Troublesome teeth

First-year molars often surface toward the end of a baby's first year. They are blunt, square teeth, used for grinding and chewing.

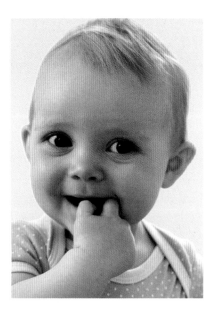

First molars can cause much pain as they erupt through the gums. Sometimes a flap of gum loosens to reveal a new white tooth, and your baby may rub the side of their face or their ear, feel the area with their tongue, and drool more. Both sides of your baby's mouth may be affected. Girls tend to teethe earlier than boys. Your baby may want to chew to ease the discomfort. Offer hard foods such as bread sticks, rice cakes, toast, or apple slices. Very cold smoothies can help soothe inflammation.

Emerging molars Your baby might rub the side of their face or put their fingers in their mouth where it's feeling tender.

ASK A DOCTOR

My baby's teeth look mottled and almost striped. Is this normal? It is normal for a baby's teeth to have mild ridging and appear bluer rather than white. If there are distinct marks on their teeth, there are a few possible causes. Some antibiotics, particularly tetracycline, shouldn't be prescribed in pregnancy because they can cause baby teeth to become mottled as they form in your baby's mouth early in pregnancy. There may also be problems with the enamel if it has formed unevenly. Ask your dentist to check their teeth if you are worried, but rest assured that most problems will not affect your baby's permanent teeth.

How clean?

Your baby is exposed to many germs during their daily activities, so is there any need to continue sterilizing their feeding equipment?

The simple answer is, for the most part, no. Your baby's mobility means their hands make contact with the floor wherever they go, and if they go to play groups or have siblings, they frequently play with toys handled by other children. They put their fingers and toys in their mouth all the time. However, do wash plastic toys in warm, soapy water regularly and put cuddly toys through the washing machine on the hot cycle occasionally to minimize risk.

Wash plastic spoons and bowls in hot, soapy water, or in a normal dishwasher cycle, but don't worry about sterilizing them now. Consider sterilizing bottles and cups that have had formula or breast milk in them, because the fatty deposits on the insides of the bottles can be hard to remove from washing alone, and residue can cause tummy upsets.

Keep your floors clear of debris and wash wood and tile floors regularly. Also, wash your baby's hands after petting animals. Don't be too anxious—your baby has to be exposed to germs to build their immunity.

Encouraging independence

To support your baby's development and ease separation anxiety give them the opportunity to explore their world without you always guiding them.

Ensure that wherever your baby can go is safe, of course, and free from hazards, but then let them travel from room to room, without you if they'll let you hang back. Talk to them as they move so they know you are near. Slowly, their confidence in the idea that in fact they are okay without you for a little while will grow, along with their independence.

Playtime leader

Give your baby a basket containing a few suitable toys and let them choose what to play with. Once they have selected one, engage with them in play to show them that you are interested in the choices they make and that you will follow their lead.

There are certain toys that are particularly good for encouraging independent thinking. Shape sorters, stacking cups, and building blocks will all help your baby try to solve problems on their own.

Self-feeder

At mealtimes, allow your baby to have a spoon of their own so they can try to feed themself, even if you have another spoon so you can ensure some of the food actually finds its way into their stomach! Finger foods are great for independent feeding.

What to eat

As your baby gets older, you will relish the days when you could choose their food without them making any objection. You can give a little independence by offering two healthy choices for a snack, encouraging them to point to the one they prefer. Whatever they choose, they get to eat. If they then want the other snack, too, let them have it, as the exercise should be fun and will help them feel as if they have a degree of control over their own life, which, in turn, helps them understand the advantages of independence.

DEVELOPMENT ACTIVITY: HIDE AND SEEK

Your baby has understood the concept of object permanence (see p.233) for some time now. Playing peekaboo (see p.136) has helped them realize that you are still there even when they can't see you, and hide and seek is the perfect progression for a mobile baby, as it encourages trust in your presence and absence. Play it in one room only and as a family first to allow your baby to get the idea of how it works. One of you hides while your baby and the other parent count and then "seek" together. Next time, you and your partner swap roles, so your baby knows that either one of you may disappear but you will always come back. Once your baby understands the concept of the game, they can play it with just one of you hiding while they seek. The first few times, call from your hiding place to give them a clue and, more importantly, to reassure them that you're still there close by. Then, encourage your baby to "hide" (often unconvincingly!) while you pretend to find them.

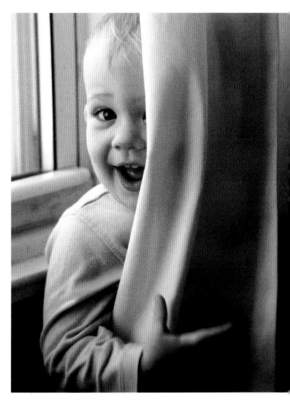

Ready or not! Your baby will love playing hide and seek with you, and learning not to panic when they can't see you.

Constant colds

Your active, social baby contracts lots of germs from many people and environments. It may seem as if they have a constantly runny nose.

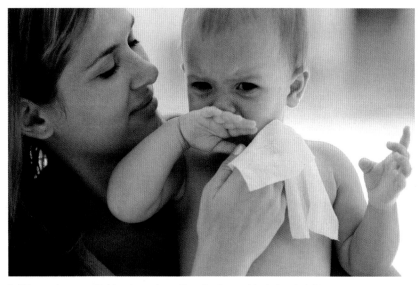

Sniffles and sneezes Babies do tend to suffer a lot from colds during their first year—but each minor illness helps build their immunity so they can fight off similar viruses in the future.

While a cold may disturb your baby's sleep, contracting relatively harmless bugs is an important part of building immunity. Your baby will inevitably be exposed to germs through toys at the homes of friends or at playgroups, which is fine. However, avoid clearly very ill children, especially those with infections such as croup or a chest infection. Ideally, you don't want your baby catching anything more serious than a common cold.

Treating colds

It is normal for your baby to have up to eight or more colds a year. The majority pass in a week or two. Make your baby as comfortable as possible. If they have a fever (around 101°F/ 38°C) and they are very fussy or uncomfortable you could give fever reducing medicine, but the fever may be helping fight the infection. The dosage should be based on your baby's weight.

Give plenty of fluids to help prevent dehydration, and make sure they get lots of time to rest and sleep when they need to. Don't force them to eat if they don't want to—babies often lose their appetite if sick. Offer them small amounts of food often.

DANGER SIGNS

If your baby has a cold and shows any of the following complications, contact your pediatrician.

Fever A temperature of 103°F (39.4°C) or higher, or one above 98.6°F (37°C) that persists for more than two days, should be checked by your pediatrician.

Drowsiness We all feel a bit more sleepy when we are trying to beat infection, but if your baby is hard to rouse from naps, or floppy or unresponsive, seek medical help urgently.

Dehydration Babies need fluids to fight infection, so if they have refused their bottle, the breast, or water for more than eight hours, seek advice. See p.215 for signs of dehydration.

Rash While some rashes are relatively harmless symptoms of a virus, any rash is worthy of medical attention.

Ear rubbing If your baby is rubbing their ear and seems very unhappy, they may have an ear infection.

Persistent cough If they have a cough that lasts more than a week, they may have a chest infection.

Labored breathing If your baby is struggling for breath at any time, go immediately to the doctor.

Showing caution

Your baby's life is full of new experiences and not all are to their liking, so they'll naturally show caution and even distress at times.

Just a couple weeks ago, your baby may have been fearless in their curiosity and exploration but now, after a few tumbles and one too many startling discoveries, some babies will be a little more cautious in their exploration. Separation anxiety can mean they're more easily distressed in new situations, especially if they think you may be leaving. This is a natural progression as they learn about the world, and may vary from day to day or week by week as they gain confidence in each situation.

Encourage your baby to keep exploring and engaging in new situations. Stay with them while they scan the room or begin to investigate a new toy or play equipment, for example, or push them in a ride-on car, but keep talking so they know you are there, even if they can't see you.

You may find they startle easily at loud or unfamiliar noises; these often can't be avoided so handle this with plenty of cuddling and reassurance, and very simply explain, "Oh, that's a car going 'beep beep.'"

Gradually, they will become accustomed to most sounds as they experience them but, of course, being startled is a natural response to keep us safe, so it's bound to occur occasionally when there's an unexpected noise. Don't make fun of your baby's wariness or reluctance to do something, or use the phrase "Don't be silly!" It's important to keep reassuring them until they feel more comfortable in any new situation.

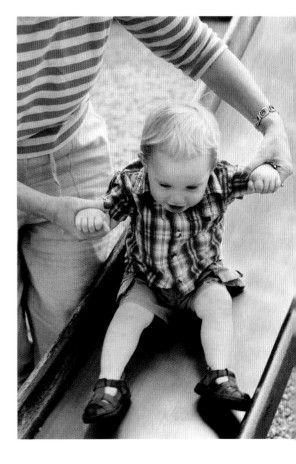

Building confidence If the height of the slide is an issue, help them come down it slowly and reassure them that you've got them and it's safe.

ASK A CHILD PSYCHOLOGIST

My baby doesn't seem to like the dark. How can I help them get used to it? For some babies, being in total or almost total darkness can be frightening (even some adults prefer to sleep with some light at night). A small nightlight may be enough to reassure your baby that all is well if they wake up, and allow them to recognize their surroundings quickly. This reluctance to be in the dark does not need to be changed or "treated"—trying to force them to sleep in total darkness is more likely to cause distress than teach them that darkness is okay. If your baby insists on having the light on at night, then use a dimmer switch to turn the light down over a period of a week or two.

Eating out

It's never too soon to get your baby used to being in a restaurant with you, but certain things can help make the experience easier.

A good indicator of a baby-friendly restaurant is that it has high chairs, baby-changing facilities, a children's menu, and kiddie activity packs. If you're unsure, call ahead to check. If you want to bring your own baby food, ask about facilities for warming it. Also, it's a good idea to reserve a table by the window so your baby has quick distractions to look at throughout the meal, if necessary.

Take plenty of tabletop activities with you. A few building blocks, board books with flaps, and a small shape sorter will keep your baby occupied while in the high chair. Time your reservation to coincide with your baby's lunchtime so they are preoccupied with eating while you are (even if you have to feed both of you simultaneously). This should also give you plenty of time before they become tired and needs their nap.

Finally, try to plan short visits with a baby this age. Sitting at a table for a long restaurant meal might be too much to ask of a little one.

ASK A PEDIATRICIAN

How do I clean my baby's ears? The ear is self cleaning—ear wax removes dust and debris from the inner ear. It may look unsightly but it's beneficial, so don't remove any lumps of wax while they are still in your baby's ear cavity. You can wipe away wax from the outer ear with a damp cotton pad. Never put a cotton swab in their ear. It will push the wax farther in, and you could poke too far and damage their eardrum.

Learning through touch

Your baby's senses teach them everything they need to know; now that they are more aware, capitalize on their ability to learn through touch.

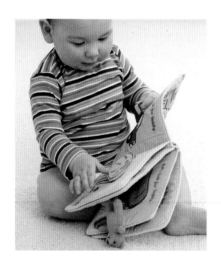

Support this learning through touch by offering different textures to feel and experiment with.

Put your baby in the high chair and present two or three bowls of different textures to get their fingers into. Make sure the contents are safe for mouthing. Some mashed-up banana, a bowl of cereal loops, some pasta shapes, and a bowl of cooked rice are all interesting textures for

Exploring textures Books that feature a variety of textures allow your baby to explore and learn through the sense of touch.

them to explore with their fingers. Keep an eye on what goes into their mouth (to prevent choking) and be ready with a clean washcloth to wipe any gooey fingers.

Give your baby books that feature a variety of fabrics and textures aimed at teaching babies the meaning of words such as silky, soft, squishy, rough, and so on. Sit with them and read these books together, and encourage your baby to touch the different textures in the book and say the words that describe them.

Using objects correctly

Your baby can associate objects with actions and anticipate sequences of events, which inspires them to use objects as they see you doing.

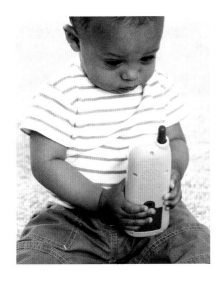

Your baby now understands that their cup holds water or juice, and is able to bring it to their mouth. They know what their toothbrush and washcloth are for, and they may try to use their spoon correctly. They will enjoy practicing these skills on a regular basis, as they learn from you.

Let your baby take a turn at squeezing the toothpaste onto their toothbrush. Let them brush their teeth alongside you, put your socks on together, and let them stir the cake batter with the wooden spoon. Trying things enhances understanding of the relationships between objects and activities. Prompt this understanding by giving them the words for the objects they use and the things you do with them. Soon your baby will point to named items, and even retrieve them.

Ask your baby to pass you their washcloth in the tub, or their cup at dinner. If they hear an instruction and the correct words often enough, while watching you point to and use objects, they'll soon make the connections necessary to understand your requests.

Who to call? As your baby gains control over their hands and fingers, they'll be eager to employ them "correctly" when using objects.

THE PINCER GRIP

The pincer grip is a fine motor skill that begins developing at around eight months of age, and becomes increasingly sophisticated as your baby grows older. To perform it, they use their index finger and thumb together to pick up and hold items. It is this grip (or grasp) that will allow them to button a shirt, use a pencil, play musical instruments, and operate a mouse on a computer in years to come. Being able to perform the pincer grip is a developmental milestone that indicates that your baby's brain, nervous system, and muscles have become much more coordinated and synchronized. It also opens up a world of possibilities for them. With a pincer grip, your baby can stack blocks, feed themself, manage a shape-sorter, and much more.

You'll notice that your baby began to pick up objects by brushing their hand over a toy, then curling their palm and fingers around it. Then they'll grasp things using all four fingers and thumb, which is still a bit awkward. As they approach 12 months, the ability to hold something between a forefinger and thumb in a pincer grip enables them to pick up and maneuver objects much more easily and precisely. To encourage the refinement of your baby's pincer grip, give them small things to pick up from the high-chair tray at mealtimes, such as cereal loops and vegetable puffs, or give them a simple lift-out puzzle to tackle. Avoid small objects that might pose a choking hazard if they put them into their mouth.

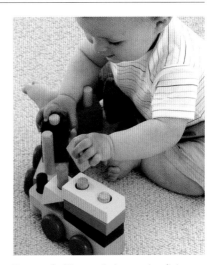

Better grip Give your baby toys that fit in their hand to help improve their whole-hand grip and, eventually, their pincer grip.

311

Encouraging self-feeding

Your baby loves to put their fingers in their food and transfer it to their mouth. Although messy, this is the start of feeding themself.

Many babies want to be independent and feed themselves but, at this age, most lack the hand–eye coordination to get food onto a spoon and into their mouths. Finger foods come into their own at this point since they allow your baby to enjoy more independence.

Use this to try to introduce a wider variety of tastes and textures now: crunchy foods, such as bread sticks, rice cakes, toast, and dry breakfast cereals are all ideal finger foods. Also try cucumber sticks, cubes of mild cheese, and cooked pasta shapes. As your baby gets better at feeding themself, you can introduce a daily meal of "small bites"—for example, mini sandwiches, pita bread, or toast cut into strips with cheese; veggie sticks with hummus; chunks of cheese or finely grated cheese; cooked vegetables; some chopped grapes, apple, pear, or banana.

Make sure that your baby's finger-food meals are balanced and healthy (see Good nutrition for babies, p.193).

You could encourage them to try new foods by adding just one new item to their finger-food meal among others you know they like.

All this practice with finger foods is great for their fine motor skills and coordination, which will help when they start to use a spoon (see p.339).

Fun with animals

Young children adore animals and soak up everything to do with them, whether looking at animal pictures, or meeting the real thing.

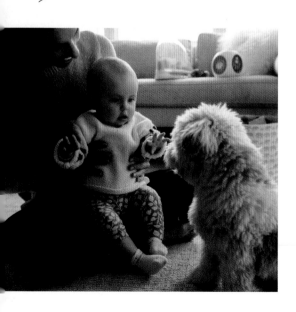

Learning about animals is a natural part of your baby's development. Familiarize by looking at pictures in books, and watching programs about animals. Talk about the animals, pointing out each one by name with the noise it makes. Sing nursery rhymes, too, that have animal noises, like Old MacDonald."

If you have a yard, consider putting up a bird feeder and let your baby watch the birds eating. Or point out regular visitors such as squirrels. On outings, point out birds, cats and dogs, and ducks and geese in ponds or rivers. Or take them to a children's petting zoo. While they may be too young to pet the animals, their senses will take in everything, and they will build confidence around them. Hygiene is of course essential to remember when handling animals. Wash hands well after being with farm or domestic animals, and make it routine to wash hands after playing in the sandpit or yard and before mealtimes. Teach your baby, even now, to ask before petting a dog.

Family pets Contact with pets increases your baby's confidence around animals. Supervise animals around your baby at all times.

The importance of affection

Showing your baby love and attention is probably second nature by now and they will thrive on as much physical affection as you can give.

Some of the most important work on babies' need for affection and attention was done by psychologist John Bowlby in the 1960s, and it has defined our way of nurturing and creating security for children ever since.

His attachment theory taught us that the bond between parent and child is the foundation for your baby's security and creates a positive pattern they will repeat in the relationships they go on to make.

A baby who has been brought up in a secure, loving environment where affection is given and received freely through hugs and kisses, pats and snuggles, is more likely to grow up to be an affectionate adult.

There have been plenty of different ideas about the "best" way to raise your baby, from the old adage that children should be "seen and not heard" through to schedule-based and more baby-led methods. Whichever approach you prefer, there's no doubt that fundamentally your baby needs your love, attention, and affection in order to develop a sense of security, stability, and confidence. When you comfort your baby, offer them lots of warm physical affection. They also need your consistency, so they can predict what reaction they will get and what pleases you. As they get older, it will be important for them to know what behavior is preferred by you and what is unacceptable.

Undivided attention

Laughing with your baby, tickling them, giggling, and giving them undivided attention is another way to show how much you love them. Studies have shown that if you are watching them playing but doing something else, too, such as reading or talking on the phone, your baby's play will be less complex than if you watch them with your full focus.

Follow their lead at playtime—sometimes they will want to be held, at other times, to get down because they want some freedom. Sometimes all they need is a gentle stroke on the cheek or head to know that you love them. By responding to, and respecting, the peaks and valleys in your baby's need for affection, you show them that you value their feelings, which means that they learn to value them themself.

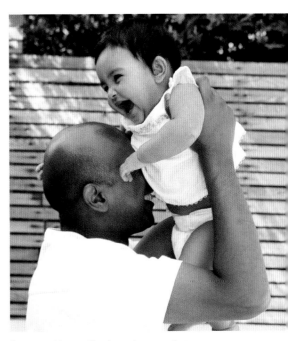

Secure and happy Consistent love, comfort, and protection from parents and caregivers helps babies develop good mental health.

BEING GENTLE

A 10-month-old baby doesn't have any real sense of their strength, and still lacks the necessary coordination to monitor how hard they pat or hold on to things. However, it is never too early to teach them to be as gentle as they can be. Encourage your baby to stroke their cuddly toys or dolls, gently holding their hand so they get a sense of the lightness of touch. Choose one special toy, perhaps a teddy bear, and give it a hug in front of your baby, then encourage them to do the same, saying "Ahhhh, teddy bear." Gently put the bear down, cover them in a blanket, and give them a kiss, then encourage your baby to do the same. Such role play reinforces a baby's understanding of the need for care and kindness with others.

11 months

MANY BABIES HAVE A FAVORITE COMFORT OBJECT THEY WANT TO TAKE EVERYWHERE. As your baby becomes more mobile, they will develop greater self-confidence and be very clear about what they do and don't want to do. Be patient but firm about the limits you've set. From their first smile at about six weeks, your baby may have progressed to fits of full-blown laughter. Enjoy!

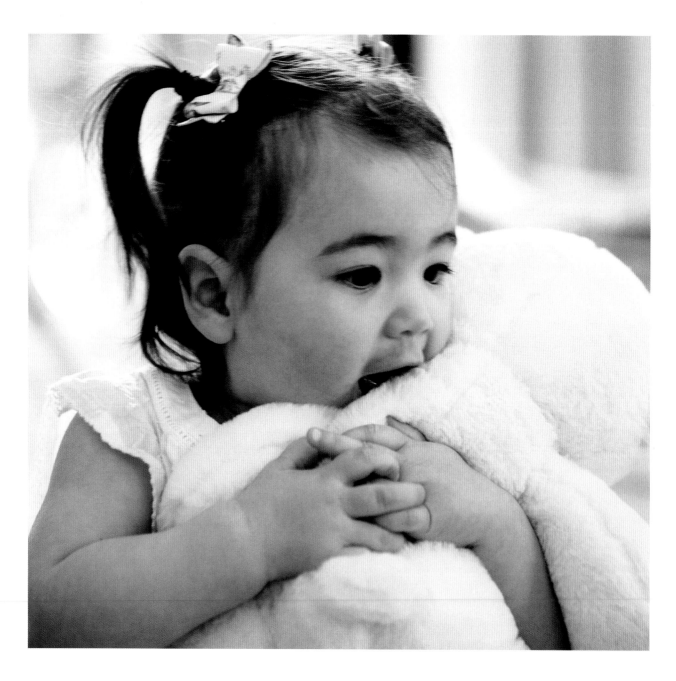

Letting your baby help

Your baby might enjoy giving you a little "help" with some small tasks, and will think it's fun to be just like you.

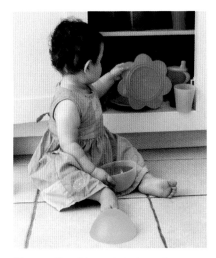

Clean up time Ask your baby to perform simple tasks, such as putting their clean bowls and plates away.

The simplest and most useful thing your baby can do for you is help you put their toys back into the toy boxes at the end of the day. If you make this activity part of the end-of-day routine, you may also find that, by the time your baby reaches toddlerhood, this behavior has become second nature. Empty a toy box in the middle of a room and turn cleaning up into a game: "Can you find the rabbit? Great! Now put the rabbit in the box." Give them lots of praise and even take turns—"Now I can find the train. Here it is! Into the box." Use the time as an opportunity to reinforce colors, shapes, animals, and so on in your baby's experience and learning.

Slowly, but surely, the straightening up will be done, if a little slowly!

Cleaning

Give your baby a clean duster and let them wipe the surfaces they can reach as they cruise around the house. Even if wiping down the sofa is not altogether very helpful, give lots of praise and encouragement for helping out. Similarly, give them a damp cloth after mealtimes and ask them to help you wipe the table— although their wipes will be in one area back and forth in front of where they're sitting, they'll get the idea, and in years to come, perhaps they'll even do it truly helpfully!

DEVELOPMENT ACTIVITY: STACKING FUN

Stacking helps develop your baby's hand–eye coordination, encourages them to figure out logic puzzles, and reinforces what they have learned about cause and effect. Good stacking toys include cups that fit inside one another and also sit on top of one another if turned upside-down (plastic measuring cups will do the job just as well), colored bricks, and hoops that go over a central cone.

To stack cups and hoops appropriately, your baby has to figure out their shapes and relative sizes and pass the objects from one hand to the other. The bricks require skill with balance, fine motor skills, and the gentle touch that's needed to get items of the same size to rest securely one

on top of the other. With either type of toy, these tasks introduce your baby to the beginnings of mathematical problem-solving, which gives them a head start with mathematical skills for later in life.

Start your baby off by showing them how the stacking is done, then tell them it's their turn. Watch as they carefully try to figure out which item goes next and give them a hand if they need it. If the toy falls over, that doesn't matter—it's all part of the learning process, and your baby will love building things back up again.

Early maths Stacking toys introduce your baby to math skills, all in the name of fun.

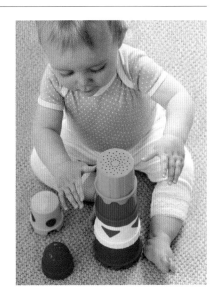

Meeting other children

Your baby will benefit from growing up with children of all ages—babies their own age will play in parallel; older children will encourage interaction.

Older children will enjoy reading to your baby and crawling around "forts" in a way adults might find awkward. Your baby might find it easier to engage with children, with whom they can play nearby, rather than with new adults who may want to interact, or interfere with their play. Children may also love the chance to "take care of" your baby and—given clear guidelines—can be surprisingly good

helpers. Even though you have to be there, it will help your baby feel more independent. Older siblings make home-grown playmates. But if your baby is your first or only, look for opportunities for them to interact with others. If you have nephews and nieces, ask them to visit or supervise a visit to their home. Meeting regularly, if practical, can build close family ties beyond your immediate circle.

If you want, you could consider going on vacation with friends with children. However, make sure there's enough space within your accommodations and that you know the other family well enough to be able to speak freely about your wishes for your baby and yourselves.

Time to yourselves

You and your partner need some time to focus on each other, and to pursue some of your favorite individual activities again.

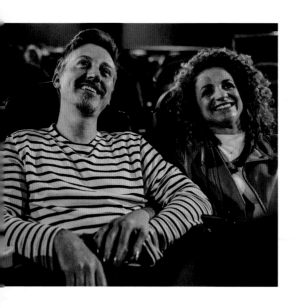

You might pay a babysitter for the evening to go out together, or schedule a night or two away, leaving your baby with a trusted friend or family member. You could set up a babysitting circle with your friends with babies so you can take turns caring for each other's babies once in a while. However you manage it, your relationship will thrive on having time to enjoy each other's company, taking in favorite activities, or treating yourselves. You can also

Just the two of you You and your partner need time away from your baby to relax and enjoy being on your own together.

give yourselves permission to resume individual activities you used to enjoy. You may want to restart a sport you have put on hold. Seeing friends socially can be a boost; whether it's shopping, going to a movie together, grabbing a coffee, or attending organized activities, this gives you time to recharge your batteries. Whatever the activity, the important thing is that you both have some time and space to do the things you enjoy and that make you each feel special, both together and as individuals.

Home comforts

There's no doubt that a comfort object is helpful, especially when your baby is anxious, but what if it starts running your life?

Your baby encounters new experiences every day. The bombardment of learning and understanding comes thick and fast at 11 months, and the whole process can be both exciting and unsettling for a baby just getting used to the notion that they are independent from you. It's little wonder, then, that comfort objects (sometimes called transitional or security objects) provide a constant. They represent your love; they smell of home; and they have positive, safe associations. Your baby will need their comfort object when you are not nearby, when they experience something new, or when they feel ill or tired. Sometimes, they may rely on their comfort object so heavily they can't bear to let it go.

This is all very well, but can start to fray the most patient parent's nerves after a while. It's difficult enough to remember everything you need when you go out, but simply frustrating if you're halfway down the road with baby safely in the car seat when they start wailing—because you've left their "best friend" behind! Plus, you are saddled with the huge responsibility of keeping track of—and never, ever losing—your baby's most precious possession.

Go with the flow

There's little you can do about this situation other than accept it and make contingency plans. Once your baby has formed an attachment to a particular thing, taking it away will make them feel insecure and upset. So ideally, they should be able to reach their comfort object whenever they need it, wherever they happen to be. Eventually, they'll either grow out of it, or you'll need to help them let go of the object gradually, but not until they're older. For the time being, do all you can to protect it. If possible, buy a couple of spares in case it gets lost. If your baby is attached to an irreplaceable blanket, consider cutting it in half so you can wash one half, while the other is being used. Try to wash it before it becomes too deeply embedded with your baby's scent so they don't reject it when clean (and are less likely to notice when you swap it for one of the spares while the original is in the laundry).

DEVELOPMENT ACTIVITY: TUNNEL TIME

Babies of this age love playing in toy tunnels. Nylon tunnels are readily available from most good toy stores. However, a tunnel made from three cardboard boxes taped together with their ends open can work just as well. Customize it with peepholes along its length so your baby can see you. Encourage them to crawl inside the tunnel, perhaps by placing a few toys inside, and play peekaboo as they emerge from one end. Or surprise them yourself by appearing "magically" at the opposite end. If they seem confident within it, you could hang a blanket over one end for them to peek out. Don't force them to play with the tunnel if they seem nervous about going inside—just leave it on the floor until they are ready to explore.

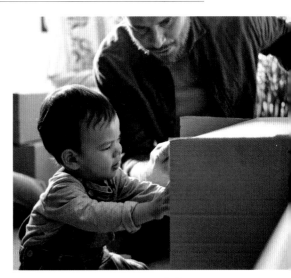

Tunnel play Exploring in a toy tunnel helps develop your baby's gross motor skills and powers of anticipation.

Story and rhyme sessions

As well as enjoying books at home, it can be fun to join in with story and rhyme activities with other babies and parents.

Most libraries now offer membership to children from birth, and actively encourage babies and toddlers to make the most of their facilities, including dedicated activity sessions for babies, using rhymes, stories, songs, and possibly pictures and puppets, to help keep little ones entertained and interested. Not only is this sociable and interactive for your baby, it also provides an opportunity for you to meet other parents and explore the wealth of books on offer in the library. Visiting the library from an early age and encouraging your baby to explore and enjoy books will set them up for reading activities as they grow older.

If you don't have a library close to your home, your local parent and baby group may have a story-time session that you can join—if not, why not suggest that you start one? A book club for babies!

AS A MATTER OF FACT

Babies laugh much more frequently than adults: an average baby laughs around 300 times a day, compared to an average adult, who laughs around 20 times a day—although how much we laugh also depends on personality. Between 9 and 15 months, babies understand that when Mom puts a diaper on her head or "moos" like a cow, she's doing something unexpected—and that it's funny.

Quality time

If one or both of you are out at work all day, it's important to make sure you have some one-on-one quality time with your baby.

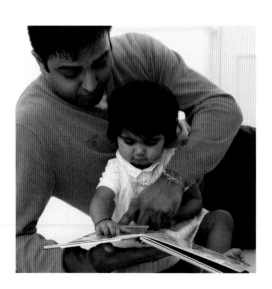

Reading style Each parent may have a unique reading style that stimulates your baby's enjoyment of story time in different ways.

Babies derive and learn different things from each parent, so it's important that your baby gets individual time with each of you if at all possible. This can be difficult to manage when one or both of you work, but your different ways of parenting are equally stimulating for your baby, which broadens their understanding of human uniqueness. One of you is often a source of comfort and peace, for example, while the other represents excitement and fun. Love and attention from you both helps promote your child's social, emotional, and intellectual development.

If you're both at home in the evenings, try to organize your routine so one of you does bath time, and one of you reads the bedtime story, then you both get to kiss your baby and say good night. Or try to plan things so at least one of you gets to sit down and have breakfast with your baby before you go out in the morning. When you do have time off together, make sure you play individually with your baby, as well as together.

On the way to walking

At this age, your baby will probably crawl, possibly pull themself up to standing, and may even cruise—but when will they walk?

It's natural to look forward with excitement to witnessing your baby's first steps—after all, as they totter unsteadily toward your waiting arms for the very first time, they're taking huge strides on the road to independence.

If your baby is by now cruising reasonably confidently along the furniture, it's possible they may take their first independent steps at any time. However, since the average age for babies to take their first steps is at 13 months, it is unusual—though not unheard of—for them to start walking this early.

Walking depends on the development of gross motor skills, coordination, and build (a baby with a long body and short legs, for example, might find it harder to get their balance). If your baby was late to hold their head up or sit unaided, they're likely also to be late to walk—their gross motor function is taking a little longer than average to reach each milestone. There's no apparent correlation between early walkers and athleticism or intelligence—some babies simply do it sooner than others.

Slowly, slowly

Your baby's first steps are more likely to be a side-to-side shuffle that gradually inches them forward rather than a striding march. Only once they have developed much better coordination and balance (often not until the age of two) will they pick up one foot to place it in front of the other. Until then, they will take lots of little steps, barely raising their feet from the floor at all. Babies also keep their feet wide apart and bend their knees, making them look bow-legged, and they tend to walk with a slightly arched back and toes pointing inward. Early walking may not look elegant, but it'll seem miraculous to you.

Once your baby starts walking, patience will be your biggest virtue. They'll need you to hold their hand and match their snail's pace as you walk to the car, or to fetch something from another room. Progress can be frustratingly slow, especially when you're in a hurry. But try to avoid scooping them up too often—they need all the practice they can get!

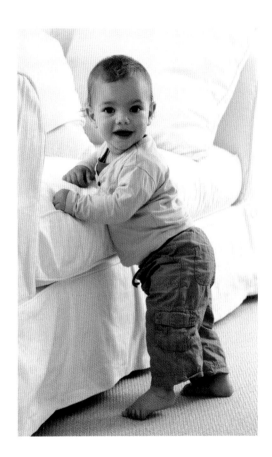

Enjoying mobility As long as your baby is moving around, it doesn't matter whether they do it on their bottom or legs for now.

DEVELOPMENT ACTIVITY: CRUISE CONTROL

If your baby is at the stage where they're pulling themself up but not quite cruising yet, you can encourage them by putting a toy a few feet away from them so they have to side-step to get it. The more stepping they do, the better their stability and coordination will become.

All this movement is good exercise for their leg muscles, making them stronger; and good practice for lifting and planting their feet. Once they're more competent at cruising, you can place the toy a little farther away, or on the next chair, to encourage your baby to move between pieces of furniture.

Parenting with confidence

As you race toward the end of your baby's first year, reflect on just how much you've learned—and be proud of yourselves as parents.

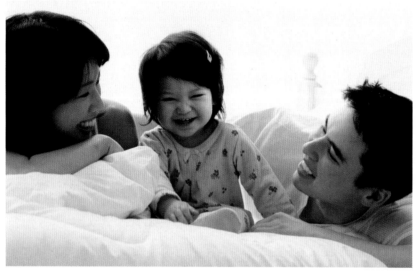

Happy family Being confident in your decisions and abilities as a parent will help you, your partner, and your baby enjoy family life that much more.

You are not alone. Your parents, your friends, and your pediatrician are all there to offer advice and support if you need it. Together, you and your partner demonstrate that confident parenting isn't solitary.

Be confident

Your baby looks to you for guidance—and will for years. No parent always gets it right, just have faith that your decisions are made with the best intentions. Believe in them, but also be able to abandon them if you realize you've made a mistake. It is a sign of strength to be able to admit when you are wrong, take responsibility for the error, and move on.

Be firm

Your self-confidence as a parent shines through in your ability to set boundaries for your baby. No matter how much they protest something you have good reason to say no to, or to prevent them from doing, hold firm. Your baby is more likely to grow up into a confident individual if they see that you mean what you say.

Be happy

Finally, love the job you're doing. Every day, as you watch your baby grow and learn something new, be proud of them—and yourself. They will feed off your delight, which means they will be happy, too.

CONFIDENT PARENTING

Do …
• **Take the positives** from your own upbringing and repeat the good practices your parents had, and learn from the best aspects of other parenting styles you see around you.
• **Think about the negative parenting** traits your parents or others might have had—and avoid repeating them.
• **Treat your baby with respect,** which doesn't mean giving in to them all the time—but instead gently setting firm boundaries.
• **Talk to your baby** as you would like to be spoken to, listen to them as you'd like to be listened to, and be there to comfort them whenever they need you.
• **Always show love**—tell your baby how much you love them, and let your actions speak louder than your words.

Don't …
• **Be hard on yourself** if your plans go awry—if your baby is growing and happy, you're doing fine.
• **Be critical of your partner**—always discuss your differing approaches and keep an open mind to the specifics of your parenting styles. Remember, you both have your baby's best interests at heart.
• **Be afraid to ask for help:** there are lots of resources available to you—use them if you need to.

Breastfeeding and your bust

Breastfeeding doesn't change the shape or size of your breasts—it's pregnancy that does that. Here is some key know-how.

During pregnancy, a surge in hormones causes your breasts to increase in size. They stay like this throughout pregnancy, and if you breastfeed, will stay this size more or less until you're baby is weaned. (If you don't breastfeed, your breasts will return to their pre-pregnancy size a few weeks after giving birth.)

Your breasts don't contain any muscle, but are attached to the muscles of your chest wall by thin ligaments. As your breasts increase in size, these supportive ligaments may stretch, which happens regardless of whether or not you breastfeed. If you gained a lot of weight during pregnancy, and go on to lose it, this can have an effect on your breasts, too. It's important to wear a properly fitting nursing bra when breastfeeding to support your breasts.

Your breasts are made up of fatty tissue, so if you gain weight your breasts will grow larger, and if you lose it, they shrink. The amount they shrink should be in proportion to your weight loss, so if you become slimmer than you were prior to pregnancy, your breasts are likely to be smaller than they were, too.

Your breasts might be a little less firm when you stop feeding, but there is some good news. In the six months or so after stopping, fatty tissue will gradually replace the milk-producing tissue in your breasts, which leaves your breasts feeling fuller. Exercising your pectoral muscles (see box, below) can help your breasts become firmer and more lifted. Well-hydrated skin has more elasticity and looks smoother, so drink plenty of water and use moisturizer to keep your neckline feeling soft and supple.

Get remeasured by a professional bra fitter when you stop nursing in case your breast size has changed.

STRENGTHENING YOUR PECTORALS FOR A FIRMER BUSTLINE

A pair of handheld weights or a couple small bottles of water will help you get the best results with some of the techniques below.

Push-ups If you're new to push-ups, place your hands on the floor, extend your legs out behind you, and rest your knees on the floor. Cross your ankles. Support yourself on your arms, keeping your back straight. Bend your elbows to lower your upper body so your nose touches the ground, then straighten your arms to raise yourself again. Repeat 10 times, rest, then do another 10 times. If you are concerned about straining your abdominals or uterus, try an inverted push-up. Stand facing a wall with your arms outstretched and palms placed on the wall at shoulder height. Gently bend your elbows to move your body toward the wall, then straighten them to return to the starting position.

Chest press Lie on your back with your arms above you, elbows slightly bent, and a weight in each hand. Slowly and deliberately lower your arms out to the sides, keeping your elbows bent, until your fists hover over the ground. Raise your arms to your starting position. Do 15 repetitions, rest, then do 15 more.

Overhead press Stay on your back with a weight in each hand, arms above you, elbows slightly bent. Gently lower your arms over your head until you feel the weight touch the floor behind your head, then bring your arms back up to the starting position. Do 15 repetitions, rest, then do 15 more.

Chest stretch To wind down, stretch the muscles you have been exercising. Sit with your back straight and hold your hands behind your back, bringing your shoulder blades together to open up your chest. Hold for a count of 10, then release.

Baby talk

Listen very carefully—your baby might be saying actual words, but you may not have noticed. Encourage them by repeating their first words

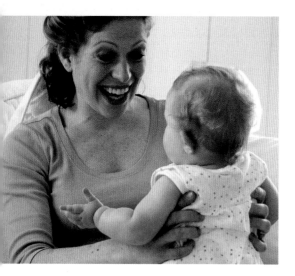

In some cases, it's not easy to recognize the words your baby says, but at other times, they may be obvious. Perhaps if they like trains, they might say "choo-choo," or they might say "meow" when they see a cat. Their increased vocabulary doesn't have to be full of the actual nouns that we attribute to objects.

Consider, too, that your baby's words might lack an ending. It is perfectly normal for babies to be

Clever! Your baby loves to babble, but if you listen carefully to what they're saying, you might hear some actual words!

unable to make the hard sounds at the ends of words when they first begin to talk. In which case, a horn noise might be more a "too" than a "toot," a cat might be a "cah," and a dog, a "doh."

Although your baby might be closer to two years old before they have a real knack for finishing their words, you can help the process along by keeping background noise to a minimum when you talk to them, so they can hear you clearly. Also, be careful to finish your words. From time to time, feel free to exaggerate the hard sounds at the ends of words a little to help them focus on them.

Sheer determination

Babies are remarkably resilient and steadfastly tenacious when it comes to achieving something they have set their minds on doing.

The utter determination of babies is what drives them to learn new skills and develop the ones they already have every single day. Of course, if there is a downside to your baby's will to try it again and again, it is that they might be unwilling to let you help them, which can mean that some practical tasks—such as putting on a hat so you can go out—take significantly longer than they might if you stepped in.

Teachers increasingly report a pattern that suggests that when students struggle, they are unwilling to go back to a task to see it through to its conclusion. Try to encourage stickability in your baby by praising their willingness to keep trying, and giving them lots of chances to repeat until they succeed, have had enough and turn away naturally, or allow you to help them. Above all, give them lots of praise for their continued efforts.

ASK A MOM

My baby has started biting me and it hurts. How do I stop them? Your baby has no idea they're hurting you, but it's not a habit that you want to encourage! Make sure you don't react too strongly but do say "Ouch, that hurts" and give a matching expression. Sit them on the floor for a minute and distract them. They'll soon get the message that this is something you don't like.

Time for playgroup

Helping your baby socialize will teach them important life skills, from communicating with peers to learning to be kind.

Now is a good time to start taking your baby to a playgroup, because they'll enjoy playing near other children and playing new games and with different toys. The closer the playgroup is to home, the better, because your baby can make friends with children who live nearby, and who one day might even go to school with them. Some groups are run by the community, others by local churches or a group of dedicated parents (who will pass the baton as their own children head off to school). Try out a few in your area, finding one (or more) that feels the friendliest and that your baby seems to enjoy the most.

What to expect

Much of what happens at playgroups depends upon their size. A small playgroup might have a room or area for toddlers, with a few climbing toys and arts-and-crafts activities, and a separate room or area for babies. Larger playgroups will have whole rooms dedicated to aspects of play—perhaps a room for painting (or other messy play), a room for babies, and a room for active play for toddlers. Most offer soft drinks and coffee and light snacks, as well as drinks and snacks suitable for the children. At the end of the session, there is usually a circle time, when everyone joins together to sing some songs, celebrate birthdays, and give notices about activities.

As a rule, playgroups are informal and relaxed, and parents are free to play with their children and talk to other parents as they wish. Some groups will ask for a small contribution each time you visit (or periodically) and some will ask if you would be willing to help out one week—perhaps by serving snacks or doing some craft preparation at home. Getting involved is a great way to feel part of a community.

Baby doesn't want to play

The noise levels and frenzied activity at some playgroups can be quite daunting for some babies, and if your baby doesn't want to get off your lap the first few times you go, don't despair. Find an activity that the two of you can do together, or simply find a book and read to them. Once you have been several times, their natural curiosity will get the better of them, and they'll go off to explore. However, bear in mind that, at only 11 months, they will be happy playing alongside other babies, but won't necessarily want to play with them.

DEVELOPMENT ACTIVITY: FLOUR PAINTING

Find a shallow tray, ideally in a dark color. Sprinkle some flour over the tray and rock the tray back and forth so there is an even covering across its surface. Now show your baby how to trace their finger through the flour to "draw" patterns and shapes. This activity is far less messy than using paints! Flour "painting" is a great way of bringing out the budding artist in your baby, and it will help them develop their fine motor skills, which are so important for drawing and writing later on in life.

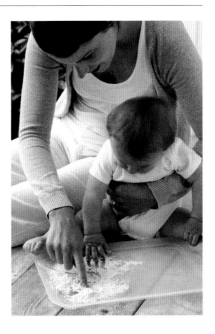

Budding artist Flour painting is a good way of introducing your baby to the concept of mark-making. They'll enjoy drawing shapes as well as the tactile quality of this activity.

Sleeping through the night

If your baby isn't sleeping through the night yet, don't worry, you are not alone. However, an 11-month-old should be capable of a good night's rest, so it's worth considering whether some of the ideas below might help you both get the sleep you need.

Your baby needs sleep so they can process the events of their day, and in order to grow. You and your partner need sleep, too. Generally, having too little sleep makes us irritable, impatient, and uncompromising—hardly a recipe for family harmony.

While it may seem hard to tackle your baby's night-waking now, any bad habits they establish will become even harder to break as they get older.

Assuming that their nap times are working well, at night an 11-month-old baby should be able to sleep for a good stretch, perhaps 10 to 12 hours. By this age, they should be eating 2–3 meals a day, possibly with snacks in between, so they shouldn't need any nighttime milk feedings.

Reasons for waking

If your baby isn't used to settling themself back to sleep during the lightest phase of the sleep cycle (which, as adults, we don't notice), they will rouse fully and call out for comfort or for milk. This can become a habit if you always comply. Babies who are between 9 and 12 months often also suffer from separation anxiety, which can become acute when they wake alone in the darkness. Other reasons for waking might be that your baby is getting too much sleep in the daytime, napping too late in the afternoon, or might just be struggling to reestablish good habits after a bout of illness or teething pain that caused nighttime waking.

The key thing is to decide which approach or approaches you feel comfortable trying, and stick to them. Keep in mind that if your baby has been consistently wakeful in the night (that is, you've never had a period during which they have slept through), breaking the habit can take up to three weeks of persistent effort. Don't give up!

Bedtime basics

Your baby will benefit from a strict but loving bedtime routine. Give plenty of positive and soothing signals that it's time for bed. Spend the last hour of the day engaged in quiet interaction together. This way, they'll get plenty of positive attention that will encourage them to feel calm. Give them a bath, get them dressed for bed, and read them a bedtime story. Saving one story specifically for bedtime is an unequivocal signal of what is coming next.

When the time comes to sleep, cuddle and kiss them, put them in the crib, settle them down, say good night, then leave the room. You can leave a nightlight on if you wish, and perhaps soothing music. Ensure the crib is a happy place to be. Avoid using it as a convenient place to confine your baby while you do something quickly. Instead, make it a place where their favorite cuddly toy sleeps, where they keep their comfort object when they aren't using it, and where they see a big smile from you last thing at night and first thing in the morning.

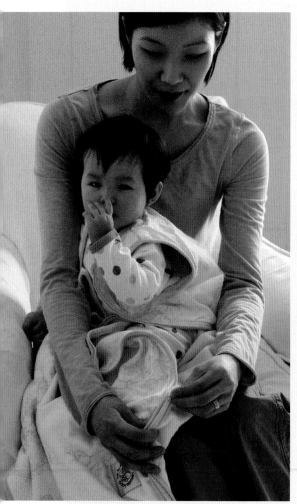

Cozy bedtime routine Keep the last hour of your baby's day restful as you prepare for bed with lots of reassuring cuddles and kisses. Encourage them to self-soothe while slumbering in their crib.

Midnight mayhem

If your baby has a tendency to wake up and want to play, you need to convince that nighttime is a time to rest. If they are crying, soothe them calmly, but don't chat with or engage them. If your baby's nap times are too long, or they're having a late afternoon nap, they may not be tired enough at bedtime to sleep through the night. You could move their afternoon nap forward by 15 minutes, and make it 15 minutes shorter, too. You don't want your baby to be overtired when they go to bed, but be ready for sleep.

Waking for a feeding

If you're in the habit of giving your baby a nighttime breast- or bottle feeding, this can be hard to give up, especially if there is a part of you that enjoys the closeness you share in the still of the night. You can try gradually reducing the amount of milk you are giving, either by reducing the time you spend breastfeeding or by gradually decreasing the amount of formula in the bottle over several nights. Or you could start offering your baby water instead of milk when they wake; over time they may not consider this worth waking up for. You'll be more confident that they are not actually hungry if you know they have eaten well and had a milk feeding before bedtime.

Waking for a cuddle

If your baby is determined to have your reassuring presence in the night, it can be hard to keep getting out of your warm bed. However, be aware that if you take them into bed with you (see box, opposite), they will not learn to settle in the crib—and that when they are a toddler they will take up a lot of room in your bed! If you prefer to have them sleep in their own space, it is best to soothe them by going to them when

they call and patting them in the crib, talking calmly or singing, rather than lifting them out to cuddle. Some babies need to have a short wind-down cry before they go to sleep, so be careful not to mistake this for a summons.

Sleep "training"

You may have heard other sleep techniques mentioned, for example gradual withdrawal or controlled crying. Gradual withdrawal is the gentler method that involves soothing your baby to sleep in the usual way, but then laying them in the crib just before they drift off, and sitting in the room (without engaging with them) until they fall asleep. Eventually they should learn to go to sleep with you at the other side of the room, and then with you out of the room altogether.

Controlled crying involves soothing your baby in the crib by stroking and patting them when they wake, but each time they cry leaving them to wait a little longer before you go to them, the idea being that eventually they learn to soothe themself back to sleep. Many experts, though, feel controlled crying

is not advisable on the grounds that it is stressful for babies and parents.

With all the different methods, consistency is essential.

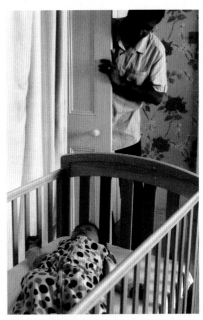

Restful sleep Babies need a good night's sleep so the brain can consolidate the day's learning and the body can recharge for more action.

IN BED TOGETHER

There's little doubt that a baby in their parents' bed is less likely to wake up crying or be difficult to settle at night. However, even if at this point you are all getting a good night's sleep, as your baby gets older your nights are likely to be less peaceful. As your baby gets bigger (and stronger), they'll move more, kick, and make a noise at night. There are also risks associated with co-sleeping, and it is not advised in certain circumstances (see pp.30–31). If you or your baby are not co-sleeping as soundly as before, you may wish to think about moving them into their own bed sooner rather than later. Some babies make the transition easily, others need to get used to the idea—you may have to keep your baby's crib in your room for a while, for example. Even if your baby moves out, your bed can still be a great place for cuddles in the morning!

Toy time

Choosing appropriate toys for your baby can be mind-boggling. Observe them at play to help you select toys that will interest them.

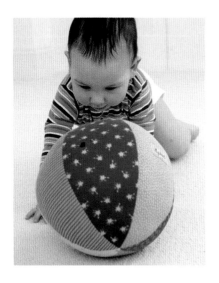

Your baby's thinking and problem solving are geared to fun and discovery. Books, balls, building blocks, and stacking cups are all great for honing their ability to understand cause and effect and shape and size, and to develop their problem-solving skills. Make sure items are of a size that your baby can hold and pass from one hand to the other easily.

Any toys that encourage movement, or support your baby as they pull to

Fun with learning Toys designed for this stage of your baby's development will help them enjoy and be enthusiastic about learning.

stand, are also good choices. Check the age-range on new toys before you buy to make sure that they are suitable for your baby's age and stage of development. A toy should suit your baby's individual level of mobility, dexterity, and understanding. You don't need to spend a fortune on store-bought toys—make use of things you might you might have lying around the house. For example, the inner tubes of paper towel rolls or wrapping paper rolls make wonderful "trumpets," and a cardboard box is fantastic for climbing into and out of, or to use as a "net" for a thrown ball.

Shapes and sizes

You can start to introduce new concepts such as large and small now, but don't expect your baby to identify these all by themselves yet.

Comment on familiar objects and describe their properties using words such as "bigger," "smaller," "soft," and "hard." Your baby will start to grasp these concepts in the months to come.

Introduce shape-sorters and toys of different sizes and textures, and your baby will act out concepts such as in and out and large and small without realizing. Play story games with their soft toys or teddy bears, talking about little baby ted and big

mommy or daddy teddy. Then you can show them the toys and ask, "Show me the big one." Soon they'll be experimenting with these ideas intentionally. Make use of stories that contain themes about shapes and sizes, especially those with sensory panels. Talk to your baby about big, small; round, square; high, low, and so on, bringing shape and size into conversations and observations on a regular basis.

AS A MATTER OF FACT

Don't be surprised if your baby's eyes are still changing color. Although base eye color is usually established between six and nine months, subtle changes in tone may be noticed later as more dark pigment is produced in the iris (green eyes turning more hazel, for example, or hazel eyes becoming deeper brown). Eye color can keep changing into toddlerhood, and sometimes even in adulthood.

Time away from your baby

You're bound to have mixed feelings about a night away from your baby. Leaving them with caregivers you trust will make it easier.

Now that you are so accustomed to being responsible for your baby's welfare, it can be quite difficult to "let go" and hand them over to someone else, especially for a whole night. For this reason, it's important to be comfortable with whomever you choose to care for them while you are away. And it helps if they're very familiar to your baby and have an idea of their routine and preferences.

Preparing your baby

In the week leading up to your absence, spend lots of time with the person or people who'll be looking after your baby. Ideally, have them come to stay with you, so your baby has the security of their own home as they get to know each other. If you can invite the caregivers to stay for a few days before you leave, all the better. Ask them to do some feeding, nap time, bedtime, and waking routines so your baby is used to their care by the time you leave.

Preparing the caregivers

By familiarizing themselves with your routines before you leave, your baby's caregivers will be well prepared. Ensure they know which foods baby can eat (leave meals prepared meals if you can) and which snacks. While, you may prefer they kept to your schedule, let them know it's okay to make changes in order to keep your baby happy.

If your baby is staying with their caregiver, ensure they have a crib, their comfort object, and plenty of food, diapers, and changes of clothes. Prepare for a day longer than your planned absence to guarantee they will be short of nothing. Ask the caregivers to perform a quick babyproofing check with you before you leave. Always leave emergency contact details.

Preparing yourself

Agree on times to call before you go so you can check on how your baby is doing. When the time comes to leave, be cheerful, brave, and purposeful. If you sneak off, they may worry that you won't be back. Give them a wave, and hit the road.

ASK A CHILD PSYCHOLOGIST

Will my baby get out of their routine with another caregiver overnight?
It can be unsettling for your baby to be in a different environment, and their routine is bound to change, at least a little bit. However, your baby is able to tolerate brief variations to the usual schedule as long as the routine at home is well established. Once they're home, quickly settle back into the usual pattern and don't be tempted to keep them up late or change things because you want extra time or want to "treat" them because you've been away.

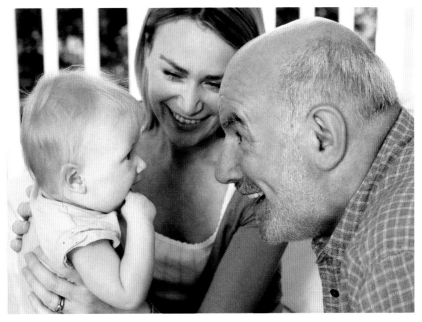

Preparation for your absence In the week before you go away, make sure your baby spends plenty of time with whomever will be taking care of them during your absence.

Building language skills

Around this time, you might want to use a bit less "parentese," start to lower your pitch, and make your intonation more adult in style.

At this stage, encourage all forms of communication between you and your baby. Whether your baby uses words you can understand or not, give them the space to say what they want to say, even if it appears to be gibberish. When your baby pauses in their babbling, respond with adult language. What they need to hear back from you is the correct way of saying things.

Try to refine your understanding of what they are saying. For example, ask, "Are you asking me for a drink?" or,

"Would you like to go out?" or, "Would you like the teddy?" Don't worry if you can't immediately tell what they mean; keep trying and you may get a smile to show you've got it right. Listen and respond to their sounds and first words, and show your delight so they'll know they're on the right track. Allowing your baby to speak, and then listening and responding to them, encourages their language skills and builds their communication confidence.

ASK A PEDIATRICIAN

My baby wakes during the night and wants a bottle of formula. How can I discourage this? Your baby shouldn't be hungry during the night now; they should have taken in all the calories they require during the day. Often, the only reason babies of this age demand a feeding at night is for comfort. Make sure they have a good last feeding before bedtime and offer water if they wake in case they are thirsty.

Muscle development

Your baby's fine and gross motor skills have come a long way, but there's still plenty you can do to encourage their development.

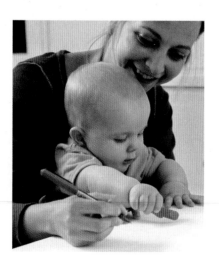

Gripping a crayon Scribbling is fun and improves your baby's fine motor skills.

The muscles of your baby's legs and arms continue to strengthen with every physical challenge. Encourage your baby to climb over and under soft pieces of furniture (with a soft landing), up stairs (with supervision), and in a soft-play environment. Playing games such as "Row, Row, Row Your Boat" helps to develop good upper-body strength. Also, try dancing with your baby by holding their body or hands as they

stand and bounce, which is great for developing their leg muscles.

Your baby is now more able to control their smaller muscles, such as those in the fingers. Get them used to paint and paper by making handprints, or guiding paint-covered fingers across paper to create their first painting. You can try giving them a fat crayon if you think they'll hold it and guiding their hand to make a mark across the paper. It might be a bit early to grapple with this yet, but you'll probably find that they have a strong grip—if you try to take the crayon away, they may not let go willingly!

Encouraging healthy eating

Help your baby develop a taste for healthy foods before they start to develop any particularly strong likes or dislikes.

Although your baby is too young to stir or chop, they can sit with you as you prepare their food and talk them through the process of what you're doing. If you can spark their interest in what they're eating and make them feel part of the preparation process, they're more likely to be open-minded about enjoying it.

Allow them to experience the textures of what you're feeding them before and after cooking and talk to them about the colors of the foods. For instance, say to them, "This is a carrot—look how orange it is! Shall I peel the carrot?"

Make it visually appealing

If you were presented with a plate of food in a restaurant that looked unappealing, it's unlikely you would want to eat it. Your baby's response to food is no different. Babies love bright colors, different shapes, and, once they can cope with small, soft lumps, a variety of textures. Use these facts to make the healthy foods you offer your baby look interesting and appetizing.

Arrange different types of foods in little piles on your baby's plate—for instance, put gently steamed vegetables they can pick up with their fingers in one area, and chicken casserole in another. Try serving your baby's meals on plates that have separate compartments—these are often brightly colored and decorated to appeal especially to babies and toddlers.

If you are feeling artistic, you can use finger foods to create fun faces, or make a train out of mini sandwiches. Use shaped cookie cutters to make shaped sandwiches—your baby will love eating a star or flower!

Another good trick is to create swirls or other shapes of colorful fruit compote in a bowl of otherwise bland-looking oatmeal.

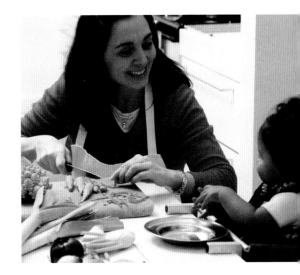

Sous chef Spark your baby's interest in meals by talking to them about how they are made and getting them to "help" you.

FINGER-FOOD DUNKERS

Your baby loves to feed themselves, so encourage this developing skill with finger-food dunkers. They'll enjoy this fun way of eating healthy foods. Below are ideas to get you started, but be warned—they are messy!
• **Homemade baby guacamole** Mix chopped tomatoes with mashed avocado and a teaspoon of lemon juice; serve with whole-grain toast.
• **Tomato sauce and pasta** Make a simple tomato pasta sauce and offer your baby a few very softly cooked pasta twists (chopped into smaller chunks, if necessary) to dunk in it.
• **Cheese fondue** Make a cheese fondue: in a pan ,gently heat 1oz (25g) butter, 1oz (25g) cream cheese, and 2oz (50g) grated

mild cheddar cheese until melted. Serve with chunks of bread or toast and lightly steamed vegetables for dipping (halved new potatoes are good).
• **Pancake dippers** Strips of pancake or pieces of banana can be dipped into plain yogurt.
• **Meatball dippers** Dip meatballs into a fresh tomato sauce.
• **Yogurt dippers** Dip chunks of steamed fish (check for bones), or chicken into a minty yogurt dip made of creamy Greek yogurt and chopped fresh mint.
• **Homemade fish fingers** Dip in a homemade tomato sauce.

Work vs. home?

There are positives both to going back to work and to staying at home, so it's a good idea to remind yourself of these occasionally.

Going back to work is beneficial for more than just your finances:
• You will quickly relearn all the important information and skills you need to do your job.
• It can be a confidence boost in your independence beyond your home.
• It can be a nice change to dress up in your work clothes.
• It allows you to socialize and see the colleagues whose company you enjoy but may have missed for a while.

Benefits to staying at home are:
• You're around to witness your baby's every milestone.
• You have time to reassess your career and look at new work opportunities.
• You have the opportunity to connect to your local community and network with parents.
• You have more time to get active, enjoying exercise on your own or together with your baby.

A NEW CAR SEAT

Your baby may outgrow their infant-only car seat between 9 and 12 months. (Requirements vary by model and by the baby's height and weight.) Convertible car seats can be used first in the rear-facing position and later facing forward. (This isn't recommended at least until age two.) Requirements vary by model, but a convertible car seat may bring your child all the way through preschool.

What's that noise?

Your baby is interested in all the sounds they hear around them, so help them learn about the different noises in their world.

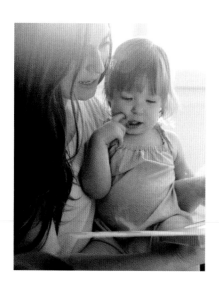

Say it out loud Sound out the noises of objects and animals in your baby's picture books.

You can have lots of fun teaching your baby about the many different noises they're likely to encounter. From cars to animals to the telephone or doorbell ringing, there's plenty of scope to hone your skills of imitation or engineer it so your baby hears the real thing.

Play with toy animals with your baby and demonstrate the noises they make. If barking, mooing, and meowing all gets a bit much, think about buying, or borrowing from the library, an animal sounds book so you can help your baby push the animal buttons to hear "baas" or birdsong. Or you can download an app designed to teach babies about animal noises.

You can teach your baby about everyday household noises, too, so they aren't startled when there's a knock at the door, or you turn on the vacuum cleaner. Help them push the doorbell so they can hear the noise it makes. They'll soon start to remember who or what makes the noises they hear.

Extended breastfeeding

Extended or long-term breastfeeding means breastfeeding beyond your baby's first year—so is it for you?

The longer you breastfeed your baby, the longer they will benefit from the goodness in your breast milk. Breast milk becomes more concentrated in its nutritional benefits when your baby is feeding less often, and continues to provide them with vitamins A, C, B12, and large amounts of folate, calories, protein, and calcium. However, it is also true that by the time your baby reaches their first birthday, their primary source of nutrients will be the food they eat.

The World Health Organization (WHO) has identified that toddlers between the ages of 16 and 30 months who breastfed have been found to have fewer illnesses, as well as illnesses of shorter duration than non-breast-feeding toddlers.

Extended breastfeeding has benefits for your health and well-being, too. There is a reduced risk of developing certain cancers, including breast, ovarian, uterine, and endometrial cancer. The WHO also suggests that it may reduce the risk of osteoporosis.

A decision for you

How long you choose to breastfeed should be entirely dependent on what feels right for you and your baby, because the experience of breastfeeding is a very personal and individual one. You may encounter negative opinions about the benefits of breastfeeding beyond six months or a year. If you experience negative comments from those whose opinions matter to you, simply explain why you are continuing to breastfeed, giving particular emphasis to the benefits for your baby—cited as a greater sense of security and confidence.

Many parents of older babies continue to partially breastfeed—offering breast milk in the morning and evening as a comforting start and end to the day. This can be ideal because your baby shouldn't need regular nursing during the day if they are properly established on solids.

Still breastfeeding While it's more unusual in the West, breastfeeding older babies and toddlers is normal in many cultures.

AS A MATTER OF FACT

In Western culture, breastfeeding much beyond infancy is now relatively rare, despite the fact that the World Health Organization (WHO) actively recommends breastfeeding for at least the first two years of a child's life.

Up until the 1960s, women in many cultures, including in Kenya, Mongolia, and New Guinea, routinely breastfed their babies until they were three to five years old. However, this practice is becoming less prevalent as more women in these countries enter the workforce. Today, there are few societies where children are routinely breastfed until they are three or four years old, and these communities tend to be found in low-income countries, such as the Sirionó people in Bolivia. In the US, initial breastfeeding rates have risen—75 percent of new moms breastfed according to 2019 Centers for Disease Control and Prevention (CDC) figures. However, the number still breastfeeding at six months drops to 55 percent.

Leading by example

By watching and copying you, your baby is starting to use you as a role model to follow. Keep setting them good examples.

FOCUS ON TWINS: TWIN TALK

Do your twins give the impression that they understand each other's babbling? Most experts agree that twins don't share a "language" as such, but rather a "code," or series of shortcuts they develop when conversing with each other. This usually starts in infancy, when twins copy one another's immature speech patterns, such as jumbled sounds and made-up words. Because both twins are developing at the same rate, they often reinforce each others' communicative attempts and increase their own language. Although "twin talk" may be cute, you should help your children learn to use correct language when speaking. You can do this by speaking to your twins individually rather than together, and reading to them so they hear plenty of words.

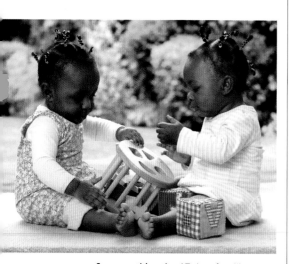

Say something then! Twins often like to copy each other's babble.

Your baby may not have uttered their first word yet, but may be shaking their head to say "no," pointing at items they want or want you to notice, and waving bye-bye. These are all actions we use as we communicate with our babies every day, and they have picked them up from you. If your baby isn't waving yet, don't worry—some babies don't do this until well into their second year.

Capitalize on their copying behavior by pointing things out, or expressing your meaning with actions as well as words. If you're telling them something is big, open your arms wide. If you are telling them it's lunch time, make an eating action.

Mimicking chores

Your baby will also want to play with the things they see you hold and use, from a harmless measuring cup to a dangerous kitchen knife. (Hazardous items should all be locked away by now, but it's always good to double-check you haven't become complacent and left anything lying around the house.)

Give your baby toy versions of grown-up tools. A toy iron allows them to be just like you, but without the danger of burns; a toy mobile phone makes your own far less appealing if it's left in reach.

You are the ultimate learning tool

Maximize on your baby's wonderfully suggestible nature. If they see you respond happily to a given situation,

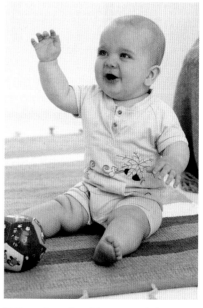

Hello and goodbye Wave to your baby and they may wave back .

they are much more likely to respond happily in a similar situation, too. And if they see you using utensils to eat your food, they'll want to use their spoon, too. Even if they don't mimic you immediately, they may well have processed what they've seen and do it another time—psychologists call this deferred imitation.

All this does put parents in the spotlight—observing your behavior takes precedence over any other kind of learning your baby will experience at this age. So whatever you do, be good!

Upside down

Your baby's increased coordination allows them to maneuver themself into different positions to gain new perspectives on their world.

At this age, your baby will probably pull up to standing, but getting down is more problematic as they still haven't figured out how to bend their knees. If they see a toy on the floor that they want, they will either bend down from the waist with legs straight to grab it, or will simply sit down with a thud (although slightly less of a thud than before!). When leaning down from standing, they may peek between their legs and try to reach through them to grab toys and other objects. In fact, they have no real sense of their own abilities and limitations, and will try all sorts of approaches to get what they want, and may be surprised to end up in an unexpected position!

Help your baby practice their balance and coordination by encouraging them to bend forward and pick up toys on the floor from a standing position.

They may also push themself up on their legs when they're in a crawling position, and peek backward. Every new position provides a new angle on the world, and they're developing spatial awareness. Encourage them to point to things they see from their new vantage point, and watch them giggle with delight when they see their favorite items upside down.

Now that your baby is probably a very competent crawler, you can help them master coming down the stairs (far harder than going up)—on their tummy, feet first, and sliding backward. The same movement is used for sliding off the sofa.

SAFETY OUTDOORS

Once your baby is on the move, they will want to explore the great outdoors—starting with your yard! Plenty of outdoor play is hugely beneficial for your baby's health and well-being, but before you let them loose, take a good look around any outdoor space and ensure it's safe for your inquisitive, mobile baby. The following guidelines will help keep your baby safe:

• **Check that there are no poisonous plants your baby could reach.** If you're unsure whether something is poisonous—perhaps flowers were planted by a previous owner—take a cutting or photo to your local garden center to see if they can identify it.

• **Keep potted plants out of your baby's reach** so they don't eat the soil or pebbles, which are a choking hazard.

• **Watch your baby all the time near water.** Be careful around bird baths, water tables, wading pools, and swimming pools. Drowning can happen in very little water.

• **Make sure any play equipment is sturdily built.** If you are assembling it yourself, follow the instructions exactly. Keep play equipment away from fences and walls.

• **Cover the sandbox** when not in use to prevent cats from using it as a litter box. Check the rest of the yard for cat and other animal feces.

• **Most importantly, supervise your baby** at all times in the yard.

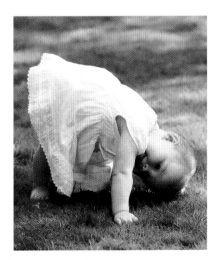

A different view The world looks different from various angles, and your baby now has the maneuverability to try out new positions as they straighten their legs and pivot down.

Getting baby's attention

Your busy baby may be so intent on exploring at times that they don't pay attention to your guidance or warnings.

Usually your baby will hang upon your every word, eager to interact, listen, and respond. Of course, they'll also spend time engrossed in play and it'll be more of a challenge to get them to listen, especially if you're asking them to stop or want to divert them onto something else. If you need to interrupt, you'll get their attention most effectively if you get down to their level and make eye contact. Say their name first and then give a short, simple statement. For example, if they're annoying the cat and you can see a scratch coming, say, "[Name], stop poking the cat" and guide them away to reinforce the instruction. Avoid long sentences or multiple requests and always guide them gently to move if needed. There's no point listing dangers; they can't imagine the possible hazards that come so readily to your mind. Instead, if there's a problem, mime the consequences, for example if you need to show your drink is hot, mime touching the cup and say, "Ouch, hot, don't touch" while waving your fingers as if they're burned. It will take many repetitions to teach this danger awareness so don't expect them to remember for quite a while.

If your baby consistently doesn't respond when you talk out of their eyeline, it's worth asking your doctor to check their hearing.

No more bottles

Your baby is now able to master a sippy cup and take milk this way. Dropping the bottle early can help protect their teeth.

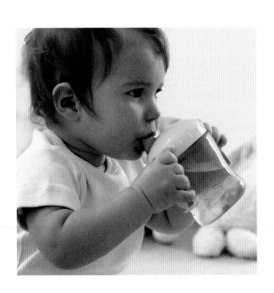

The longer your baby drinks from a bottle, the harder it will be for them to move onto a cup and fall asleep without sucking. The sucking action causes milk to swirl around their mouth, bathing the teeth in the sugars contained in milk, causing tooth decay. If you wean them onto a cup early on, they won't be as likely to associate milk with comfort, so will be less likely to comfort eat later in life.

Drinking from a cup Get your baby into the habit of drinking their milk and other fluids in a cup to prevent tooth decay.

To make the transition, switch the nipple on their bottle to a spout so they become used to drinking rather than sucking. Buy colorful cups and let them choose which one they'd like to drink from. Habits can be established quickly in babies under a year, and if they feel they have a choice, the disappointment of not having a bottle will soon be forgotten.

If you're breastfeeding, work toward giving one or two smaller feeds a day and offering expressed breast milk in a cup to make up the difference. Suckling breast milk does not cause tooth decay.

Your child's first teacher

You are your baby's first teacher. Your guidance and actions are their benchmarks for understanding the world around them.

Your baby looks to you for guidance and information and will learn how to behave, interact, and negotiate their world by watching and listening to you. For this reason, it's important to do your best to model the type of behavior you want your baby to learn, and present your family values to them through your actions.

While they are still too young to display any table manners (and digging in and making a mess is an important part of learning to eat), you can exhibit good manners yourself. Sit and eat with your baby whenever you can. Studies show that the more frequently families eat together, the better their relationships. Your baby will learn that mealtimes are sociable, and will see how you and your partner listen when others are speaking and wait your turn to talk. This teaches them about relationships, respect, and acceptable behavior.

Determine healthy ways to control your frustration when things go wrong or you're stressed. There's no doubt that setting a positive example for your baby is beneficial; when they see you socializing, reading, being organized and active, and enjoying fulfilling relationships, they will be likely to absorb these qualities, too. However, while the example you set is important, it's also healthy to recognize that there's no such thing as a perfect parent, and that

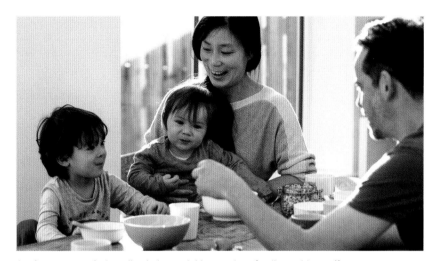

Setting an example As well as being sociable occasions, family mealtimes offer the perfect opportunity to model good table manners.

parenting is a constant learning process.

Don't be too hard on yourself if you don't manage to get everything right, whether leaving a messy kitchen, ignoring a phone call, letting routines slip, or being petty with your partner. Babies can cope with things not always being ideal. As long as you're in tune with your baby's needs, put these first, and give consistent care, then you're good enough. Providing a secure environment is the best thing you can do for your child.

ASK A CHILD PSYCHOLOGIST

My baby has temper tantrums already! Is this normal? While your baby is not yet emotionally capable of a true toddler-style tantrum, babies can appear to lose their tempers. This is a sign that they are frustrated at being unable to express their needs. Try to remain calm and patient yourself. Many babies respond to being held and comforted when feeling out of sorts; sing a familiar song to calm them and try to distract from the situation. Speak quietly so your baby is reassured that everything in their world is not out of control, and show them how to master whatever it was they were trying to do, or gently move them to another room where the trigger will no longer upset them.

Growing appetite

The more mobile your baby becomes, the more their appetite increases. They may need more food and regular snacks to sustain their energy.

By now your baby is eating two or three meals a day. They should be getting plenty of whole-grain carbohydrates, fresh vegetables and fruits, lean meats and fish, eggs, dairy products, and beans. While some babies can become picky eaters at this age, continue to serve a variety of healthy foods, revisiting the foods that have been rejected every few days or so until they become familiar.

Don't offer your baby unhealthy snacks between meals. Snacks should contribute to their overall diet and make up for any shortfalls. If they learn to satisfy hunger with fruits, whole-grain toast, yogurt, squares of cheese, strips of fresh vegetables, a hard-boiled egg, or a few spoonfuls of tuna, they will develop healthy eating habits and associate good, fresh food with mealtimes and snack times.

Encourage your baby to taste new, appropriate foods from your plate.

Show them different foods when shopping or preparing meals, and let them touch, smell, and taste them so they become familiar. Let your baby eat until they feel full; they may eat lots at each sitting for a few days, then seem to want less for a while. Allow their hunger to decide how much they eat: while it is important that they get regular, healthy meals, these can be smaller or larger, as long as your baby's weight remains stable (see p.278).

A different approach

Instead of racing to do the chores when your baby is asleep, slow down and let them join in. You may be surprised to find you both have fun.

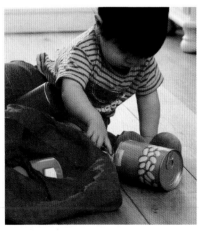

Little helper Unpacking the groceries doesn't have to be quick when it's this interesting.

When your baby begins a play session, you may have a few minutes to make a phone call, check emails, or make a list before they demand your attention. You may also be able to get a few things done while they nap. However, these small windows of opportunity are unlikely to provide all the time you need for chores.

Although it may take much longer, letting them participate in your practical activities will keep them occupied and teach them about the way in which a household runs. Let them sit on a pile of laundry while you sort the clothes and name the different colors; or make a game out of refilling your diaper changing stations and repacking your diaper bag, letting them handle the items.

You might even want to include your baby in some of your other daily routines—for example, sharing a bath together. If you read your book or your emails out loud when they are happily playing on the floor, they'll love the sound of your voice as you catch up with your reading. You may get less done than you would like, but you'll have the satisfaction of working with your baby as a positive part of your day, leaving you more time for rest after their bedtime.

Outdoor play

It's important that your baby has plenty of outdoor playtime to ensure they get fresh air, sunlight, and lots of exercise.

Gross and fine motor skills, coordination, balance, and imagination are developed when children are given plenty of opportunities to climb and play, and to respond to the natural world with its multitude of textures, smells, activities, and possibilities.

Being outdoors is also helpful in letting your child experience a different field of vision and new sensory stimulation. Seeing into the distance, feeling the wind on their skin, and noticing changes in the light all offer the senses new information.

Time spent outdoors in a natural environment is known to improve adults' moods, so taking your baby outside regularly will probably give you a boost and start a habit for your baby that will be good for them as they grow. Time spent in sunlight also encourages the production of vitamin D in your baby's body (see p.221), which helps them build healthy bones and teeth. Be sure to take steps to prevent sunburn.

Make an effort to get outside at least once a day, and in nice weather, let your baby sit in the grass, crawl in the park, or amuse themself in the sandbox in your local playground. Push them on the baby swings, play ball, point out the squirrels, and take a bag of frozen peas to feed the ducks. Give them a safe place to explore; hold their hands so they can stand supported and splash in puddles; and let them crawl and get their hands dirty. Once they're on their feet, hold their hand and enjoy "mini" explorations of your local park or neighborhood, letting them take their time and stop to examine nature along the way. Have their stroller at the ready so they can rest when they get tired.

Spending quality time outside with your baby will do wonders for your perspective and it will give them a new view of the outdoors, your neighborhood, and the world.

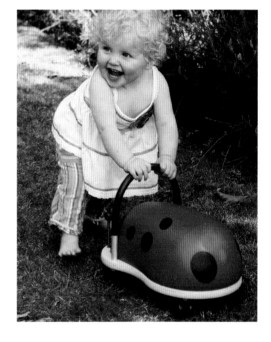

Outdoor fun Playing outdoors allows for exuberant fun and a change of scenery.

DEVELOPMENT ACTIVITY: RAINY-DAY FUN

Your baby needs some time each day to move their body freely so they can make those gross motor movements that teach them so much about what they can do with their body.

If you can't venture out due to rainy days or cold weather, think of ways in which you can keep them active at home. Encourage them to crawl up and down the stairs next to you, and have a crawling race across the living room floor. Hold their hands and dance to lively music; and set up an obstacle course with cushions, pillows, folded towels, and their favorite toys for them to climb up, over, and around.

You could make a drum kit with kitchen pots and pans and wooden spoons, or play a game of tag, chasing them as they crawl around the living room, and playing action rhymes when you catch them.

As long as they get a little out of breath and, ideally, is giggling, too, they'll be using up energy and, of course, having plenty of fun.

12 months

AT FIRST, BABIES BELIEVE THAT THE IMPORTANCE OF A POINTING FINGER IS THE FINGER ITSELF. Your baby's manual dexterity has come a long way and they are now adept at using their index finger to point to items of interest. They're also getting better at using a spoon to feed themself, but as hand–eye coordination is not yet fully developed, mealtimes are bound to be messy!

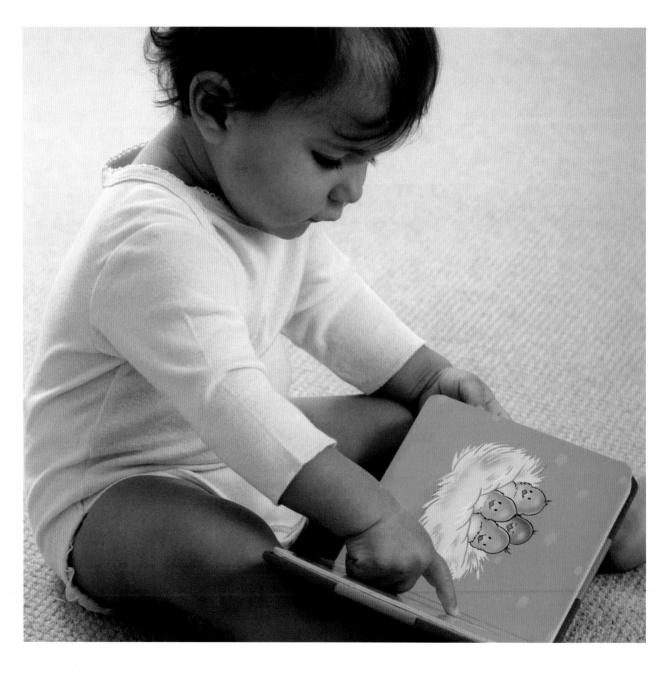

Practice makes perfect

It'll be a while before your baby can successfully feed themselves with a spoon, but they'll enjoy trying to eat with one, just like the rest of you.

By now, your baby may want to feed themselves, even though they don't yet have the motor skills and coordination to bring a spoon easily to their mouth. However, practice makes perfect. To make it easier, give them a short-handled plastic spoon rather than a long-handled weaning one. Give them a bowl, preferably one with a suction cup on the base which will hold the bowl in place as your baby dips their spoon into it. As they negotiate the spoon and bowl of food, offer spoonfuls from a second bowl that you hold. They will eventually learn the art of picking up and holding a spoon, filling it with food, and placing it in their mouth.

Forget about etiquette

To begin with, your baby is likely to hold the spoon in one hand and use the other hand to scoop what's in front of them into their mouth. At this stage, let them do as they please. If they want to grip the spoon and eat with their fingers, that's fine—they'll get around to spooning it in when their coordination has improved. Give them a bib (a wipe-clean one will save on laundry), and you may also want to put some newspaper or a splash mat on the floor under the high chair.

Even if most of the food ends up in their hair, don't discourage them from experimenting with the spoon. You can hold their fist as they grip the spoon and help them move it to their mouth, but remember that they don't yet have the coordination or the flexibility in their wrist to be able to do this themselves. Don't

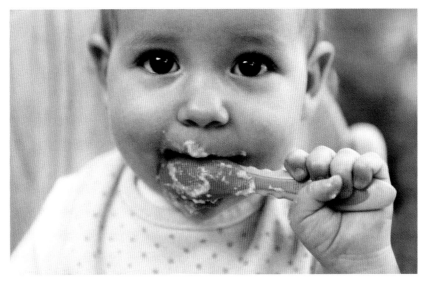

Self-feeding with a spoon Be prepared for a good portion of the contents of your baby's bowl to end up in their lap, on the floor, and all over their face—even in their hair!

underestimate the importance of providing your baby with guidance and a model to copy. Sit down to eat with them at mealtimes so they see how you operate your own cutlery.

The most important thing at the moment is that your baby is encouraged to get food into their tummy in the easiest way possible and that they enjoy themself at mealtimes. Successful self-feeding is a big developmental step for your baby. Now it's all about confidence—they will be unlikely to be able to feed themself a full meal without any help until they are about three, so mealtimes need to be fun, positive, and full of praise in the meantime.

ASK A NUTRITIONIST

Why isn't my baby hungry at mealtimes?
At this age, they need only 17 fl oz–1 pint (500–600 ml) of milk a day. While it's still too early for cow's milk, small amounts of cheese or yogurt are acceptable. Offer solids before milk feedings so meals start on an empty stomach. Also, cut down daytime bottles or milk feedings. They can now manage on a feeding in the morning and at night, with a little milk alongside meals. Ensure they don't have constant access to other drinks, especially juice. Avoid offering too many snacks: they should be small, and give plenty of time to digest before mealtime.

Patting, poking, and pinching

Your baby's hand-eye coordination is improving constantly, and they are now capable of pointing and poking, and may even pinch, too!

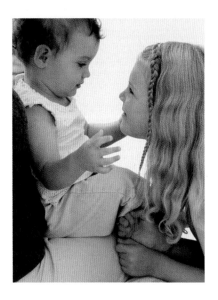

Being gentle Teach your baby how to treat siblings with gentleness.

Your baby will begin to test their own strength and abilities and you may find them prodding, poking, pushing, and even pinching pets, toys, and people. In fact, any activity that offers a resounding reaction will attract their repeated interest.

Your baby's unwelcome behavior is nothing more than an exercise undertaken to satisfy curiosity and gauge the response they get. They're not being malicious, but trying out their skills and experimenting. When they do poke or hit, show them how to interact more gently. Show them how to pat or stroke your family pet. Provide words for these actions, such as "Nice cat, pet the cat," so they learn to understand the terminology for the actions you want to see. Soon enough you will be able to say the words, "Pet-pet" to get your baby to stroke rather than hit.

If they continue being too physical, distract. Find opportunities to put your baby's skilled little fingers to better use. Give them an activity board with buttons to push, dials to turn, and strings to pull.

When they won't go to bed

Your baby equates bedtime with being away from parents—and all the fun—and may resist attempts to settle them down at night.

Babies need less sleep as they get older. If your baby starts to put up a fight at bedtime, make sure their evening routine continues to be relaxing and comforting so they look forward to this time and associate it with enjoying close, quiet time with you.

Throughout the day, ensure your baby gets plenty of physical exercise and stimulation so they are tired enough to go to sleep at bedtime. Consider moving their nap to an earlier slot, or their bedtime later, so they are ready to settle down.

Try not to become frustrated with a reluctant sleeper, especially if they start to learn that reluctance leads to attention. Simply settle them in the crib as usual and return when they call you. Stroke and pat them, sing a familiar nighttime song or say the usual "good night," then leave. Be upbeat so they don't feel that bedtime is a punishment. Keep other noise to a minimum during this phase so your baby isn't distracted by what's going on elsewhere.

If all else fails, at bedtime put your baby in the crib with a few toys and the usual comfort items, and allow them to occupy themself quietly until sleep descends, then remove the toys.

Limits and boundaries

As your baby's first birthday approaches, you may be wondering what you can expect of their behavior, and what parenting style to develop.

Most parents are concerned about what sort of parent they will be, and most aim for a middle ground focused on being warm and loving, and firm, but fair, when it comes to guiding their child's behavior. The challenge is often to get the right balance between giving your child the freedom to explore the world, yet ensure that they grow up to be well-behaved individuals with a real sense of right and wrong.

You are already setting boundaries, by moving your baby away or distracting them if they snatch toys from another child. You probably also hold their hands firmly and say "no" if they do something they shouldn't. So by 12 months, your baby may have figured out that "no" means "stop," but hasn't grasped the ideas of right and wrong, and may not heed your instructions simply because curiosity has got the better of them.

Types of discipline

Discipline tends to fall into two main categories—that needed for safety and that needed for good behavior.

When it comes to safety, it's important to remove your child physically from danger. If, for example, they go to touch the oven door, or grab a lamp from the table, move them away, hold their hands firmly, and, kneeling at eye level, tell them "no" and explain why—"The oven is hot, it will burn you. Ow!" or "The lamp is heavy, it will bump you."

Once won't be enough with explanations, but repetition and consistent responses will help your baby get the message.

When it comes to good behavior, don't expect too much. Your baby still considers themself to be the center of the world and has only the shakiest idea that they could upset others. At this age, they learn by watching, and you are their key role model. When you show good manners and speak calmly, they'll absorb this and start to show this behavior, too, as they

develop. They don't understand the concept of saying sorry yet, but it's not too early to demonstrate how it's done so they get to know what's expected.

Whatever parenting style you develop, there are some key points to remember. Your child will be more responsive if you are consistent; spend more time and energy praising and encouraging rather than scolding; and, when the time comes to use discipline and consequences, you do so calmly and without anger.

DEVELOPMENT ACTIVITY: SOFT AND HARD

Help your baby understand the different properties of the objects they encounter each day. Give them different textured toys and household items to hold and handle, and describe each one, talking about whether it is smooth, hard, soft, or furry, as well as what color it is. Talking to them in this way helps them expand their vocabulary and understand that not only do things have names, but they also have different characteristics. This in turn helps your baby start to make connections and comparisons. They're not ready to name all these items themself, but you are helping them understand.

Exploring through touch Fill a basket with different textured toys and objects, and encourage them to dive in and explore.

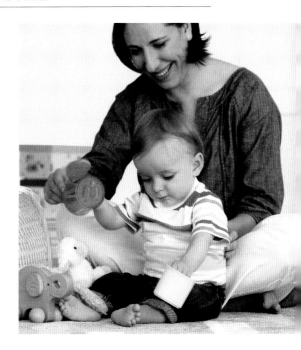

In your baby's own time

It can be tempting to want your baby to meet the same milestones as their peers, but remember that every baby is different.

Milestones are designed to give you a rough idea of when your baby will be physically, mentally, and/or emotionally ready to master those challenges or skills that are acquired across infancy and childhood. They are not, however, tests to establish intelligence or define future prowess in different areas. In fact, achieving milestones such as walking or sleeping through the night early is no indication that your baby will continue to "achieve" at a high level, nor do everything else early. It's important to realize, too, that just as milestones act as a guide rather than a rule, the order in which they are reached can vary from baby to baby. Some leap ahead physically and are slower to talk. Others gain hand–eye coordination earlier, while walking happens further into the second year. So while your friend's baby of the same age may be busy climbing stairs, yours may be far more preoccupied with making different sounds.

Your baby is unique, with their own personality. They will meet milestones when they're ready, and unless they are obviously lagging well behind peers of the same age, there is no reason for you to be concerned. If you genuinely think there could be a problem, you should check with your pediatrician.

It's me!

Your baby is developing a sense of independence, and in the coming months, their self-awareness will grow.

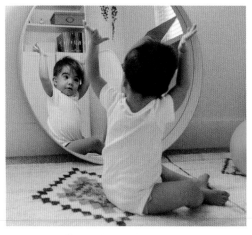

Hello! Your baby will enjoy using a mirror to explore their senses, particularly their visual sense.

Your baby is showing signs of beginning to understand that you are separate from them. The earliest signal of this was a few months ago, around the time they realized you aren't always there and sometimes move out of sight. This is when they grasped the concept of person permanence: the idea that you exist even when they can't see or hear you.

As they discovered their own body, their self-awareness grew, alongside their increasing control over, and consciousness of, how their body moved. They are also developing a mental picture of themself and others. At around 12 months, they'll be able to tell the difference between a photograph of themself and that of another baby, and from 15 months comes the revelation that the image in the mirror is their reflection.

Your baby's involvement in some basic fantasy play is another sign that they're aware of themself and others. When the two of you act out cuddling a teddy, or pretend to give it a drink, they're copying others' behavior.

As they move through their second year, their awareness that they're a separate person from you will grow, so watch for them asserting their personality. Soon, "no" will be their favorite word!

Working parent

Juggling work and parenting can be stressful, and you may feel that you aren't able to give 100 percent to either. These feelings are normal.

Despite any concerns you may have as a working parent, be assured that you can most certainly raise a healthy, happy baby and enjoy your work. The secret is to be organized and flexible, and to get your priorities straight. If you put your job first when you are at work, and your baby and family first at home, you are bound to get things right. The other parts of your life that surround this, including household chores and socializing, may need to move to the back burner for a while—certainly until you establish a routine that works for everyone—and it is equally important that you lower the expectations you hold for yourself. If you are just about keeping all of the balls in the air, then well done!

Work–life balance

While it's undeniably tricky to keep work and family life running smoothly, there are several things you can do to help your days go well. First, get organized. Make sure you know what needs to happen when, and stick to the same routine each day so you can streamline events and your baby knows what's going on, which will help them feel secure. Set out everything required for the morning the night before so you can relax knowing that everything is ready, no matter what happens the following morning. Batch cooking and bulk-buying are other organizational helpers that save you a great deal of

Your baby will be just as excited by a big, empty box into which he can crawl or tip over as he will be by the latest and most expensive new toys. Scrunch up paper into balls to fill the box, then encourage him to tip the contents out and reload the box. Drop in a few toys for him to discover while he plays. Similarly, a sturdy laundry basket makes a great toy car or train—your baby will enjoy playing the part of the driver or passenger when you push him around.

These games will help to stretch your baby's imagination and improve his gross and fine motor skills. What's more, they'll keep him occupied for stretches of time!

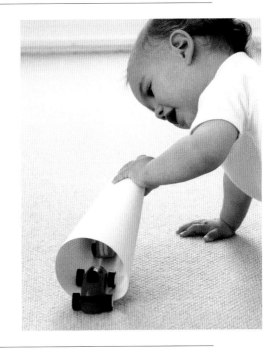

Improvised toys Even a piece of paper taped into a cone shape will be "useful."

time in the long run—and probably some money, too.

It's important to have backup plans, too, in case your baby is sick or your caregiver is away. Try to organize a support network that you can turn to for dealing with the unexpected.

If at times you feel overwhelmed, focus on the positives. Feeling guilty for not being there to see all of your baby's "firsts" or tend to their daily needs won't help you. Instead, celebrate the fact that your baby is healthy and happy and you're able to

go out and earn a living. Concentrate on the most important areas and only agree to things that enhance your life. An exhausted, unhealthy, and emotional parent isn't going to be effective in any area of life.

Lastly, don't feel guilty about relaxing work ambitions for the time being if you find a young family isn't conducive to a go-getting mentality. There will be plenty of time to chase those goals when your baby is more independent.

New skills

In addition to their milk feedings, your baby should now be eating three meals a day, and an occasional snack when they are particularly active.

Your little one's fine motor control is improving all the time and they are becoming adept at manipulating objects accurately. They are also more interested in trying to use tools, such as a spoon or fork, for their intended purpose.

Preload a spoon with food, then support your baby in bringing the spoon to their mouth. Let your baby do the rest of the work, putting the spoon into their mouth themself. It may get messy! Use sticky or lumpy foods like mashed potato or oatmeal. Remember to praise your baby when they successfully feed themself.

Self-feeding Be patient while your baby learns and explores. They may not get it right every time.

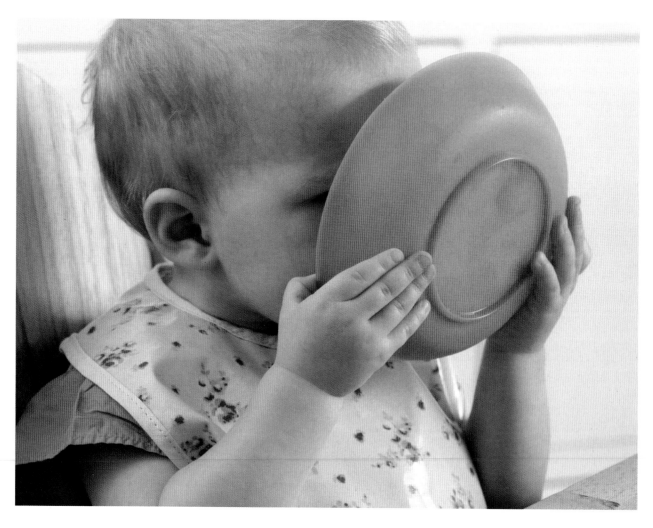

Figuring it out

Your baby now shows an increased ability to solve problems, and enjoys creative activities and toys that test their developing skills.

DEVELOPMENT ACTIVITY: ARTS AND CRAFTS

Encourage your baby's creativity as well as their hand–eye coordination and fine motor skills with regular arts-and-crafts sessions. Purchase some chunky nontoxic crayons, tape a large piece of paper to the kitchen floor, and show them how to make marks with their crayons. Create patterns and scribbles. Talk about the colors you are using and guide your baby's hand to make straight lines or circles, naming all the different shapes you make. Every couple of months, save one of their creations in a scrapbook or art portfolio so you can see how their skills progress over the coming years. In the summer, go outside and use chalk to create pictures and scribbles on the sidewalk or deck.

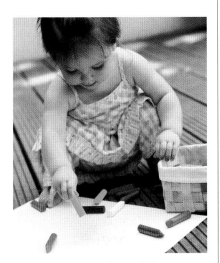

Free flow Your baby will enjoy being expressive with colors and shapes.

Toys such as shape-sorters, simple first jigsaw puzzles, musical instruments, and building blocks help your baby improve their analytical thinking, which, in turn, will develop their ability to figure out how things in their environment operate. They will encourage your baby to reason, deduce, analyze, and use logical thought, and then to put their ideas to the test. They are also learning to problem solve when their ideas do not work immediately. For example, if they have chosen a slot in which to fit their wooden puzzle piece and it doesn't fit, they may persevere to create the right match. Although they can become frustrated, most babies enjoy a challenge and repeat things until they get them right.

To encourage your baby to develop and hone their problem-solving skills, give them puzzles and activities they can master before moving them on to more challenging toys. Early successes breed confidence for the harder tasks. If they struggle to master a new toy, bring back simpler toys to rebuild their confidence first.

Observation and imitation

Your baby will solve problems by observing and copying. This is one reason why it's worth spending lots of time playing with them and showing them how things work. Demonstrate new toys and then let them try, applauding their efforts.

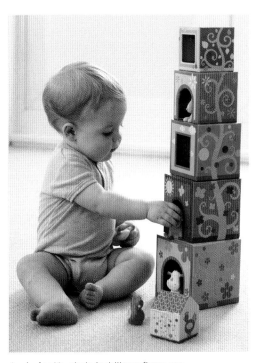

Analyzing Your baby's ability to figure out what fits, and their new fine motor skills, allow them to solve more complex puzzles.

Encourage your baby's socialization skills; give them the chance to play alongside other children on a regular basis. Seek out local playgroups, or a community playground, so they get used to being with other babies. Or arrange a regular get-together with parents and babies you've met, rotating who hosts. All of these opportunities offer your baby the chance to observe other babies doing things in different ways, allowing your baby to observe and learn.

Planning your baby's birthday

You may wish to celebrate your baby's first birthday with a party. But don't be surprised if they don't show much interest in the proceedings!

Keep your baby's first birthday party simple—you can't celebrate their transition to toddlerhood if you are busy serving appetizers or clearing up spills, and they will prefer to have you by their side, particularly if there are more people than usual in your home. On that note: choose a few people your baby knows well.

Forget about themes and party games—your baby will have no interest in them. Balloons may be fun, but tape them out of reach to prevent your baby from popping them (the scare could ruin the day!). Or use helium balloons and cut the strings so the little ones can't reach them.

Keep the party short—an hour or 90 minutes is likely the extent of your baby's attention span. Aim to start the party half an hour after they wake from their nap so they're refreshed, but not too grumpy, and ensure they have something to eat and drink before the guests arrive. Ensure food intended for adults is out of reach.

Don't be worried if your baby finds the colorful wrapping paper more exciting than the gifts! If guests ask for gift ideas, a good choice is books to build up your baby's library. If there are lots of gifts, open them over several days to prolong the fun.

Sleeping less

Your baby may resist settling down at bedtime and need much less sleep than before, but it's important they get enough to stay healthy.

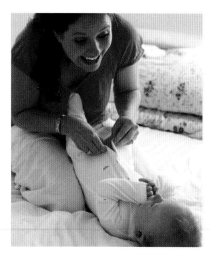

Routine A consistent bedtime ritual helps your baby prepare for impending sleep.

As they approach one year, your baby needs about 14 hours of sleep in a 24-hour period. They may have one long nap of around two hours, but may continue to need two daily naps totaling 2–3 hours, which is fine. Don't worry about meeting a specific sleep goal.

Your baby will benefit now from having a comfort object, which will help soothe them if they wake in the night. You can also place a few crib-safe toys at the end of their crib: they may be happier to settle in their crib if they can see something fun to keep them occupied. They'll likely fall asleep mid-activity.

Figure out the best nap system for your baby. A late-afternoon nap might make it hard for them to settle at night—a quiet, gentle playtime instead may relax them. One longer nap around lunchtime may keep them going all afternoon, as long as they're in bed early.

Consistency is key with bedtime. Be aware, though, that if you settle them down before 6 p.m., they're going to rise before 6 a.m. the next morning! If you're a night owl rather than an early bird, you may need to adjust your baby's bedtime accordingly to fit in with yours.

Outdoor pursuits

Now that your baby is one year old, you can start to introduce some new outdoor activities that you will both enjoy doing together.

Your baby is old enough to enjoy taking part in some of the outdoor activities you enjoyed before they were born, but may have avoided for practical reasons since.

If you like to walk or hike, buy a baby backpack carrier. Take your baby with you to buy it so you're happy that you both find it comfortable. It needs to have adequate back support for you, with a sturdy, front-closing strap, and to be the right size for your baby, with sufficient head support if they fall asleep. Most are waterproof with sun and rain shields, and have a pouch to carry essentials such as a drink, snack, diaper-changing kit, and sunscreen. Check that it is certified by the Juvenile Products Manufacturers Association, and inspect all straps and fixtures regularly for wear and tear. Ideally, walk with at least one other adult so someone can check on your baby and help get the carrier on and off, as well as share the carrying. A sturdy, thick-wheeled stroller is good for longer walks over uneven terrain.

Cycling as a family

If you're looking to get back on your bicycle, you can fit a bike trailer to your bike. Look for a label that says it meets Snell, ANSI, or CPSC safety requirements. A baby should be at least 12 months old and should have been sitting well without support for at least two months before riding in a trailer or a bike seat. All children should wear a bike helmet securely on their head, whether in a trailer or in a baby bike seat. Avoid putting your baby in a bike seat until they are at least one year, because they won't have sufficient muscle strength before then to support their head while wearing a helmet.

To get your baby used to the sensation of being in a trailer, and help you to adjust to pulling them behind you, start with short rides on smooth paths to avoid jolts, and steer clear of roads. Take your partner or a friend with you at first, and build up to longer trips.

Don't put your baby in a backpack or a trailer if it's very hot or cold as it will be difficult to regulate their temperature. On longer trips, take frequent breaks to check on them, and take them out at intervals so they can move freely.

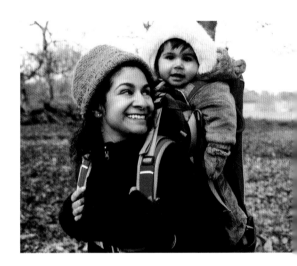

Easy rider Baby carriers are a great way to enjoy walking with your baby—and they get to see the world on your level.

ASK A NUTRITIONIST

Should I encourage my baby to eat everything in front of them? It's best to let your baby's appetite be the guide. Encouraging them to finish up their plate may lead to negative food associations and increase resistance. At this age, the appetite of some babies wanes slightly. In the first year, your baby tripled their birth weight, but they gain weight more slowly in their second year, so while more active, they may not need to eat as often. Keep in mind, too, that they still gain a proportion of their calories from milk. Also, as they are more mobile, it may be harder to get them to stay still long enough to finish every last morsel. On the other hand, if your baby is less interested in milk now, you may find that they wolf down their food. Either way, as long as you offer a variety of healthy foods (ideally concentrated around mealtimes), your baby will gain the nutrients they need to thrive.

Mind those Ps and Qs

This is the ideal time to demonstrate good manners to your baby by showing them the polite responses you would like them to mimic.

Your baby will pick up on phrases you use regularly and start to understand their meaning, so being polite and considerate toward them and other people can only have a positive effect.

Say "thank you" when your baby hands you a toy, and "please" when you ask for something from them so they get used to the sounds of these words. It doesn't matter that they won't be saying "please" or "thank you" themself

for a while, just hearing them as part of conversation will help them begin to make sense. Say "excuse me," "you're welcome," and even "I'm sorry" appropriately as you go about your activities. They'll understand that these words are part of normal behavior, and will adopt them more easily when they start to talk more.

Be polite to people around you, too, including your partner. Be generous

with praise and appreciation, and always show empathy for others. On those occasions when you can't be a perfect example, just be aware that your baby may be listening—try to keep rude remarks to a minimum!

As your baby's vocabulary expands, prompt them to say "please" and "thank you" by asking, "What do you say?" and repeating either "please" or "thank you" so they get into the habit.

Dressing for the weather

While your baby's clothing needs are fairly modest, there are a few wardrobe basics that will equip them for all weather conditions.

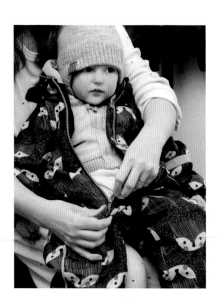

Comfortable clothing Opt for simple styles that are easy to add or remove to keep them the right temperature in all weathers.

Layer your baby's clothing so you can adapt what they're wearing as conditions change, or they move between inside and outdoors.

In colder months, dress them in several layers, including a onesie, top, and then warmer fleece or sweater. They'll need a warm outer jacket (waterproof if it's wet) for outdoors, as well as mittens and a warm hat. All-in-one snowsuits are perfect for especially cold days. If they're sitting in the stroller, they'll need a fleecy cover

or blanket to keep them cozy. If you go into a store, remove the blanket and hat, and remove layers and hats indoors at home.

In the warmer months, a few light layers are sufficient, with a summer cardigan to put on and take off as needed. A sunhat is essential: opt for a floppy one or a hat with a brim and back flap to cover their neck. Always protect their shoulders from the sun. Keep a long-sleeve t-shirt on them, and, on the beach, buy a baby lycra swimsuit that covers them and blocks most UVA rays. When they're indoors on a hot day, a diaper may be all they need.

348

Too sick for child care?

It can be tempting for working parents to dose up an unwell baby with medicine and send them to daycare, but they should be kept at home.

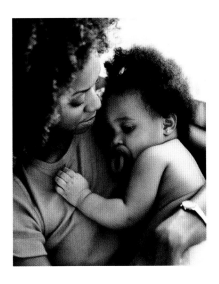

A child's immune system gradually builds up antibodies to unencountered infections; meanwhile, your baby may well catch whatever bug is going around at the childcare center, and may succumb again a short time later. For this reason, parents have an obligation to keep children who are ill away from that environment until they are no longer contagious, or it will become a veritable breeding ground for infections.

Feeling unwell An under-the-weather baby should remain at home until they're better.

If your baby is ill, be honest—staff caring for them will soon know if they are unwell! Have a back-up plan, with a list of family members or friends who can step in to care for your baby; or aim to work from home or temporarily swap hours.

Ensure your baby is comfortable at home and gets plenty of fluids to flush out infection. Expect some fussing, tearfulness, and irritability, as well as a few broken nights, and be patient. When in doubt, call your doctor who can assess the situation, reassure you, and provide guidance about the right time for a return to daycare.

ASK A PEDIATRICIAN

When should I keep my baby at home?

• Most babies and children suffer from regular colds (you can expect anywhere between one and eight a year in the early years). If nasal discharge is thick and sticky, your baby may be more susceptible to further infections, including ear infections. It's best to keep them at home until they are feeling good enough to play, eat, and sleep well.

• If your baby has a fever, they should stay at home for at least 24 hours after it has ended. Not only will they be irritable, sleepy, and uncomfortable, making the childcare experience distressing, but they will need plenty of rest and fluids to recover.

• Most rashes can be treated at home after a consultation. Rashes have many causes, including infectious diseases; check in with your pediatrician before sending your child to daycare with a new rash.

• Flu and other respiratory illnesses can become serious in babies if they are not monitored, so call your pediatrician if your baby has flu symptoms (see p.376). These illnesses can easily spread around a childcare center, so a baby with the flu must stay home.

• A baby with diarrhea or vomiting should always be kept at home. Your baby will be sent home if they experience these symptoms at the childcare center. They'll need to stay at home for at least 48 hours after the last episode, no matter how well they seem to feel.

• Bacterial eye infections, such as conjunctivitis (see p.370), are highly contagious. Keep your baby at home until symptoms clear.

• Keep your baby at home if they catch whooping cough, or another childhood illness such as measles, rubella, or mumps. Although in the early months whooping cough is routinely vaccinated against, it's still possible to catch, but is less severe. Keep them at home, too, with chickenpox; roseola; scarlet fever; and hand, foot, and mouth disease.

• If your baby has impetigo or another contagious skin disease, keep them at home for at least 48 hours after starting antibiotics. Scabies needs to be treated before your baby can return.

Making savings

Having a baby is an expensive business, as you certainly know by now, but there are ways to save money as you go along.

You might think twice in your baby's second year about buying things you won't use for long. Items like the bassinet, clothing, blankets and sheets, and baby bathtub are probably no longer useful to you. If you're thinking about extending your family, they may come in handy the next time around; if not, you might want to think about selling them to raise a little cash for the next phase ,or donating them to charity, possibly a group like Goodwill. Then, think about buying secondhand for the next phase— especially for clothing, which your baby will quickly outgrow and is likely to get dirty with all that play! If buying new, make the most of sales—and consider bargains that future proof your growing baby. Collect coupons and offers that come with baby products for future purchases—they can add up to considerable savings.

AS A MATTER OF FACT
Your baby grows more in the first year of life than they will ever again. How they continue to grow after this time is partly influenced by genetics, namely the height of their parents, but also by their environment. So if they are well nourished, loved, and cared for, they will almost certainly reach, their growth potential.

Sibling support

Older siblings may feel a little sidelined by a baby who is demanding of your attention, so make sure they get special time with you, too.

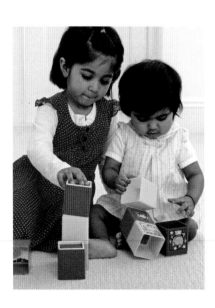

See how it's done Older siblings will enjoy helping their new brother or sister play, but do supervise them when they're together.

Older siblings may adore their little sibling and be thrilled to be involved in caring for them and playing with them. However, as baby gets older and more interested in their sibling's toys and games, they become a nuisance. At times, they may get grumpy or frustrated, even physically unkind. If this happens, intervene right away and reinforce the notion that hitting, pushing, biting, or hair-pulling, for example, is not the way to behave toward other people.

As your baby demands more, their sibling's needs will also increase. The closer in age they are, the more difficult they might find it to have to share you. However, even much older siblings can feel left out.

Make time to be with your older children on a one-to-one basis. When your baby is asleep, avoid rushing around getting jobs done. Instead, spend time playing with their siblings. Regularly arrange a time when someone can look take care of your baby, and plan a treat or activity with your older children in advance so they can look forward to their special time with you.

Toys for 11 months up

As your baby approaches their first birthday, they'll be ready for some exciting new toys that will stimulate growing curiosity and confidence.

FOCUS ON TWINS: PLAYTIME

Entertaining two babies is definitely challenging, but not impossible. Make sure you put out enough toys for both of them. This doesn't mean dragging everything out (which would be overwhelming) or going overboard purchasing twice as many toys, but ensuring there are enough toys to keep both occupied. Toys that can be easily split, such as soft blocks, are perfect, too. It's important to treat your twins as individuals. Be aware of each twin's likes and dislikes, and provide toys to suit their different needs. Lastly, enjoy one-on-one time with each baby. Don't assume that because they have each other, they have less need for you. You are their number-one playmate and teacher, so it's vital that you and your partner spend quality time with each baby.

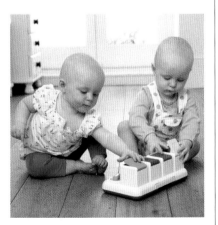

Side by side As with other babies this age, your twins will be happily preoccupied in their own pursuits.

Your baby may have outgrown many of their old toys by now. If you are having a party to celebrate their first birthday, you may be thinking of gift ideas and, no doubt, you'd like to get them one or two age-appropriate toys. There are many toys on the market that are suitable for one-year-olds, so you've plenty to choose from. Try to give a variety of toys to help your baby develop different skills.

Toys that encourage physical activity are a good idea, as your baby's motor skills are developing rapidly. Babies make the most of push-along baby walkers, which support them as they push them around, but make sure your baby doesn't become over-reliant on them for walking. Balls are also popular now; your baby may enjoy batting one and passing it back and forth to you.

This is also a good age for sorting toys, such as shape-sorters and stacking cups, which help your baby to hone their problem-solving skills and explore how smaller objects fit into bigger ones.

Very basic and sturdy wooden puzzles with knobs to lift the pieces in and out of position will appeal to your older baby, and they may spend a long time turning them to try to make them fit into the different holes. Choose simple shapes and show your baby how the puzzle pieces fit.

Toys with a string to pull will also delight your baby as they can grasp and pull quite easily now. Try a toy

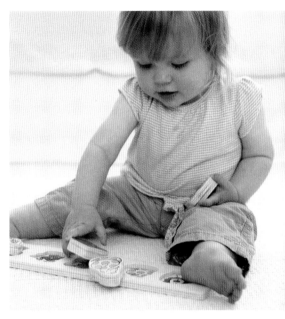

Puzzles Chunky puzzles with simple shapes will appeal to your one-year-old baby.

that climbs up its string, or makes a sound, or plays a song when its string is pulled.

If it's warm outside, water or sand tables or pits provide endless enjoyment as your baby fills buckets, empties them, and makes a real mess! Never leave your baby unsupervised near water.

Finding a balance

Happy, fulfilled parents are good for babies, so you both need to have time and space for all those aspects of your lives that are important.

By now, you and your partner may both be back at work, on a full- or part-time basis, having arranged additional care for your baby. Or one of you may have decided to stay at home to care for your baby while the other one works. Or you may both be working part-time and juggling the sharing of childcare between you. Whatever you have decided to do will probably be the result of planning and discussion between you.

There's no doubt that life now is different from your life before your baby. If one of you is caring for your baby at home, you may be thrilled with your new role of raising them the way you want, sharing activities with them each day, and proudly watching them grow and develop. However, you may also miss some aspects of your pre-baby life.

A different person

If you have given up work, you may feel that your image of yourself has changed and that you feel like a different person. It's easy for your confidence to falter, even though you are doing what you chose to do and recognize the valuable role you are playing. It's important that you don't give yourself selflessly over to what you think your baby needs. You need to develop a new life for yourself in which you find a routine that works for you and to feel confident in your parenting.

Take some time for yourself each week, perhaps asking your partner or a relative to watch your baby for a morning or a few hours on the weekend so you can do something you enjoy. You may decide to hire a babysitter or employ a part-time nanny to give yourself a break. Never feel guilty about this. Being happy and fulfilled as a person will make you a better, more evenly balanced parent.

Most of all, nurture friendships with other parents with babies of a similar age. You will be an invaluable support to each other. If you feel isolated, use playgroups to meet other parents. Your pediatrician or local library will have details of what's available in your area.

If you have gone back to work, you may miss your baby or feel guilty that you're not at home. Rest assured: your baby will be fine. Create special times together when you aren't at work. If your partner is the main caregiver, make sure you have time to talk each day. Your partner will need to tell you everything your baby is up to; this will boost your partner's sense of achievement and ensure you feel part of your baby's development.

At this stage, try not to be too rigid. You may find one or the other of you does not have the work or childcare options they expected, or changes their mind about their role. Discuss anything that doesn't feel right for either of you, and be open to making changes.

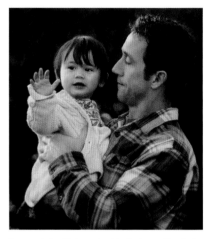

See you later It's important to find a routine that works for both you and your partner, and one that offers a life with and away from your baby.

ASK A PARENT

I keep having to get up at night to replace my baby's pacifier. Is now a good time to wean them off it? Yes, it is generally recommended that babies stop using pacifiers by the age of one, partly because habits are less ingrained before then and partly because of concerns that relying too much on pacifiers when babies start babbling could affect their speech development. Start by limiting its use: let your baby have it to fall asleep, then take it out of their mouth so they get used to it not being there when they wake. When you get rid of the pacifier, offer another comfort item, such as a blanket or toy, to distract them. Your baby might object for a night or two, but most adapt quickly.

Changing tastes

Your baby's palate is becoming more sophisticated, so this is the ideal age to expand their diet and get them interested in family meals.

If you haven't already, let your baby join in eating what the rest of the family is having; it's one of the best ways to encourage healthy eating habits. They'll learn to enjoy the flavors of the food they'll grow up on, and will also enjoy feeling part of the social experience of eating as a family.

Although your baby is still learning to feed themselves, offer a plate of their own with foods customized from your meal. (Separate their portion before adding any salt when cooking.) Soups, casseroles, pasta, meatballs, and family roasts are perfect for older babies. If your baby is a picky eater, you can hide a selection of vegetables in sauces and soups , but do not offer other, sweeter options.

If using wine, ensure that you cook it off long enough for the alcohol to evaporate. Leave salt and whole nuts off the menu still, but you can add new seasonings and cheeses to flavor their food.

If your baby is still reluctant to eat very lumpy foods, offer finger foods as well as regular foods in a lumpier form. Give finely chopped poached chicken and mashed vegetables with chunks and strips of each to encourage experimentation.

When your baby dreams

At this age, your baby begins to dream a little less than they used to, but their brain is still consolidating what it has learned during the day.

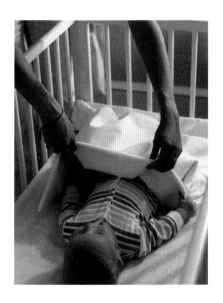

Sleep tight Throughout the night, your baby has periods of deep, restful sleep, and phases of lighter sleep, during which they dream.

As your baby approaches one year of age, they will have less "REM" or dream sleep (see p.109) than before. It is during this phase of sleep that your baby's brain works hard to process and consolidate information acquired during that day. (Premature babies still have more dream sleep than babies born at full term, and continue to need more for several more months.) When your baby dreams, their central nervous system enters an "active" state and their temperature may rise a little, while their brain-wave activity and heart rate both increase. During this lightest stage of sleep, they may wake up briefly, or seem restless in their sleep.

Try to avoid responding too quickly if they cry slightly or sound disturbed in their sleep; they will usually settle themself. Periods of dream sleep are followed by phases of deep sleep, and most babies have about five periods of each type of sleep, occurring in a cycle, throughout the night. In deep sleep, your baby's breathing will be regular, and they may sigh and make sucking motions.

A little reader

Your baby will have definite favorites on the bookshelf now, and will love having the same stories read to them over and over again.

Books keep babies occupied for long periods of time, with pages to peruse, and then turn to see what's next—but they offer much more than just a way of passing time. Books enhance vocabulary, language acquisition, and concentration. As the months pass, your baby will be more able to follow a story—a skill that will one day help them read on their own.

Babies love to have familiar stories read to them. Research has found that every time you read the same story to a baby, they pick up new information from the narrative, and their memory is improved. You may find that your baby "follows" the story with you when you read a familiar book to them, as they anticipate what is coming next and begin to respond to what is about to happen. If you miss a page—or even a sentence or a word—they'll probably look perplexed!

Old and new

Old favorites encourage your baby's development, but it's important, too, to introduce a variety of books and, once they are able, to encourage your baby to choose their own stories.

Keep books on a safe, low shelf in an accessible bookcase or basket, so they can dig them out themself and select the ones they would like to look at. Pack a few books, too, for long car rides and shopping trips. Give your baby as many opportunities as you can to use books as a distraction and to keep themself occupied. When reading with your baby, engage them in the story. Ask them to point to different elements, and make noises or sounds for the characters. As well as stories, find books with a single word on a page to encourage word recognition. Offer interactive books with flaps, textures, or buttons.

Consider creating a special book for your baby full of photographs of their favorite people, places, toys, and activities. Use an online provider or simply laminate the pages and sew them together. As they get older, encourage them to tell stories about what they see in their special book.

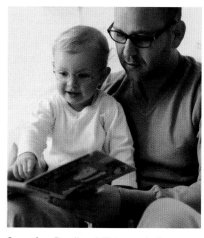

Story time Reading daily to your baby will help develop their language and communication skills.

DEVELOPMENT ACTIVITY : SPLISH, SPLASH, SPLOSH!

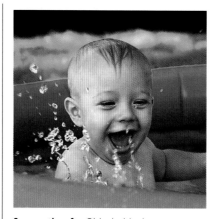

Summertime fun Older babies love to splash around in small pools in warm weather. Make sure, though, that you never leave them unattended in the water, even for a few seconds.

Once your baby is on their feet, it's time to invest in some rain boots. Babies love nothing better than a good splash in a puddle on an outdoor walk! Or get a baby pool out in the summer and supervise while they learn about how water moves in response to their actions, and how things float. Playing with water makes swimming fun for your baby and develops their senses and confidence. Best of all, it allows them to explore their environment while making a splendidly satisfying splash! However, never leave your baby unattended near any pond, kiddie pool, or swimming pool.

Becoming more mobile

Mobility is a part of every toddler's development, and even the most reluctant crawlers or walkers will make a move in the coming months.

Early walkers may now move on to running, but most babies are still working toward their first steps.

Once you baby does start to walk, they will test their skills by trying to walk backward, sideways, and up and down the stairs, before lurching forward at speed—and usually taking plenty of tumbles on the way.

Try to spend some time outdoors on grass, which will cushion your baby's falls and help them develop balance on a slightly uneven surface. They will have no sense of distance, nor will their depth perception be mature (so they may walk off the end of landings and porches), so keep a close eye on them.

Multiples mayhem

As with all babies, give your twins or other multiples a safe environment to practice walking—often in different directions! Remember that they may develop at different rates to each other. This simply reflects different developmental traits.

Full steam ahead! Your baby may find it difficult to stop once they get going, so ensure your home is fully toddler-proofed!

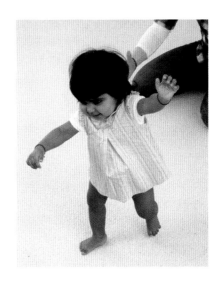

Changing the routine

Over the coming months, your baby will need slightly less sleep. Let their needs, not their routine, dictate how much sleep they get.

Over the coming year, your baby will need to sleep for between 10 and 13 hours in a 24-hour period. Whether this requirement is met entirely during the night, or is divided between daytime and nighttime sleeps, will be determined by your baby's individual needs. However, very few babies manage a whole day without at least one restorative nap.

You may also find that your baby is more tired on some days than on others, and will need a morning nap just a few hours after they wake up. They may also develop a habit of sleeping through lunchtime, so you'll need to tweak your routine to ensure they get a good meal before settling down so they don't wake early through hunger.

Whenever your baby is ready for their afternoon nap is fine. If your baby is showing signs of being sleepy, settle them down and wake them only if they sleep past 4 p.m.—the point at which daytime sleep usually interferes with a good night's sleep.

If your baby fares better with a nap during the day, ensure they get some physical activity beforehand to help them settle well, and continue with your usual pre-nap routine. Beware that at this age, they're likely to wake up and want to play, and may make an attempt to escape, too, so ensure that the crib is safe (see p.279), with the base on its lowest setting.

Cow's milk as a drink

Once your baby is one year old, they are old enough to have cow's milk. Choose whole milk until they're two, after which you can give 2 percent.

Up until now, breast and formula milk have been the most suitable to meet your baby's particular nutritional needs. Once your baby is a year old, though, it is safe for them to drink cow's milk, which will provide them with healthy fats, protein, calcium, vitamin A, and essential fatty acids (EFAs), along with other key minerals.

If you are raising your baby as a vegetarian, or if they are a picky eater,

consider a "growing up" formula, which contains extra iron and vitamins. Aim to expand their food repertoire so their food alongside whole cow's milk meets their nutritional needs.

All dairy products are high in the nutrients contained in cow's milk, so don't panic if your baby doesn't take to it. Simply increase their intake of other dairy products and calcium-containing foods, such as leafy green

vegetables, beans, tofu, and soy.

Babies need a great deal more fat in their diets than adults, so give your baby whole milk and yogurt. This provides the energy and fat-soluble vitamins needed for growth. Under the age of two, fats should make up about half their calorie intake. After that, alongside a varied, nutritious diet, you may consider changing to lower-fat milk.

Baby still wants to breastfeed

Whether or not you have other ideas, your baby may want to continue breastfeeding and show no signs of being ready to stop.

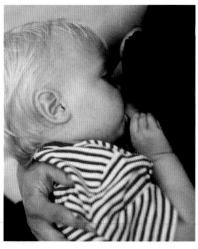

Still natural For a one-year-old, breastfeeding still feels natural and comforting.

There's no right time to stop breastfeeding. Many parents find that their babies often "wean" themselves around now as they get distracted by the world around them. Others seem happy to continue. This is fine, too—unless you would like to stop.

Take your time weaning your older baby off the breast as this is a well-established habit for them that provides much comfort. Give them cuddles and reassurance. Replace breastfeedings with formula (until they are one year old, see above) because they still need 17–20 fl oz (500–600 ml) of milk a day, even once they're on solids. However, they'll

probably get what they need in two feedings a day, plus some milk with meals if necessary. If you want to keep the morning or evening breastfeedings, this is good for you both on every level (see p.331).

For an older baby, breast milk can be a valuable source of nutrients. One study found that in a baby's second year, just 15 fl oz (450 ml) of breast milk can provide 29 percent of a baby's energy needs; 43 percent of protein; 36 percent of calcium; 75 percent of vitamin A; 94 percent of vitamin B12; and 60 percent of vitamin C needs each day.

First times

Your baby will face many new experiences in the coming months. A little preparation will help them negotiate them comfortably.

At some point over the coming year, your baby will have their first visit to the dentist or hairdresser, or perhaps their first sleepover at Grandma's. Some babies happily adjust to new experiences; others need a little warming up. Either way, if your baby knows what to expect from a new situation, they'll feel more secure about it.

If you need to go to the dentist, doctor, or hairdresser yourself—or are taking an older sibling—take your baby along, too, to get them used to the surroundings.

While the hairdresser is cutting your hair, hold your baby on your lap and explain what's being done in an upbeat tone of voice. Let them see the dentist examining your teeth, or the doctor taking your blood pressure, while you sit back calmly.

If you think your baby might be fazed by a new upcoming experience, borrow a library book that tells them all about it. If they're going to stay at Grandma's or Grandpa's on their own, plan a trip or two in advance for the pair of you to enjoy together so they get used to being there with you first (see also p.327).

On the day

When the time comes for your baby's first haircut or other new experience, make sure they're not hungry or tired, and give them their comfort object or a toy or book to distract them if they look a little worried. Explain very

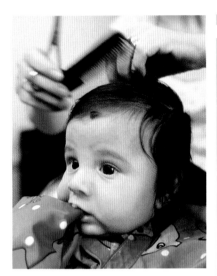

Hair raising A first haircut shouldn't worry your baby if they've visited the salon with you.

simply where you are going and what's going to happen. Remind them of the story you read about the scenario they're going to encounter, or recall that just like Mommy or Daddy had their hair cut, now it's their turn to be fussed over and look neat. Let them know that afterward you plan to wrap up the experience with something fun, such as a trip to the local playground. This will help create positive associations with the event. Above all, stay calm and upbeat yourself—if you show a fear of the dentist, for example, your baby will quickly pick up on this and be worried for themself.

ASK A PEDIATRICIAN

When does my baby need their first dental appointment? It's a good idea to have your baby's teeth checked at around six months, or whenever the first teeth emerge, so they become accustomed to the experience of visiting the dentist, and to check that all is well. They won't need a full checkup until around their first birthday. Your dentist will give you plenty of advice about your baby's oral health, including brushing and using fluoride toothpastes, and will check that there are no signs of early decay.

Treat the first appointment like a social occasion, getting your baby used to the new environment and different smell. At first, and maybe for the first few appointments, your baby can sit in your lap while the dentist looks at their teeth. Your baby will probably love the attention. Try not to panic, though, if this isn't the case and they make a fuss; you can always reschedule an appointment for a later date.

My baby was distraught after getting their shots. Does this mean they'll be terrified of future vaccinations? Your baby won't remember their first sets of shots, so rest assured they won't have developed a fear of the pediatrician! However, it may be in their nature to react loudly: some babies do scream loudly, while others are quiet or more easily comforted.

YOUR BABY IS **TWELVE MONTHS OLD**

Words with meaning

By now, many babies have a small repertoire of words they can use with meaning, and a rapidly increasing vocabulary.

First words tend to be those that have the most meaning for your baby, such as "mama," "dada," and "bottle" (which often comes out as "baba"). Your baby may not be able to say many of these words accurately, but you'll know what they mean. Don't be surprised if your baby changes their words for various people and items. They may call their bottle a "baba" one week, then "bobo," or "mik" (milk), the next.

Your baby learns language by listening and, at this point, they'll understand far more than they can say. Continue to chat with them and offer the correct words for items. However, being able to repeat words doesn't mean using them in the right way. Listen and watch when your baby speaks—their intonation and gestures may give you a clue to the intended meaning.

Some babies don't use their first words until well into their second year, but by around 20 months, you can expect your baby to have 30–40 words in their repertoire. These will be mixed in with a stream of babbling. After 20 months, they'll begin to pick up words at an amazing rate—sometimes one or two a day—and you'll have no doubt about what they're saying—and what they want!

Reflecting on your year

So have you loved the past year—or barely survived it? All parents are different and some are more "ga-ga" about babies than others …

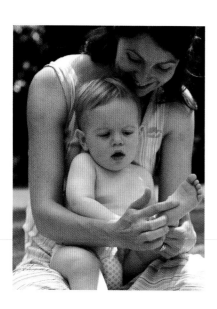

Now you have almost 12 months' experience under your belt, how would you describe yourself as a parent? Has it been an otherworldly, sublime experience in each and every way, or are you finding the mountain of diapers a constant battle? Or, more likely, a mixture of both?

If you haven't enjoyed the past year as much as you had hoped, try not to feel disheartened—loving your baby themselves doesn't mean you have to love the baby "stage." For some,

Apple of your eye Your baby is adorable, but can be hard work at times, too!

parenthood becomes more rewarding as babies become better able to interact. As your child's personality develops, you'll probably find that the more mundane practicalities of parenting are outweighed by the joy of the little person who is emerging. It's a cliché, but babies really do grow up incredibly fast: one day you have a toddler, the next thing you know you're taking them to kindergarten—so try to appreciate every moment. There will always be weak spots and hard times, but the bond you share with your child is precious and unique—wherever you happen to be on the parenting journey.

Your baby is one today

Congratulations—your baby is officially a toddler! You have many exciting changes to look forward to in the coming year.

Your baby's first birthday can be a time of mixed emotions for you—they are becoming more independent, and will depend less on you for feeding and even getting around. They may have clear ideas of what they can and want to do, and for the first time you may find yourself locking horns with a contrary little person. As they head toward the age of two, you can expect them to become much more reluctant to accept your intervention!

Paradoxically, separation anxiety continues well into your toddler's second, or even third, year, and they will seek out your presence and find security in their routines. Continue to reassure them with regular physical affection and enjoy plenty of activities together to reinforce your bond.

Their speech will develop hugely in the coming year, and you will soon have the knack of working out what they're saying. Reading, singing, and chatting will continue to support their language acquisition. Over the next year, they'll start to string together short sentences and, with a combination of gestures and words, make their needs easily known.

Your toddler's safety remains a top priority, and you will have to check their environment and activities continually to ensure they aren't putting themself in danger as they explore their expanding world. Make sure they understand the basics of stair safety, and keep an eye on them always when you are out and about.

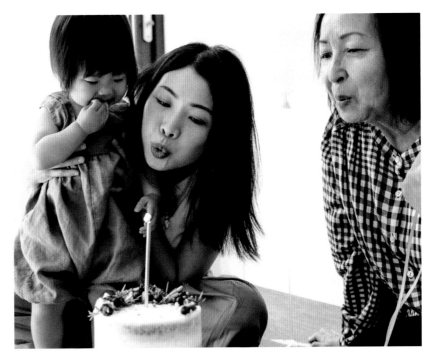

Happy birthday! Your baby's birthday marks the end of a miraculous year of development, and you may choose to celebrate this wonderful journey with your family and closest friends.

Support their developmental skills with games and pursuits that keep them entertained and stimulated. Your input remains crucial to their continued development.

Your baby will hold their own at the dinner table now, and the more often you can eat together, the better their food choices, table manners, and social skills will become. Try not to pass on your own dislikes—a varied diet will give them the best chance of good health and development.

Take time to stop and enjoy the small things—write down their amazing firsts, capture their activities on camera, save their first artistic creations, and record their attempts at speech. The coming years will pass with lightning speed. You've created a unique little person with a world of opportunity in front of them. Take pride in their achievements and rest assured that all of your hard work has produced the best possible results.

YOUR BABY'S
HEALTH

The health and well-being of your baby are prime concerns, and the more informed and confident you feel about recognizing and treating illness when it happens, the easier it is to manage. Most babies experience at least one bout of sickness in their first year, so this chapter clearly explains all the common illnesses and how best to treat your child. Of course, there's no substitute for a parent's instinct, so if you are worried about your baby's health, call your pediatrician right away.

Your unwell baby

THE BETTER INFORMED YOU ARE, THE MORE CONFIDENT YOU WILL FEEL CARING FOR YOUR SICK BABY. Your baby's immune system is still developing, so they are susceptible to a number of illnesses during this first year. Most of these will be minor, but occasionally a more serious illness may develop. It's vital that you know what to look for so you can take the right action.

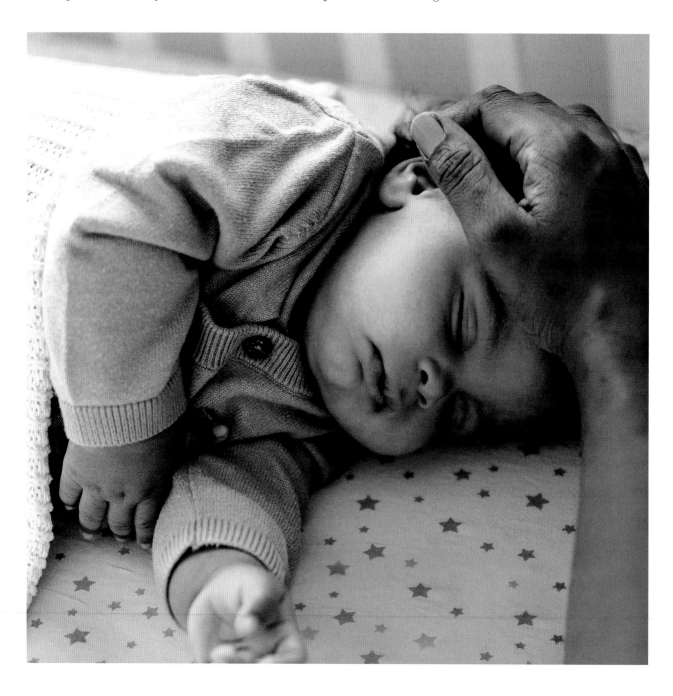

When your baby is ill

As a new parent, it can be hard to tell if your baby is sick, but as you get to know them, you'll recognize when something is wrong.

Prolonged crying can be a sign that your baby feels unwell or has pain, especially if you can't pacify them. Listen for a hoarse cry or one of a higher pitch than usual. Conversely, a very ill baby may cry much less than usual, so take note if your baby is unusually quiet and subdued, especially if they also have other symptoms (see p.369).

Your baby may lose interest in feeding when they're not feeling well, or they may take in less than usual. Vomiting is a common symptom, too, and it doesn't always mean the problem is with your baby's tummy.

Once your baby starts smiling, they're likely to smile a lot of the time. If your baby looks grumpy or won't smile at you when you talk, there may be something wrong. In much the same way, older babies often lose interest in playing when they're not well. Instead, your baby may become more clingy, hanging onto you when you are nearby and not wanting you to leave the room. If your baby's breathing is noisier or faster than usual, there's likely to be something wrong. A slightly ill baby may also sleep more than usual. However, you should be able to rouse them; if they're unresponsive, call an ambulance or take them to the hospital yourself if you can get there quickly.

Dehydration

Many common illnesses cause serious fluid loss, and fever compounds the problem. Babies can quickly become dehydrated, which is a major concern, so it's vital to recognize the signs.

• At first, dry lips may be the only symptom.
• As dehydration worsens, your baby's diapers may be drier than usual. Their skin may feel dry and loose. Your baby may be a bit lethargic. You may also notice that their fontanel (the soft spot on top of the head) looks slightly sunken. Contact your pediatrician immediately. With severe dehydration, your baby may pass dark yellow urine, have fewer wet diapers, and their eyes may appear sunken. Your baby may have a fast heart rate or be breathing rapidly. They need urgent treatment: call your pediatrician, or go to a pediatric emergency facility.

To avoid dehydration, offer plenty of breast- or formula milk. They will need extra fluids to replace those lost, especially if they have diarrhea or vomiting. If your baby is under six months and formula-fed, you can also offer them oral rehydration solution. If your baby is vomiting, ask your doctor about how to give an oral rehydration solution, which is easier for them to keep down. This replaces fluids, and the sugars and salts lost due to an upset tummy.

TAKE YOUR BABY'S TEMPERATURE

Fever is the body's response to infection, so a raised temperature can tell you if your baby is ill. Normal body temperature is 98.6°F (37°C) and about 1°F (0.5°C) lower when taken in the armpit. The best way to take your baby's temperature is from the ear or armpit, although the latter can be hard because they need to hold still for at least a couple minutes to get a reading. Oral thermometers can't be used for babies because they might bite them. When you talk to your doctor, tell them the temperature that you read, and how you took it.

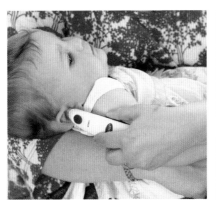 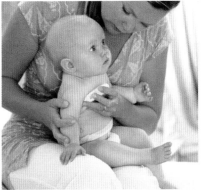

Ear thermometer Hold your baby firmly and place the thermometer in your baby's ear, following the instructions to make sure you position it correctly (left). **Under-arm thermometer** Place your baby on your lap and hold them still to get a more accurate reading.

Getting medical help

If your baby is ill, you may need to take them to the doctor's or—if you are seriously concerned about their health—to the hospital.

Seeing the doctor

The American Academy of Pediatrics recommends taking your child to the pediatrician at least nine times during the first three years. Most practices fit in sick babies between appointments and offer emergency appointments. When you call to make an appointment, let the receptionist know your baby's

WHEN TO CALL THE DOCTOR

As you get to know your baby, you'll find it easier to recognize when they need medical help. Seek advice if you think your baby may be sick. Babies can become critically ill quickly. Call your doctor if your baby:
• Runs a fever of over 100.4°F (38°C) for newborns; over 101°F (38.3°C) for babies under 6 months; or over 103°F (39.4°C) for babies over 6 months.
• Has a fever that persists for longer than five days.
• Refuses to feed.
• Appears drowsy and off-color.
• Vomits persistently, bringing up green or blood-streaked vomit.
• Shows signs of severe dehydration (see p.363).
• Has six or more episodes of diarrhea in a period of 24 hours, or continues to have diarrhea for longer than five days.
• Passes blood or mucus in their stools.
• Has bleeding that will not stop.
• Produced discharge from their ears, eyes, or genitals in the past 24 hours.
• Has difficulty breathing, or is panting or breathing rapidly.
• Has a rash
• Has a seizure (convulsion)
• Has a minor burn or scald.

age. If your baby has a rash, mention this—an infection may put others at risk, so the doctor may prioritize you. Take a spare diaper with you, since you will probably want to put a clean one on after the doctor examines your baby. If your baby has diarrhea, it can also be useful to take a dirty diaper with you in case your doctor needs a sample for testing. Many pediatricians have someone on call for advice 24 hours a day, so call their number first if you feel it is urgent.

Getting the most from your visit

Describe your baby's symptoms clearly, not forgetting the details of their temperature and any medicines or home remedies you have already tried. Always tell your doctor what's on your mind, whether you're concerned about a cough or worried about the possibility of meningitis. This will ensure you are both on the same wavelength.

Make sure you understand any instructions as to what to do, and how to give any medicines. Your doctor should also tell you what to watch for and what to do if your baby doesn't improve, and when to return for follow-up. Don't worry about being a bit of a nuisance; occasional false alarms are inevitable when you're finding your way as a parent. Many doctors have children themselves and can identify with your situation. They

Making an appointment Talk to your pediatrician if your baby is showing signs of illness, or you are not sure of their condition.

should understand your concerns about your precious little bundle, and will know that one or two unnecessary consultations are far better than letting things go unchecked for too long.

If you feel you can't communicate with your doctor, perhaps this isn't the right doctor for your family. Every professional has different interests and skills, and after a few consultations you may decide you would be better with a different doctor, either within the same practice or an entirely new one.

If you just want advice

Some local hospitals offer 24-hour hotlines with pediatric health advice

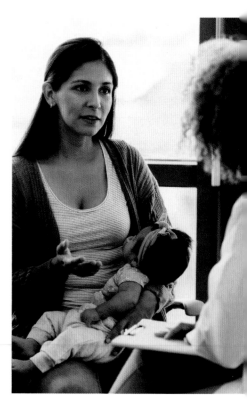

for parents. Try your pediatrician for issues such as breastfeeding and minor concerns like colic, or your pharmacist for advice on treating minor ailments such as diaper rash. Many areas have walk-in centers or urgent care facilities, where you can drop in any time of day and see a nurse, but before you go, check that they have facilities for babies. If you need to see a doctor when the office is closed, call and their service will arrange an appointment or have the doctor call you.

Going to the ER

Most parents take their little one to the ER at some point. In the majority of cases, there's nothing seriously wrong. Occasionally, though, worries about a baby's health may mean they need to stay in the hospital.

However worried you feel, try to stay calm. When you arrive at the ER, find your way to reception. You may be redirected to a children's emergency room if there is one; otherwise there should be a dedicated children's nurse to assess your child. Be as clear as you can about what has happened and your baby's symptoms. The nurse will assess the severity of your child's illness, and you will either be seen by a doctor right away or asked to wait.

If you aren't seen immediately by a doctor, it can be difficult to predict how long you will have to wait, since priority in an ER is given to the most urgent cases. However, as a general rule, young babies are usually seen within a few hours at the most. Because you may be waiting some time, don't forget to take your baby's comfort object, a pacifier, if needed, plus any milk, bottles, or diapers.

WHEN TO CALL 911

Call 911 for an ambulance, or take your baby to the hospital yourself (if you can get there quickly) if your baby:
• has stopped breathing or is having difficulty breathing; has blue skin, lips, or tongue
• is unresponsive, floppy, drowsy, or will not wake up
• has had a fit (convulsion) or febrile seizure
• has severe bleeding that will not stop
• has a purple-red spotty rash that doesn't fade when a glass is rolled over it
• has a severe allergic reaction (anaphylaxis)
• has severe scalds or burns
• appears to become unwell after swallowing something harmful, such as a household product or medication.

STAYING IN THE HOSPITAL

Children's hospital units are now much brighter, friendlier, and less formal places than they used to be. Pediatricians don't wear white coats and are often the most approachable of all hospital specialists.

Staying with your baby If your baby has to stay in the hospital, you can almost always stay too, though expect facilities for parents to be basic in many units. From your baby's point of view, the most important thing is that you can be there to reassure them throughout most tests and procedures. If they have to have blood taken, an anesthetic cream is usually applied first to make the test painless. If your baby needs a surgery under local anesthesia, your presence is usually welcome. You won't be allowed in for procedures under general anesthesia, but you can be there holding your baby

until they are fast asleep. Bringing in favorite toys, a comfort object, or a blanket may help settle your baby.

Planned hospital admissions If an older baby needs to go into the hospital, there'll be time to warn them. Tell them a little about it so it doesn't come as a huge surprise. Babies are very aware of their parents' moods and emotions, so try to stay positive no matter what's happening. If you have negative feelings about hospitals or needles, do your best to keep them to yourself. Use a soft voice to help calm your baby. You can also sing favorite songs or nursery rhymes.

Being informed Understanding the treatment your child is being given will help prevent unnecessary anxiety. If you're not sure what's happening, ask, and never

feel intimidated. There are usually doctors and nurses on hand who will be happy to answer your questions. It can be useful to write down any questions you have, since it's easy to forget when there is so much going on.

When it's time for your baby to go home, make sure you understand the discharge plan and have contact details if you need to seek help.

Taking care of your sick baby

Your baby is likely to need all your attention when they're feeling ill. Knowing what to do can make all the difference in their recovery.

YOUR HOME MEDICINE CABINET

Stocking a cabinet with essential medical supplies will enable you to deal with common ailments quickly and effectively. Keep medicines out of your baby's reach—ideally in a cool, dark place—and check expiration dates. Make sure medicines are right for your baby's age.
• Liquid baby acetaminophen
• Baby ibuprofen
• Calamine lotion, for bites and rashes
• Rehydrating solution/sachets
• Antibacterial ointment for cuts and scrapes
• Infant topical pain-relief gel, to relieve teething discomfort
• Medicine syringe and/or spoon
• Thermometer
• Self-stick bandages

ADMINISTER DROPS

In all cases, wash your hands, make sure the medicine dropper does not come into direct contact with your baby, and sterilize it between uses.

Nose drops Lay your baby on their back on your lap, tilting their head back gently if they are an older baby. Be sure to support your baby's head and drip the nose drops into each nostril.

Eye drops Lay your baby down on your lap and hold their head steady with one arm. Gently pull down the lower eyelid and squeeze the bulb so drops go into the space between the lid and the eyeball. Then wipe the excess drops off their cheek. If you have trouble managing this, get another adult to help hold your baby.

Ear drops Warm the ear drops by holding in your palm for a few minutes, then lay your baby down on their side on your lap. They need to be comfortable since they will have to stay in this position for a little while. Hold their head firmly, yet gently, and let the drops fall from the dropper into the ear. Keep them still for a few minutes since you don't want the drops to spill out right away. When your baby sits up again, a little excess may leak out, so have a tissue ready to catch it.

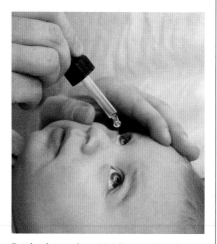

Putting in eye drops Holding your hand steady, squeeze the bulb of the dropper to infuse the medication behind the lower lid.

You can expect babies who are sick to be demanding and to need your presence. Prioritize things so you can spend time cuddling your little one, or at least sitting with them. A good babysitter or trusted relative can fit the bill, but your baby will prefer to have the reassurance of a parent.

A sick baby may still want to play simple games, or to hear you tell a favorite story. Often this is the same story over and over again. They may also enjoy listening to recorded stories and rhymes, though it's your voice that has special significance for them.

Keep an eye on their temperature (see p.363) and check it if they feel especially warm or are miserable. There's no need to treat every fever, but try to lower it if they are uncomfortable, the temperature is very high, or your doctor has advised you to do so. Infant acetaminophen or ibuprofen may be suitable (read the instructions). Use one of these medicines only, not both together.

Babies usually need extra fluids when they're ill, especially if they're feverish. Fever is a normal response to infection, but it contributes to dehydration. This in turn can make fever worse, so it's something of a vicious circle. If you're breastfeeding, continue with this. They may or may not need water, too—check with your pediatrician. Older babies may need encouragement to drink. Make sure there's always a drink within reach.

If your baby is on solids, don't worry too much if they won't eat much while they're not well. Right now fluids matter more than food.

There's no need for your baby to be in the crib when ill, though it may be convenient to keep them in nighttime clothing since this is often simpler to change in and out of. At night, it's a good idea to keep your baby close by. If they already sleep in their own room, you might want to move the crib into your room as a temporary measure. This makes it easier to attend to them if they need anything at night, and you may sleep more easily knowing that they are near you.

While your baby is ill, you could skip bath time in favor of sponge bathing, or a simple cleaning with a washcloth. It all depends on how sick they are and how much they enjoy a bath. Some older babies relax in the bath. You can then put them into fresh clothing, which could make them feel a lot better. Lukewarm sponging is no longer recommended as a treatment for fever.

It can be tiring taking care of a baby who is sick, so put your feet up and rest when your baby sleeps. Don't spend too much time rushing around doing chores. If you need help, don't be afraid to ask friends or relatives to take over for a little while so you can get some rest. However tired you are, never fall asleep on the sofa with your sick baby in your arms.

Giving medication

If your baby has been prescribed medication, such as antibiotics, it's very important to give the correct dosages and to finish the full course as directed. This applies to topical treatments, such as steroid creams, too. You'll need to give any medications to your baby in liquid form and there are several different methods for doing this (see below).

GIVE YOUR BABY MEDICINE

There are several techniques for giving a baby medicine by mouth, whether it's a prescription from your doctor or an over-the-counter remedy. Wash your hands before you start, and make sure you know what the dose is supposed to be. An overdose can be dangerous, especially for young babies. When giving medicine, hold your baby so they are slightly upright. Don't lay them down flat because there's a risk they may inhale the medicine into their lungs.

Using a syringe This is probably the best method for very young babies, who haven't learned to swallow from a spoon, and for medicines for which small, precise doses are needed. For a baby under six months, sterilize the syringe before use. Fill the syringe from the bottle, then pick up and hold your baby in the crook of your arm. Put the mouthpiece of the medicine syringe on your baby's lower lip and gently push the plunger so the medicine goes into their mouth.

Using a dropper Sterilize first, for a baby under six months, then draw in the right amount of medicine in the dropper before picking your baby up. Lean your baby back slightly, and place the tip of the dropper into the corner of their mouth, or just inside the lower lip. Squeeze the medicine out, making sure the dropper empties completely into your baby's mouth and that they swallow the liquid.

Using a spoon This is the most common method for babies over 12 weeks or so of age, especially if the dose is at least 2.5 ml. Measure the dose before picking up your baby. Holding your baby upright, touch the lower part of the spoon to their bottom lip, then gently tip the spoon up so the medicine goes into their mouth.

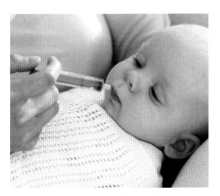

Syringe For very young babies, you'll probably find it easiest to give medicines with a syringe.

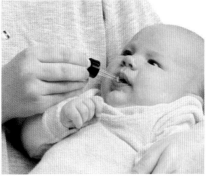

Dropper When using a dropper, make sure all the medicine goes into your baby's mouth.

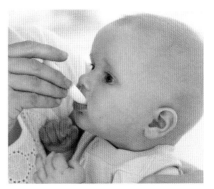

Spoon Babies over 12 weeks can usually manage a spoon.

Illnesses & injuries

AN ILL OR INJURED BABY NEEDS LOTS OF COMFORT COMBINED WITH THE RIGHT ACTION.
When your baby isn't well or has fallen and bumped themself, it's important that you know
when it's fine to treat them at home, which measures are appropriate, and when you need to
seek medical advice. If you're confident about what to do, you'll be calmer and more effective.

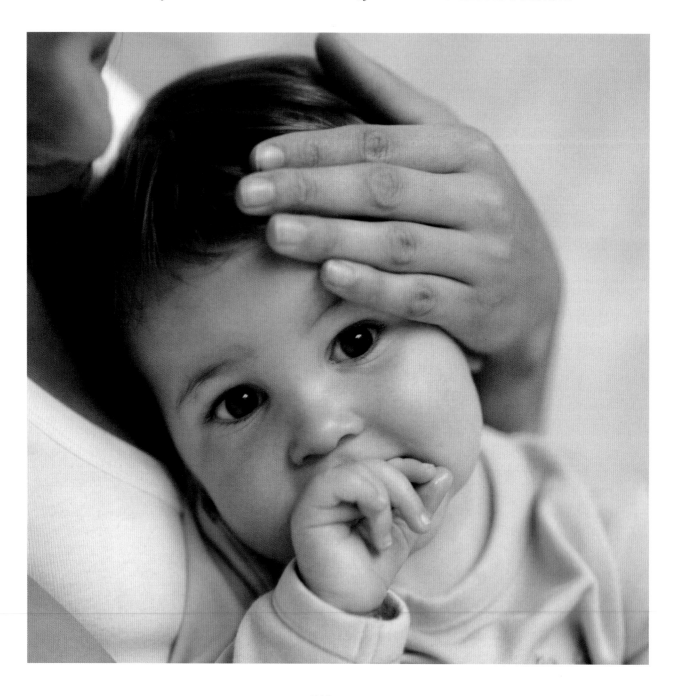

Common conditions

When your baby isn't feeling her best, it could be any one of a number of conditions. Babies often can't signal what's wrong.

Fever

Fever is not an illness, but a symptom. It is the body's normal response to infection or inflammation, so always take note of a fever, especially if your baby is under six months old.

Causes include the flu, chest infection, gastroenteritis, urinary tract infection, and infectious diseases such as roseola (see p.374). A fever can also occur after a routine immunization.

You may suspect your baby has a fever from touch, especially if the back of the neck feels hot or sweaty, but you can only know for sure by taking their temperature (see p.363).

Dealing with fever Fever can have a dehydrating effect. That's why it's important to give plenty of fluids when a baby or child is feverish, and to watch for signs of dehydration (see p.363).

Don't overdress your baby since this makes it harder for body temperature to drop back down to normal. When indoors, a diaper and a onesie may be enough, but keep watch; babies aren't good at controlling body temperature and can also get cold quickly.

There's no point in sponge bathing your baby or giving a bath since it is likely to make them miserable. It's perfectly alright to let the fever run its course without medication, but if your child is especially fussy, you can relieve fever in babies over three months with baby acetaminophen or ibuprofen if your doctor says it's okay. (Ask for the proper dosage.) Do not give both at the same time. However, if one of them doesn't work, you can try the other one.

When to see the doctor In young babies, fever is less common and therefore more significant. As a rule, the younger your baby, the more quickly you need to get medical attention, but use your instincts, too. In older babies, their actual temperature or how long they have had it often does not indicate how sick they are. Contact your doctor if:
• Your baby has a temperature of 102.2°F (39°C) or more (100.4°F/38°C or more if under three months old).
• Your baby seems unwell, even if the fever is mild
• There are any worrying symptoms such as vomiting or trouble breathing
• Your baby is unresponsive.

Your doctor may ask for a urine sample because a urinary tract infection is relatively common in babies yet does not cause any of the typical symptoms adults get (see p.409).

Get medical attention urgently if:
• Your baby has a rash that doesn't fade with pressure (see p.410)
• Your baby has a seizure
• Their general condition worsens.

Reflux

Gastroesophageal reflux (GOR) is a condition in which the stomach contents flow up the esophagus and cause symptoms. It's estimated that around half of all babies under three months have it, but few have severe symptoms. Both breastfed and formula-fed babies may be affected. Reflux occurs because the valve at the lower end of the esophagus is lax. However, this corrects itself in time.

FEBRILE SEIZURES

In babies over six months and young children, a high fever can lead to a seizure (convulsion) known as a febrile seizure.

Fever can be stressful for a baby or child's brain and can temporarily disrupt the signals between brain cells, in some cases triggering a seizure. This usually occurs at a time when body temperature rises rapidly. Your baby is more likely to be affected if there is a family history of febrile seizures or other types of seizures.

A seizure can be frightening to see even though it usually lasts less than two minutes. The baby loses consciousness, stops breathing momentarily, and tends to wet or soil themselves. The limbs and face may twitch and the eyes often roll upward. When it stops, the baby regains consciousness, but may be very sleepy.

During a seizure, lie them on their side and don't try to restrain them, but make sure they are safe and cannot fall. If possible, note the time of onset of the seizure. Call an ambulance if your baby's seizure lasts more than 15 minutes: any seizure lasting longer than this is likely to be more serious than a febrile convulsion.

If your baby has had a seizure, call your doctor. If this is their first seizure, they are likely to need hospital tests to rule out a serious cause. For any subsequent seizures, they should still have a checkup to find the cause of their high fever.

The symptoms to look out for include:
• bringing up large amounts of milk
• vomiting
• coughing
• irritability
• feeding poorly
• rarely, blood in the stools or vomit (seek urgent medical help).

You may suspect reflux in your baby if they scream during feedings as if in pain, or spit up a lot. However, many babies spit up without having reflux. Occasionally, reflux has more serious effects such as breathing problems or poor growth because a baby is unable to keep down feedings.

Giving smaller, more frequent feedings can help reflux. Burping and holding your baby upright for 20 minutes after being fed can also relieve symptoms.

Your doctor may prescribe a thickened formula or a thickener that you add to feedings, and also an infant antacid, which helps the action of the valve in the esophagus. If neither of these approaches helps or your baby has severe symptoms, your pediatrician may suggest tests or a different prescription.

Tongue-tie

There is normally a strip of tissue between the floor of the mouth and the underside of the tongue (this is called the frenulum). In tongue-tie, this strip is shorter and often thicker than usual, which can restrict tongue movements. Most cases of tongue-tie are mild, but in some babies it may prevent successful breastfeeding.

It's debatable whether tongue-tie can hinder learning to speak. Most experts don't think so, mainly because it has often improved by the time speech starts. However, if you think your baby has tongue-tie, see your doctor. A few babies need a minor procedure, using a local anesthetic, to release the tie.

Conjunctivitis

This is inflammation of the lining of the eyeball and/or eyelids. It can be bacterial, viral, or allergic. Bacterial conjunctivitis is the most common type in babies under six months. They often get conjunctivitis because their tear ducts are still immature, so germs can easily collect and set up an infection.

You may notice that your baby's eyelids are crusty in the morning or after a nap, or there may be a blob of pus in the corner of the eye. Your baby's eyes can also become bloodshot and the eyelids may be swollen.

If symptoms are mild, and the white of the eye isn't red, wipe your baby's eyes with cotton balls dipped in cooled, boiled water or your own breast milk. Wash your hands before you begin, and wipe from the nose toward the outer side of the eye, using a clean cotton ball for each eye. Be careful not to touch the eyeball.

If pus accumulates again, consult your pediatrician. Your baby may need a prescription for eye drops or ointment containing antibiotic. Conjunctivitis can affect one eye or both, but it's usual to treat both eyes if you are given drops, even if only one eye is affected.

If your baby has frequent episodes of conjunctivitis, your pediatrician

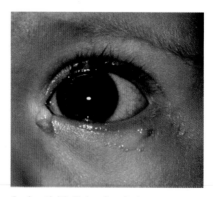

Conjunctivitis Blobs of pus in the corner a baby's eyes, as seen here, are often a sign of conjunctivitis caused by bacterial infection.

may show you how to massage the tear ducts to help the flow of tears.

Vomiting

All babies spit up—bring up a little milk—but in vomiting the stomach contracts, and the amount brought up is much greater. Vomiting is most often related to a problem with feeding or something affecting the stomach or intestines, as in:
• overfeeding
• gastroenteritis (see opposite)
• allergy to food (see p.372)
• reflux (see p.369)
• pyloric stenosis (see below)
• bowel obstruction (see right).

However, vomiting doesn't necessarily mean the trouble is anywhere near the tummy. Babies can also vomit when they're sick with an infection, especially a serious one like a urinary tract infection (see p.377), meningitis (see p.377), middle ear infection (see p.378), or chest infection (see p.377). Whooping cough also causes vomiting, most often at the end of a bout of coughing.

If your baby is sick and only vomits once, you may not need the doctor. However, babies get dehydrated easily and can become ill quickly, so as a rule consult your doctor if your baby vomits more than once or twice. Specific treatment depends on the cause.

Pyloric stenosis In this condition, there is overgrowth of the muscle of the pylorus, the valve at the stomach outlet. As a result, the outlet is too narrow for stomach contents to pass through and instead they are vomited out. Around 1 baby in 400 develops the condition. It's most common in boys between four and six weeks old.

Vomiting occurs right after a feeding and can be so forceful that the regurgitated feeding shoots across the room—so-called projectile vomiting. The baby is usually hungry and may

INTUSSUSCEPTION

In this condition, part of the bowel telescopes into itself, as if being swallowed. This creates a blockage. Symptoms include:
• screaming from pain (often intermittent)
• fever
• vomiting
• dehydration or shock
• blood and mucus in the stools (often described as looking like raspberry jelly).

It's a rare condition that affects babies 3–12 months old, sometimes just when they're recovering from gastroenteritis. However, it's worth knowing about since it can be very serious if untreated. It is often possible to treat without surgery, but some babies need an operation.

appear well, but dehydration sets in as the condition progresses. Pediatricians sometimes check for a lump in the stomach area after a feeding, but ultrasound scanning is a much more reliable test. Treatment is a small operation to release the overgrown muscle. This can sometimes be done laparoscopically.

Bowel obstruction This is not common, but it is very serious. Normally vomit looks like milk or food, but in bowel obstruction the vomit is bile stained, so it looks green. If your baby's vomit is green, contact your doctor immediately or go to the ER.

Gastroenteritis

This means inflammation or infection in the stomach or intestines, and can be caused by bacteria or viruses. It causes vomiting and often diarrhea, too, though some infections, such as norovirus ("winter vomiting disease"),

cause vomiting without diarrhea.

Rotavirus infection is the most common cause of gastroenteritis in babies. Bacterial causes include E. coli, salmonella, shigella, and campylobacter. In general, gastroenteritis is more common in bottle-fed babies. Possible symptoms are:
• vomiting and/or diarrhea
• stomach ache, especially before a bowel movement
• fever.

Always talk to your doctor if you think your baby has gastroenteritis, since babies get dehydrated very quickly. Seek help urgently if your baby has had any blood in the stool. This can occur with some types of gastroenteritis, but it is also typical of intussusception (see left), a form of bowel blockage in babies under a year. In an episode of gastroenteritis, it isn't usually essential to know which bacteria or viruses started it off. However, occasionally your doctor will ask you to provide a sample for analysis.

The main goal of treatment is to replace lost fluids and, in many cases, your doctor will tell you to treat your baby at home. Your doctor will probably advise you to give your baby an oral rehydration solution, which contains the right balance of salts and sugar to prevent dehydration. Give small sips at a time, or your baby won't keep it down. If you're breastfeeding, you can continue. If your baby is bottle-fed, use rehydration solution instead of formula.

Keep plenty of paper towels on hand, and possibly a bowl for an older baby. Maintain good hygiene, washing hands often, and keep away from other people. Most causes of gastroenteritis are very contagious. Keep a close eye on your baby's progress. If they don't improve, a hospital visit may be needed.

Diarrhea

Every baby has loose bowel movements sometimes. Breastfed babies often have loose stool, and this is normal. Diarrhea means the frequent passing of stool that is looser than usual. In some cases, the motion will be very runny and may leak out of the diaper. Causes include:
• gastroenteritis (see left)
• allergy or milk intolerance (see p.372)
• cystic fibrosis.

The most common cause of diarrhea is gastroenteritis, but in babies almost any feverish illness, even an ear infection, can trigger diarrhea. Some antibiotics can cause diarrhea, since they can kill off some of the beneficial bacteria in the intestinal tract. As with vomiting, diarrhea can make your baby dehydrated very quickly, so call your doctor if your baby has more than four to six runny bowel movements in 24 hours, or has other symptoms that concern you. Watch for signs of dehydration (see p.363), keeping in mind that when a baby in diapers has diarrhea, you can't tell whether they're urinating. You'll probably be advised to:
• Give rehydration solution. You can continue breastfeeding. If your baby is bottle-fed, you may also be able to continue, but this depends on how bad the diarrhea is. Your pediatrician will guide you.
• Keep a close eye on your baby.
• Take strict hygiene precautions and keep away from others.
• Avoid taking your baby to a swimming pool for 14 days after the last episode of diarrhea.

Constipation

This means the passage of hard, infrequent stool. Breastfed babies can pass stool less often, but if the bowel movement looks normal, then it's not constipation. The most common causes of constipation in babies are:
• Starting on solid food

• lack of fiber in the diet
• lack of fluid (for example, during an illness)
• incorrectly made formula feeds.

In very young babies, constipation can be caused by a rare congenital condition called Hirschsprung's disease in which there is an abnormal segment of bowel.

When a baby is constipated, they may only move their bowels two or three times a week. The motions may be hard and pellet-like or much bulkier. They can be painful to pass, and may even tear the edge of the anal canal, causing bleeding. As a result, the baby avoids bowel movements, constipation worsens, and pain can develop.

Consult your pediatrician if your baby is constipated. Avoid home remedies or laxatives for older children or adults, which are often unsuitable for babies.

Hirschsprung's disease may be suspected if your baby did not pass meconium (black sticky stool) in the first day of life. More tests and surgery may be needed. However, in older infants, the cause is more likely to be dehydration or a diet low in fruit and vegetables. Your doctor may prescribe a mild laxative to begin with, but the long-term answer is for your baby to have a well-balanced diet.

Jaundice

Jaundice means a yellow tinge to the skin and the whites of the eyes caused by a buildup of a chemical called bilirubin in the blood. Bilirubin comes from the breakdown of red blood cells—it's the reason why bruises go through a yellow phase.

Normally the liver clears bilirubin from the bloodstream, but the liver is immature in newborn babies and they also have more red blood cells. That's why more than half of all babies develop slight jaundice during the first week after birth. In most

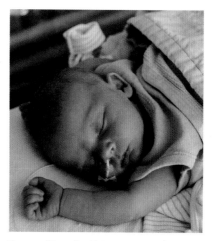

Neonatal jaundice This is a common and usually harmless condition. Look for a yellow discoloration of your baby's skin and eyes.

cases, no treatment is needed and the jaundice gets better on its own within a few weeks. Premature babies are more likely to become jaundiced because their livers cope less easily with bilirubin. This can occasionally cause problems, so if your baby is born prematurely, they may be placed under a blue light (phototherapy) which speeds up the removal of bilirubin. Breastfed babies are more likely to get jaundiced—factors in the milk seem to block enzymes in the liver, and it can run in families. It does not need treatment.

Jaundice can be serious:
• If it begins before 24 hours; causes include bleeding due to a difficult delivery, infections, and blood group incompatibility. Urgent treatment in a neonatal intensive care unit (NICU) will be needed.
• If it lasts longer than two weeks. See the doctor promptly to rule out a possibly serious liver problem. Watch, also, for pale stools and dark yellow urine because these are also very significant symptoms.

Allergy

Allergies are increasingly common, and if there are allergies in your family, your baby is more likely to develop them. However, there's more to it than genetics, because identical twins don't necessarily have the same allergies. The most common symptoms include: swollen lips and throat; runny or blocked nose; coughing and wheezing; itchy skin or rash; reflux, nausea, and vomiting; diarrhea and abdominal pain; blood and mucus in stools.

Occasionally, an allergy can cause a severe reaction called anaphylaxis (see below).

Eczema (see p.375) is the most common allergic reaction in babies. It often starts around 3–12 months. In 1 in 10 children, eczema is linked to an underlying food allergy even though the food allergy may not be obvious yet.

The most common food allergy in babies is cow's milk (specifically to

ANAPHYLACTIC SHOCK

This is a severe, overwhelming allergic reaction. Luckily, it is rare in babies. Possible triggers include foods such as milk, nuts, and eggs, as well as insect venom and drugs. There could be vomiting or a rash at first, then:
• noisy breathing or wheezing
• swelling of the tongue
• a hoarse cry
• collapse
• widespread rash.

However, anaphylaxis is difficult to spot in the very young, and your baby may just become very floppy. Immediate hospital care is vital. If you have been prescribed an adrenaline (epinephrine) injection for your baby, give it right away.

cow's milk protein). About 2−7 percent of babies under a year have it. A reaction can occur immediately after ingesting cow's milk, or it can take several days to develop.

See your doctor if you think your baby has an allergy to cow's milk. Tests can help diagnose it, but they don't always. You may be advised to change your baby's formula, or, if you are breastfeeding, to avoid dairy products yourself. Babies usually outgrow this type of allergy by the age of three. Some do not and will need to continue to avoid milk products.

Milk intolerance is not a true allergy, but an intolerance to lactose, caused by an enzyme deficiency. Symptoms include diarrhea and vomiting. An intolerance can develop after gastroenteritis and is usually resolved by changing to lactose-free milk for a month, after which your baby should be able to resume normal milk.

Other true food allergies include reactions to eggs, peanuts, tree nuts, wheat, soy, and shellfish. If your baby is allergic to eggs, they are able to receive vaccines manufactured with egg proteins. If their reaction to eggs was limited to hives, no precautions are necessary. If they also had swelling or trouble breathing from eggs, the vaccine should be administered under closer observation. Check with your doctor about these recommendations. There is no known way of preventing allergies from occurring but current advice is to exclusively breastfeed for the first six months and to wean your baby no earlier than six months, slowly introducing new foods, such as milk, eggs, peanuts, fish, soy, and gluten one at a time so you can spot any reaction.

Diaper rash

Affected skin will be inflamed and may look pimply. A wet or dirty diaper is the main cause of diaper rash, so the longer you can leave a diaper off, the better. You'll find that letting air get to the rash makes it less irritated. Try diaper-free playtime a couple of times a day for about 20 minutes or so, or as long as you can manage. Apply a little barrier cream before putting a clean diaper on.

Get advice from your pediatrician if the rash looks very angry, is weeping or blistered, or has small spots outside the main area of redness.

Chickenpox

Chickenpox is more usual in toddlers, but babies under a year can get it, too. The varicella-zoster virus that causes chickenpox is a very contagious and highly transmissible disease. The incubation period (time to develop the illness) is 14−21 days, but one episode usually gives immunity for life.

Your baby may feel sick for a day or so before the rash. Spots then appear as small red dots, mostly over the torso. They quickly develop into blisters, which may appear over a few days. Then they crust over and fall off. However, your baby remains contagious until all the spots have gone. Chickenpox is extremely itchy and your baby may be irritable and feel ill, especially if they

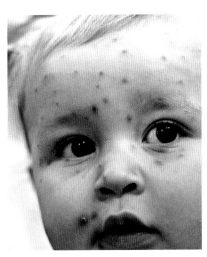

Chickenpox A chickenpox rash starts as small red dots. These turn into fluid-filled blisters with red bases, which then crust over.

also have spots inside the mouth. These are ulcers rather than blisters, and they can make feeding very uncomfortable.

In most cases, you'll be able to treat your baby at home. The following measures may help your baby feel more comfortable.
• Soothe skin with calamine lotion.
• Keep your baby's skin cool since this can help prevent more spots.
• You can try bathing your baby in lukewarm water with a tablespoon of sodium bicarbonate (baking soda).
• Keep your baby's nails short to reduce damage from scratching.
• If your baby has a sore mouth, give cooler feedings than usual, or else soft foods if they are on solids.
• Treat fever with acetaminophen or ibuprofen (always read the instructions, found inside the packaging, to ensure the medication is age appropriate. If in doubt ask the pharmacist).
• If your baby is exposed to chickenpox at under four weeks, talk to your pediatrician since they may need specialized treatment to stop them from developing severe symptoms.

Keep your baby away from anyone who hasn't had it. Chickenpox can be very serious for children and adults. It can lead to serious brain inflammation and skin infections that are resistant to treatment. Serious chickenpox is now preventable with the vaccine. It is included in the immunizations at a year of age, with a booster later. .

Thrush

This is caused by a yeast called Candida albicans (also known as monilia), which is normally present in the lower bowel. Most of the time, it causes no symptoms, but if it's present in larger amounts than usual it can cause thrush.

In babies, the most common areas for thrush are the diaper area and the mouth because these areas are warm and moist, so they encourage the growth of candida. Recent antibiotic treatment is also a factor, since some antibiotics suppress the beneficial bacteria that keep candida in check. Candida can infect your nipples if you breastfeed, causing stabbing pains, but this is no reason to stop nursing. In the diaper area, you may see:

• A red rash, often with a glazed appearance

• A scattering of small spots (satellites) outside the main area of rash.

If your baby has thrush in the mouth, there may be:

• Soreness when feeding from the breast or bottle, and poor feeding or crying during feedings

• Redness of the inside of the mouth

• White or creamy patches on the mouth or gums.

In most cases, thrush responds quickly to antifungal drops or gel prescribed by your pediatrician. Sometimes your baby needs a swab first to make sure that candida is the right diagnosis.

Roseola

This viral infection usually affects babies who are over six months old and is caused by herpesvirus 6. Its other names are roseola infantum, exanthema subitum, sixth disease, and three-day fever. Although it's common, not many parents know about it. It is highly contagious with an incubation period of 5–15 days.

• The first symptom is a high temperature, often over 104°F (40°C). There can be febrile seizures (see p.369), but despite this your baby may seem remarkably well.

• After three days of fever, a rash of pale

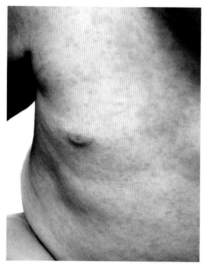

Roseola rash This common infection causes pinkish-red spots or patches, and is usually found on the tummy, chest, and back.

reddish spots appears over the torso and then spreads to the arms and legs, and sometimes the face. The spots may have a lighter halo around them. Because the rash may last only for 12 hours, it can be easy to miss.

• Your baby may also be irritable and tired, and have mild diarrhea and decreased appetite.

There's no specific treatment for roseola other than keeping your baby comfortable, giving fluids, and controlling fever. Most babies recover quickly. However, if your baby doesn't, talk to your doctor.

Laryngomalacia

Laryngomalacia (floppy larynx) is a common condition experienced in infancy and normally presents with symptoms of noisy breathing during inspiration (stridor), difficulty feeding, or increased effort breathing. If babies continue to feed well and gain weight, then no treatment or operation is necessary as the condition will usually improve by itself or go away by 18 months. If it does not and you suspect your baby has a floppy larynx, consult your doctor who may refer you to see an Ear, Nose and Throat (ENT) specialist.

THE MMR VACCINATION

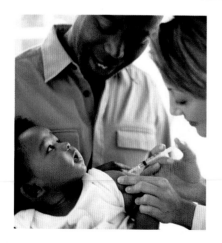

To protect against measles, mumps, and rubella, your baby will be offered the MMR vaccination between 12 and 18 months and then again between 4 and 6 years. Contact your pediatrician for advice should you suspect your baby has any one of these three infections

Measles is a highly contagious viral infection that can lead to serious complications, including pneumonia and

Getting a shot Just before the shot is given, distract your baby by calling their name or by singing their favorite nursery rhyme.

brain damage. Before the vaccine, measles caused many deaths in children. Mumps is usually a mild viral infection if contracted during childhood (it's rare in babies under two years old), but it can have serious complications, including deafness. In adults, the illness is usually much more severe and can lead to inflammation of the testes in men or ovaries in women.

Rubella (German measles) is usually a mild illness. However, immunization is important to protect pregnant women, since if they contract it, their unborn baby can be seriously affected.

Hand-foot-and-mouth disease

This is an infection caused by a type of coxsackie virus. It has no link with foot-and-mouth disease in animals. The illness is very contagious, but not usually serious. The incubation period is about 10 days. Because there are several coxsackie viruses that can cause this illness, it can recur.
• The typical rash appears on the palms, soles, and buttocks as small red spots, which can be flat or raised. Sometimes there's blistering.
• There may be ulcers in the mouth, which make feeding difficult. The spots can take two days to develop.
• Your baby may also feel unwell and run a fever.

The infection is easy to diagnose from the rash. There's no specific treatment other than keeping your baby comfortable, but it is wise to speak to your doctor, especially if your baby is very young.

Fifth disease

Also called parvovirus, slapped-cheek disease, and erythema infectiosum, fifth disease is usually mild. It's caused by parvovirus B19 and is very contagious. School-age children are

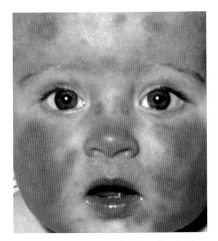

Fifth disease A bright red rash on the cheeks is characteristic of this viral infection, which is sometimes accompanied by a mild fever.

more likely to get it, but it can occur at any age. The incubation period seems to be 13–21 days, and it's no longer contagious once the rash appears.
• The typical rash is a red facial rash with a sharply defined edge on one or both cheeks. There may also be a fine, lacy rash on the arms and legs.
• Sometimes there's a mild fever.

In general, a baby or child with fifth disease will seem well. However, someone with sickle-cell disease can get very ill with parvovirus. The infection can also be dangerous if caught during pregnancy, with a small chance of miscarriage in the early stages. In adults, parvovirus can also cause joint pain, but this is transient.

Eczema

This is a common skin condition in babies. It's also known as atopic eczema, atopic referring to the tendency for the immune system to overreact. Babies affected by eczema usually have a relative with eczema or another atopic condition, such as asthma or hay fever. Eczema can clear up completely in time, but sometimes it becomes chronic.

Common sites for eczema are the ankles, elbows, wrist, face, neck, and back of the knees, but it can appear almost anywhere. The skin can look dry and cracked, or raw and weepy.

Your baby is likely to find their skin itchy, and may scratch a lot, especially at night. Keeping the nails short will help. Otherwise put scratch mittens on them before bedtime. Simple emollients are helpful for eczema.

Emollients come in the form of sprays, creams, ointments, leave-on products, and soap substitutes. You can buy these from a pharmacy without a prescription. However, if the skin condition is severe and a stronger treatment is needed, speak to your pediatrician.

Try changing to a different

(nonbiological) laundry detergent to see if this makes any difference. Your baby may also need a mild steroid cream prescribed by your pediatrician. Eczema can become infected because bacteria easily enter through small cracks. If your baby's eczema gets worse, this is a possibility, so see your doctor.

Heat rash

Also known as prickly heat, this is common in babies in warm weather. It's caused by excess sweat and is a sign that your baby is too hot. The typical small red pimples can appear almost anywhere, but most often on the neck, arms, face, torso, or near the diaper area. Your baby can find them irritating or itchy.

Cool your baby down by taking their clothes off, or changing them into lighter, cotton clothes. You can also apply calamine lotion if the rash seems to irritate your baby. The rash of prickly heat subsides within a day or two. Contact your doctor if it doesn't clear up quickly, or your baby seems unwell.

SUNBURN

Sunlight is good for babies and it helps the body produce vitamin D, but sunburn is not good. Prevention is better than cure. If your baby does get too much sun, immediately put them in the shade and give them fluids to drink. Soothe the skin with a lukewarm bath or lukewarm sponging. Make sure they don't go out in the sun again, even with sunscreen, until all the redness is gone. Call the doctor if your baby:
• Has a severe sunburn
• Has swelling on the face
• Has any signs of infection
• Starts to blister early on
• Is feverish
• Vomits, appears listless, or seems ill to you.

Colds

Babies often have colds because they are born with little immunity to the 200 or so cold viruses. Acquiring resistance is a matter of gradually becoming exposed to the range of these viruses. Colds have a short incubation period of around two days. Your baby is most likely to have a cold in the winter, when more people spend time indoors with each other.

Symptoms in babies are much the same as in older children. Your baby is likely to sneeze and have a runny or stuffed up nose, which makes feeding more difficult. Be patient during feedings and give your baby plenty of time. Your baby may also have a slight cough. This isn't usually serious, but it can develop into a chest infection (see opposite) or bronchiolitis (see right).

You can gently wipe your baby's nose; cotton balls or pads may be softer than a tissue. A couple drops of nasal saline and suctioning of the nose can help clear it and keep the mucus loose. Safely raising the head of the crib at night can help keep nasal passages clear.

Antibiotics do not treat colds, which are viral. Over the counter cold medicines are never recommended for infants. They are simply too young for them, and they may cause serious problems. A moist atmosphere makes it easier for your baby to breathe; you can buy a special baby humidifier. See your doctor if your baby:
• seems unwell
• refuses feeds
• coughs a lot
• has trouble breathing
• runs a high fever of 102.2°F (39°C) or above and that doesn't go down after giving age-appropriate acetaminophen or ibuprofen and lasts more than five days.

These may be signs of a more serious infection or that your baby has flu rather than a cold.

Bronchiolitis

This is an infection of the tiny air passages (bronchioles) in the lungs. It almost always affects babies and can be serious, especially in the very young. The most common cause is respiratory syncytial virus (RSV), but other viruses (such as adenovirus and flu virus) can cause the same symptoms. It is very contagious and often spreads in daycare centers.
• Bronchiolitis usually begins like a cold, then quickly progresses to cough, wheeze, and rapid breathing.
• Your baby's breathing may sound crackly or bubbly.
• A mild fever is usual.

Many babies with bronchiolitis seem well, but some become very ill. One sign to watch out for is indrawing of the chest between the ribs (or below the rib cage) during breathing. This suggests that your baby is fighting for breath. In severe cases, a baby may turn blue from lack of oxygen.

Always consult your doctor if you think your baby has bronchiolitis. Get medical help urgently if your baby is turning blue or fighting for breath.

In many cases, it is possible to take care of your baby at home, with your doctor's advice, but sometimes a baby with bronchiolitis needs to go to the hospital, especially if they:
• are very distressed
• are not taking fluids or become dehydrated
• are working hard to breathe
• have a very rapid respiratory rate
• turn blue.

Wheezing

Babies can wheeze and cough during or after viral infections. They may start with a cold but then develop a wheeze; cough; or noisy, rattly breathing that lasts a week or more. These symptoms occur as a result of inflammation and narrowing of the airways. Babies have narrow airways making them more likely to wheeze. It can be hard to tell the difference between this and bronchiolitis (see left). Seek urgent medical help if your baby is fighting for breath or looks blue. Wheezing

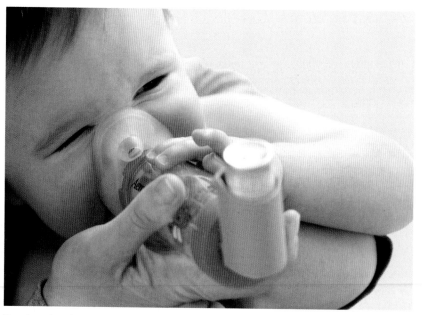

Treating wheezing Drugs to relieve symptoms by widening the airways are given to babies via a face mask and spacer attached to an inhaler.

COUGH MEDICINES

Over-the-counter cough and cold medicines should not be given to babies or children under four years old, according to the American Academy of Pediatrics.

Research has demonstrated that over-the-counter cough and cold medications are not very helpful for such young children, and in certain situations, they can actually be quite harmful.

Cold and cough medicine usually contains more than one active ingredient, so there's a danger of your baby or child overdosing if you give them, for example, baby acetaminophen after giving them a combination cold medication that also contains acetaminophen. Instead, it's better to stick with simple pain relievers and fever reducers, such as baby acetaminophen or baby ibuprofen, and give your baby plenty of liquids and love and attention.

Contact your pediatrician if your baby's symptoms worry you.

may be treated with drugs given through an inhaler to open the airways. It is too early to tell if wheezing might lead to asthma because asthma is a chronic, long-term condition that may not be diagnosed until babies are over 1 year.

Chest infection

This means any infection affecting the large air passages (bronchial tubes) leading to the lungs or the lung tissue itself. It includes pneumonia and bronchitis. Doctors often use the term "chest infection" when they can't be sure exactly where the problem lies. Both bacteria and viruses can cause chest infections. There are various symptoms that can accompany a chest infection, including:

• feeling unwell
• high fever
• rapid breathing and distress

• shortness of breath
• cough (though many youngsters with a chest infection do not have a cough)
• they may eat almost normally, or they may be off food and drink, at the risk of becoming dehydrated.

Always see your doctor if you think your baby might have this. It usually needs antibiotics and may also need oxygen and fluids in the hospital.

Croup

This is a form of laryngitis that affects babies over six months, is common in fall and winter, and is usually due to infection with para-influenza virus. Like bronchiolitis (see opposite), croup usually begins with cold symptoms and then progresses to wheezing and a typical barking cough. Your baby's voice may be hoarse. They may also have stridor—a noise when breathing in, suggesting the airways are partly blocked.

If you think your baby has croup, talk to your doctor. A baby with mild croup can often be treated at home. Your doctor may prescribe steroids, and suggest you steam the room to help reduce swelling in the airways. If your child's symptoms are severe and they are having difficulty breathing go to the hospital or call 911.

Urinary tract infections

Urinary tract infections (UTI) are surprisingly common in young babies. Most are bacterial and get into the system via the urethra—the opening that leads from the bladder to the outside. But symptoms in young babies are very different than in adults. A baby with a UTI may experience the following:

• fever
• irritability
• vomiting
• refusing feedings.

Young babies can have prolonged jaundice, or may not put on weight.

Always see your doctor if your baby has these symptoms. There is usually nothing to suggest the trouble is in the urinary system, except for the fact that your doctor will be unable to find a focus of infection when examining your baby. Only a urine sample can determine if it's a UTI.

It's vital to get a clean sample of urine for testing. You may be able to catch some urine in a sterile bottle when your baby urinates. However, this can be difficult with small babies. Your doctor will give you a special urine collector, which needs to be taped carefully over the penis or vagina until the baby urinates again. Very sick babies may have urine removed by catheter by the doctor. Make sure you deliver the sample to the doctor without delay.

UTIs need prompt treatment with antibiotics to avoid kidney damage and other complications. In most cases, a specialist will suggest a scan to rule out any abnormalities of the urinary system that could have led to infection. The doctor should give a follow-up test to make sure the infection has been eliminated after the course of antibiotics.

Meningitis

This means inflammation or infection in the meninges, the layers of tissue that wrap the brain, due to viruses or bacteria. Bacterial meningitis is more serious than viral. Many of the germs that cause meningitis live harmlessly in the back of the throat in healthy people. It's not certain exactly why they cause disease in some babies and children, but factors include overcrowding and passive smoking.

Since Hib, pneumococcal, and meningitis C immunization, many of the worst forms of meningitis have become less common. Still, meningitis is a very serious disease and it often goes hand in hand with septicemia (blood poisoning). By the time a baby has reached this stage, treatment is vital to save their life

and you must not waste a minute. That's why every parent needs to know how to recognize it and what to do. Symptoms in a baby can include:
• a high-pitched cry or moan
• refusing feedings
• irritability
• drowsiness
• limp or floppy limbs
• having a fever, but with cold hands or feet.
• a tense or bulging fontanel (soft spot on the top of the head)
• pale, blotchy, or clammy skin
• a rash of small red or brownish pin-prick spots, which can turn into

THE GLASS TEST

Rashes are common in babies, so it's hard to tell by looking at one if it's a rash linked with meningitis and septicemia (see p.377). However, the rash of meningococcal septicemia (sepsis or blood poisoning) does not fade when you press it, and a good way to check this is to carry out the glass (tumbler) test. Press the side of a glass firmly against your baby's skin where you see the rash. If you can still see the rash through the side of the glass, your baby may have meningitis/septicemia and needs urgent hospital treatment. It is harder to see on dark skin so check against paler areas.

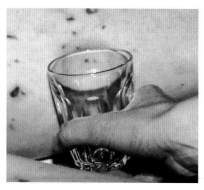

The glass test Press a glass firmly against your baby's skin where you see a rash. If the rash doesn't fade, call an ambulance.

large bruises and purplish marks. If you see this rash, it could be septicemia. Do the glass test (see below).

Call an ambulance immediately if your baby is ill with any of the above symptoms. Never wait for all the symptoms to develop. The rash and other skin changes are signs that a baby is already critically ill. Treatment is much more successful when it's given in the early stages. Tell the 911 operator as well as the ambulance and the hospital, that you suspect your baby may have meningitis.

Ear canal infection

Infection of the ear canal, also known as otitis externa, can occur when milk or food gets into the ear, or sometimes when the ear isn't dried after bath time. Babies that crawl may poke dirty fingers into their ears. Your baby may try scratching the ear, and you may see some redness or a little discharge. Generally, there's no fever and your baby remains well. See your doctor, who may prescribe ear drops. You can use baby acetaminophen or ibuprofen for pain relief, although discomfort is usually mild.

Middle ear infection

Also known as otitis media, infection of the middle ear, behind the eardrum, can be due to viruses or bacteria. It often happens after a cold when the infection spreads up the eustachian tubes that lead from the back of the nose to the ear. In babies and children, the eustachian tubes are short and run horizontally, which means they get more middle ear infections than adults. Sometimes only one ear is affected, but it's often both. Babies often have no symptoms that suggest the trouble is in the ear, but they may:
• feel very unwell
• be irritable or cry inconsolably
• have a high fever.

OTITIS MEDIA WITH EFFUSION

Otitis media with effusion is also known as glue ear. Normally, the middle ear space contains air. In otitis media with effusion, there's a buildup of sticky fluid instead. It occurs after repeated episodes of middle ear infection (see right), though there's no agreement on how many infections cause it. Some babies are more likely to develop it than others, and there can be a family history of the condition.

The most obvious symptom is hearing loss. Your baby may fail to hear you clearly, may not turn to look at you when you speak, or may look surprised when you suddenly appear over the side of the crib because they haven't heard you approach. Babies are learning all the time, and hearing is vital to most of their development. If untreated, otitis media with effusion can lead to problems with speech and behavior. Always see your doctor if you think your baby may have this or any other hearing problem.

Treatment may involve minor surgery to put in tympanostomy tubes. These tiny tubes let air in and equalize the pressure on each side of the eardrum. After a few months, the tubes usually fall out, by which time hearing is back to normal.

• refuse feedings
• vomit.
Some babies pull at the affected ear, but many babies also do this when they are tired.

If your baby has any of the symptoms above , contact your doctor promptly so decisions can be made about treatment. For infants older than 6 months, without severe symptoms, pain relief and close follow-up may be all that is needed. For others, a course of antibiotics may be required.

COMMON COMPLAINTS: QUICK REFERENCE

See a doctor if your baby's temperature is 102.2°F/39°C (100.4°F/38°C if under three months) or higher and does not go down after giving age-appropriate acetaminophen or ibuprofen, or persists for more than five days.

SYMPTOM	POSSIBLE CAUSE	WHAT TO DO
Fever	Fever is not a very specific symptom; babies can become feverish for all sorts of reasons. It is most commonly a sign of a viral or bacterial infection (see also Fever, p.369).	Offer plenty of fluids (breastfeeds, if breastfeeding); keep room cool. See your pediatrician if your baby's temperature is 102.2°F/39°C (100.4°F/38°C if under three months) or higher.
Runny nose	A runny nose, commonly producing clear mucus that thickens and turns yellow, green, or gray over about a week, is often caused by a cold (see p.376) and sometimes by flu. Other causes include allergy (see p.372), the early stages of bronchiolitis (see p.376), or croup (see p.377).	For a cold, make sure your baby has plenty of rest and fluids (breastfeeds, if breastfeeding). Ease their breathing by tilting the head end of the crib, if it's safe to do so. Ask your doctor about using saline drops.
Cough	A common symptom, it can be due to a cold (see p.376). Coughing can also be a symptom of a chest infection (see p.377); allergy (see p.372); bronchiolitis (see p.376) or wheezing (see p.376). A deep cough with a barking sound could be croup (see p.377), and bouts of coughing that end with a big breath in may indicate whooping cough.	Give plenty of fluids (breastfeeds, if breastfeeding). See a doctor if a cough persists for more than one week or is accompanied by a high fever or wheeze, if your baby is short of breath, makes a crackling breathing sound, refuses feedings, or is listless.
Rash	Once your baby is on solids, a rash around the mouth is often due to irritation from food. If their lips look swollen or they have other symptoms, suspect an allergy (see p.372). A rash can be a symptom of many common childhood viral infections, such as chickenpox (see p. 373). A rash can also occur with meningitis and septicemia (see p.377). Around the diaper area, the most likely cause is diaper rash (see p.373). Little bumps, or tiny blisters, particularly in skin folds, may be heat rash (see p.375). Eczema (see p.375) causes patches of dry skin.	Treatment depends on the cause of the rash. Do the glass test (see opposite) if the rash appears quickly or your baby is unwell. The more ill your baby seems, the more serious their rash is likely to be, so contact the doctor if you are concerned.
Vomiting	Vomiting affects most babies at some stage and is not usually serious. It is most often due to a problem in the digestive tract, but can indicate a serious infection elsewhere in the body (see also Vomiting, p.371).	Offer plenty of fluids (breastfeeds, if breastfeeding). If vomiting lasts longer than 12–24 hours, take your baby to the doctor, who may prescribe an oral rehydration solution.
Diarrhea	Diarrhea is a common symptom most often due to infection of the digestive tract (see also Diarrhea, p.370).	Treat as for vomiting (above). Use a barrier cream when changing your baby's diaper—loose stools can cause their bottom to become irritated.
Loss of appetite	Babies are sometimes reluctant to feed when teething, but other causes might be gastroenteritis (see p.371), or almost any other acute infection, including middle ear infection (see opposite).	Keep offering fluids (breastfeeds, if breastfeeding) and food, and keep checking the number of wet diapers to make sure they aren't becoming dehydrated. If they refuse several feedings in a row, contact the doctor.

Developmental concerns

Treating milestones as helpful guidelines prevents unnecessary anxiety, but seek reassurance if you do have persistent concerns.

Babies are all different, and even identical twins develop in their own unique way. Even so, there is a pattern of progression, and babies acquire new skills in the same order (see development charts, below). As a parent, you spend the most time with your baby and are often the first person to notice if they aren't developing as expected. A slight delay in one area of development isn't always significant, but delay in two or more areas is important. If your baby was born prematurely, remember to allow for that. For example, a baby born six weeks prematurely won't reach the stage of a six-week-old baby until 12 weeks after the birth.

As your baby grows up and does more, the different areas of development become increasingly interlinked. A baby may not wave bye-bye, for instance, unless they can also see, hear, and understand that someone is leaving.

It can be tempting to compare your baby with others. While other people's babies can give you an overall idea of what happens when, you can't expect your baby to do things at exactly the same time as others. If you have other children, don't expect this baby to have the same development timetable as your previous babies. Some traits do run in families. Bottom shuffling, for instance, can be familial, but most other achievements vary hugely from one child to the next. Your baby's development will be checked regularly at each of the well-care visits during their first year.

Signs to watch out for

Speak to your pediatrician if your baby displays any of the following

DEVELOPMENTAL MILESTONES

KEY

The four key areas of development are shown in different colors. Colored bands (right) are development windows, which show when your baby is most likely to acquire each skill.

- Gross motor development
- Vision and fine motor development
- Hearing and language
- Social and intellectual development

MONTH 0	MONTH 1	MONTH 2	MONTH 3	MONTH 4	MONTH 5
		Holds weight of upper body on arms when lying on front			
	Holds head up when lying on front		Grasps an object placed in the palm		
		Reaches toward moving objects			
	Tracks objects horizontally				Says
	Discovers hands			Starts making consonar	
			Turns toward you when you speak		
Startled by loud noises			Babbles fluently		
		Makes cooing sounds			
	Smiles when spoken to			Shakes a rattle to make a noise	
				Chuckles at simple game	

signs, or if they regress in any area. Your baby will be examined and if there is not a clear problem, they will be watched very closely and you may be asked to bring them back. Babies can vary from day to day, depending on their mood or whether they are hungry or tired, so it is not always easy to give a definite answer on the first consultation. Alternatively, your baby may be referred to a specialist for assessment. There may be some cause for concern if your baby:

• Has persistently crossed eyes after 6 weeks
• Isn't smiling by 9–10 weeks
• Tilts their head persistently to one side
• Doesn't make cooing sounds at about 3 months
• Makes no eye contact by 3 months
• Doesn't turn their head toward sounds by 3 months

• Has any crossed eyes after 3 months
• Still has a floppy head by 3 months (when awake)
• Doesn't reach for objects by 6 months
• Won't turn around when you speak to them at 6 months
• Isn't babbling by 10 months or stops babbling after having previously

done so (this can be a sign of deafness)
• Won't sit up by 10 months
• Won't bear weight on legs at 10 months
• Doesn't grasp objects at 10 months
• Doesn't try feeding themself at 12 months
• Has asymmetry of the limbs, or any movement, at any stage.

YOUR BABY'S VISION

Parents are often concerned about whether their baby can see properly or will need glasses. While conditions such as glaucoma, astigmatism, and near-sightedness can run in families, you don't generally need to be concerned at this stage. However, if you are in doubt or need reassurance, talk to your doctor.

A newborn baby has a very close range of vision, but you should be able to tell whether they can focus on your face at a distance of around 8–10 in (20–25 cm). Also, their pupils should be dark (or red in a flash photograph). See the doctor if you notice a white mass in either pupil.

Take note, too, if you see any abnormal eye movements, such as a squint, or any wandering or jerking movement, and talk to your doctor.

	MONTH 6	MONTH 7	MONTH 8	MONTH 9	MONTH 10	MONTH 11	MONTH 12
		Sits unsupported			Walks unaided		
		Crawls or bottom-shuffles					
			Pulls up to standing position				
	Rolls from front to back, and back to front				Cruises around furniture		
					Drops things on purpose		
		Can transfer objects from one hand to the other		Bangs blocks together			
					Can point using index finger		
d Da			Can grasp object between finger and thumb				
nds				Puts toys in and takes them out of containers			
		Sounds begin to resemble real words					
						Waves bye-bye	
such as peekaboo					Responds to own name		
		Becomes shy with strangers					

Everyday first aid

It's important you know what to do if your baby is injured. In the rare event of a major emergency, this can make all the difference.

Cuts and scrapes

Babies can become very upset if they get a cut or scrape, so reassure them while you take a look at the injury.

If it's a small scrape or cut, gently clean the area with soap and water using a gauze pad (or you can use any soft, non-fluffy material). If the wound looks dirty, rinse it under running water, pat dry with clean pieces of material, then cover with a clean dressing that is larger than the area of the wound. For a cut lip, apply an ice cube wrapped in a clean piece of burp cloth for about five minutes.

If there is a lot of bleeding, place a clean pad or piece of non-fluffy material over the cut and press down firmly on the wound. If possible, raise the injured part above the level of the heart to reduce blood flow. Keep pressing until the bleeding slows down or stops, then apply a dressing large enough to cover the wound.

Take your baby to the ER if·
• bleeding isn't under control in 10 minutes
• the wound is gaping
• there may be a foreign body in the wound.

Bites and stings

If your baby has been bitten or stung by an insect, they will be surprised and in pain, so comfort them. Bites and stings are not usually serious, but in rare cases, a bee or wasp sting can cause a serious reaction, known as anaphylactic shock (see p.372). A bite or sting in or on the mouth can be serious; if this happens, take your baby to the

hospital immediately.

If you can see a stinger left in the skin, scrape it off with your fingernail. Don't use tweezers since you'll inject more venom into the skin. You can reduce swelling and relieve itching by applying a washcloth or towel soaked in cold water, or an ice cube wrapped in a dry cloth. Hold it on for five minutes while you hug your baby. You can give your baby infant acetaminophen if they're in pain.

Falls, bumps, and bruises

Babies often fall and hurt themselves. Most of the time, all you need to do is comfort your baby and apply a cold compress to the area to relieve swelling and pain (see Bites and stings, left).

Go to the ER if your baby·
• Has a head injury
• Cannot move one of their limbs
• Is bleeding and you can't control it within 10 minutes with direct pressure, or has a gaping wound (see Cuts and scrapes, left)
• Is or was unconscious
• You're not sure if it's serious.

Burns

Fire, hot water, steam, sunlight, electricity, and chemicals can all cause burns. The damage depends on the site, size, thickness, and type of burn. The deepest burns are often fairly painless. Cool the burn under cold running water for at least 10 minutes. Remove (or cut off) clothing around the burn, unless it is stuck to the burn. After cooling, apply a clean dressing or sterile gauze and take your baby to the

hospital for assessment. If the area of the burn is small, see your doctor, but do not delay.

Take your baby to the ER right away if·
• It's a large burn (larger than the palm of your baby's hand)
• It's on the face/in the mouth, on the hands, or the genitals
• The burn is chemical or electrical (take the chemical container with you)
• Your baby seems unwell
• You're unsure what to do.

Foreign objects

Dirt, dust, or other bits can easily get into babies' eyes, and babies may push small objects, such as beans or buttons, into their ears or nose.

Object in eye Anything in the eye usually causes discomfort and crying. If it's a small speck on the surface of the eye, it can generally be washed out.

Fill a pitcher with warm water. Hold your baby with head tilted upward and pour the water into the eye, aiming for the inner corner. The eyelids need to be separated so you'll need assistance.

Take your baby to the ER if·
• An object is embedded in or stuck to the eye. Do not attempt to remove it
• You've tried to wash out an object on the surface of the eye, but have been unsuccessful
• The eye remains irritated and sore after the object has been removed.

Object in ear or nose If your baby gets something stuck in their ear or nose, stay calm and reassure them there's nothing to worry about. Do not try to remove the object even if you can see it because you risk pushing it farther in. Call your pediatrician for an appointment; they may be able to remove the object, using tiny forceps or a suction machine, or they may send you to the ER. Sometimes, a baby may not realize there's something stuck in their ears or nose. They may not hear well or one side of their nose may run or have a smelly discharge. If you have any concerns that there could be something in your baby's ear or nose, see your doctor right away.

Choking

Small objects, such as beans or coins, are often responsible for choking. Babies can also choke on food, or on mucus or milk. Coughing is nature's way of trying to dislodge an obstruction in the airway, so if your baby is choking but still coughing effectively, let them be. If, after two or three minutes, your baby continues to cough, call 911.

If your baby cannot breathe, cough, or cry, the choking is severe. They may make strange noises and their face may turn blue. You need to act immediately (see box, below).

Poisoning

If your baby has ingested something toxic, call the Poison Help Line, 1-800-222-1222. Call 911 if they have a seizure, trouble breathing, or can't be awakened. Tell the medical team what your baby has swallowed, how much, and when, and keep a sample. Do not try to make your baby vomit; this can cause more harm. Wash or wipe off any corrosive substances on or around the mouth. If they've eaten a toxic plant or berries, look in their mouth and remove any remaining pieces.

DEAL WITH CHOKING

If your baby is choking and unable to breathe, take emergency action. Have someone call 911 when you begin first aid.
• Lay the baby face down on your forearm, their head lower than their body. Support the head with your hand. Using the heel of your other hand, give up to five sharp blows to their upper back.
• If the obstruction is still there, turn baby onto their back on your thigh, keeping their head lower than their chest and give

up to five chest thrusts, pushing down with two fingers in the middle of the breastbone just below the nipples, compressing the chest $1/3$ to $1/2$ the depth of the chest.
• Continue giving a series of five back blows followed by five chest thrusts until the object dislodges or the baby becomes unconscious. Don't try removing an object from the mouth of a conscious baby.
• If your baby loses consciousness, shout for help and have someone else dial 911

while you begin infant CPR. If you are alone, call 911 after performing infant CPR for one minute. After a baby loses consciousness, you may attempt to remove an object from their mouth carefully with your finger, but only do this if you can see the object. Even if you have successfully dealt with the emergency, any baby who has had chest thrusts must be seen by a doctor to check that their delicate bones haven't been damaged.

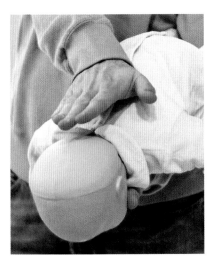

Back blows Make sure the baby's head is lower than their body. Use the heel of your hand to give back blows, making sure the blows land between the shoulder blades.

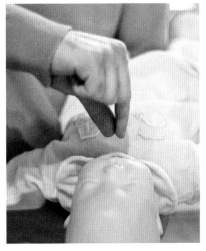

Check mouth Check unconscious baby's mouth: don't remove objects from a conscious baby's mouth. In an unconscious baby, use your fingers only if you can see the object.

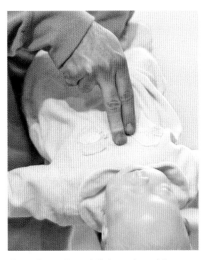

Chest thrusts To avoid injury when giving chest thrusts, your fingers should be on the breastbone, not ribs. Push inward and upward, being firm but not jerky.

Resources

Feeding

Breastfeedingusa.org
Breastfeeding support

llli.org
La Leche League
(800) LA LECHE

www.myplate.gov/life-stages/pregnancy-and-breastfeeding
MyPlate for Pregnancy & Breastfeeding

uslca.org
United States Lactation Consultant Association
(919) 861-4543

womenshealth.gov/breastfeeding/learning-to-breastfeed
Breastfeeding support
(800) 994-9662

Support groups

aafa.org
Asthma and Allergy Foundation of America
(800) 7-ASTHMA

acds.org
Association for Children with Down Syndrome
(516) 933-4700

birthdefects.org
Birth Defects Research for Children
(407) 895-0802

cff.org
Cystic Fibrosis Foundation
(800) FIGHT CF

diabetes.org
American Diabetes Association
(800) DIABETES

epilepsyfoundation.org
Epilepsy Foundation
(800) 332-1000

handtohold.org
NICU parent support site

interdys.org
The International Dyslexia Association
(410) 296-0232

marchofdimes.com
March of Dimes
(914) 997-4488

www.nad.org
National Association of the Deaf

nads.org
National Association for Down Syndrome
602-325-9112

nichcy.org
National Dissemination Center for Children with Disabilities
(800) 695-0285

nicuparentnetwork.org
NICU Parent Network

nmha.org/go/postpartum
Mental Health America
(800) 273-TALK

postpartum.net
Postpartum Support International
(800) 944-4PPD

sbaa.org
Spina Bifida Association
(800) 621-3141

shakenbaby.org
Shaken Baby Alliance
(877) 6-END-SBS

sicklecelldisease.org
Sickle Cell Disease Association of America
(800) 421-8453

sids.org
American SIDS Institute
(239) 431-5425

ucp.org
United Cerebral Palsy
(800) 872-5827

westutter.org
National Stuttering Association

Parent groups

fatherhood.gov
National Responsible Fatherhood Clearinghouse
(877) 4DAD411

meetup.com/topics/moms/
Moms Meetup Group

nationalsingleparent.org
National Single Parent Resource Center
(561) 441-8557

multiplesofamerica.org/
Multiples of America

parentswithoutpartners.org
Parents Without Partners
(800) 637-7974

Child care

childcareaware.org
National Association of Child Care Resource & Referral Agencies
(800) 424-2246

nafcc.org
National Association for Family Child Care
(800) 359-3817

nhsa.org
National Head Start Association
(703) 739-0875

Baby and child health and safety

aap.org
American Academy of Pediatrics
(847) 434-4000

americanheart.org
American Heart Association
(800) AHA-USA-1

cpsc.gov
Consumer Product Safety Commission
(800) 638-2772

nccam.nih.gov
National Center for Complementary
and Alternative Medicine
(888) 644-6226

nhtsa.gov
National Highway Traffic Safety
Adminstration
(888) 327-4236

nichd.nih.gov
National Institute of Child Health
and Human Development
(800) 370-2943

safekids.org
Safe Kids USA
(202) 662-0600

redcross.org
American Red Cross
(800) REDCROSS

Rights and benefits

www.dol.gov/whd/fmla/index.htm
US Department of Labor, Family and
Medical Leave Act

General

allaboutclothdiapers.com
All About Cloth Diapers

babycenter.com
BabyCenter

babysignlanguage.com/chart/
BabySignLanguage.com

childabuseprevention.org
Child Abuse Prevention
Association
(816) 252-8388

childwelfare.gov
Child Welfare Information
Gateway
(800) 394-3366

eatright.org
Academy of Nutrition and Dietetics
(800) 877-1600

healthychildren.org
Healthy Children, Ages & Stages
(American Academy of Pediatrics)

infantmassageusa.org
Infant Massage USA
(800) 497-5996

nichd.nih.gov/sids/
Back to Sleep Public Education
Campaign

plannedparenthood.org
Planned Parenthood
(800) 230-PLAN

smokefree.gov
Smokefree
(800) QUIT-NOW

ssa.gov/kids
Social Security Administration
(800) 772-1213

Index

INDEX

Contributors

Dr. Helen Moore, Pediatric Consultant at Chesterfield Royal Hospital, and pediatric rheumatology and critical care lead.

Dr. Aiwyne Foo, Consultant Pediatrician and former Neonatal Lead at Chesterfield Royal Hospital.

Holly Markham, BA in Global Politics from the University of Brighton; MA in Gender and Development from the Institute of Development Studies, University of Sussex.

Judy Barratt, highly experienced childcare author specializing in children's nutrition and development.

Nicola Deschamps (ANutri) dipNT, MSc, experienced author and editor with an interest in nutrition, physical activity, and public health.

Dr. Ilona Bendefy MB, BS, MRCP (Peds), former GP in London and Derbyshire, and pediatrician in Sheffield Children's Hospital. Medical graduate from St. Thomas' Hospital, London.

Bella Dale RM, midwife and infant feeding specialist with extensive experience supporting new mothers breastfeeding their babies.

Dr. Carol Cooper MA, MB, BChir, MRCP, GP, medical writer, and broadcaster. Cambridge University medical graduate and former hospital physician. Teaches at Imperial College Medical School.

Dr. Claire Halsey AFBPsS, ClinPsyD, MSc, consultant clinical psychologist. Journalist and author in the fields of child psychology, parenting, and child development.

Fiona Wilcock MSc, PGCE, RPHNut, registered Public Health Nutritionist and food writer; has written widely on diet in pregnancy and early years. Nutrition consultant to manufacturers and retailers.

Jenny Hall BSc, RGN, RN (Child), health visitor and former children's nurse.

Karen Sullivan, author and childcare expert with degrees in developmental and educational psychology.

Dr. Mary Steen RGN, RM, BHSc, PGCRM, PGDipHE, MCGI, PhD, midwife and former Professor of Midwifery at the University of Chester, with awards for original research, clinical innovation, and outstanding services to Midwifery.

Dr. Su Laurent MRCP, FRCPCH, consultant pediatrician at Barnet Hospital, London, supervising the care of children from premature babies to teenagers. Trustee of The Child Bereavement Charity.

Acknowledgments

Thanks to the models: Sarah and Kaiden Asamoa; Nina and Jamie Bradburn; Unity Brennan, Amelie Grace, and Benjamin Wolski; Selina Chand and Faith Lucy O'Brien; Narae Cho and Alex Park; Nicola and Freya Church; Anna and Eliana Clarke; Archie Clements; Philippa and Noah Dovar; Joe and Dagan Drahota; Jenny and Harry Duggin; Laura and Zoe Forrest; Rachael and Samuel Grady; Kate Heavenor and Nicolas Diaz; Olga and Mia Gelev; Beatriz de Lemos and Isabel Walker; Jordan McRobie, Jenny Parr and Reuben McRobie; Eden Martin-Osakwe; Poppy Mitchell and Oaklee Wealands; Amelie Victoria Morris; Victoria and Arthur Morton; Oreke Mosheshe and Carter Mbamali; Gabriela and Alba Nardi; Miriam Nelken and Mala Shahi; Laura and Charlie Nickoll; Amie and Rosie Niland; Lauren Overs and Grayson Andrews; Yoan Petkov; Suzy Richards and Max Snead; Heidi Robinson and Elias Crosby; Jenny Sharp and Joshua Tyler; Matthew, Angela, and Jacob Smith; Eve Spaughton and Genevieve Long; Rose and Brooke Thunberg; Anggayasti Trikanti and Carissa Afila; Rachel Weaver and Jacob Marcus; Karen and Milly Westropp; Georgie and Harriet Willock.

Picture credits

The publisher would like to thank the following for their kind permission to reproduce their photographs:

(Key: a-above; b-below/bottom; c-center; f-far; l-left; r-right; t-top)

2 Alamy Stock Photo: Cultura Creative RF / Sporrer / Rupp (cra). Getty Images: DigitalVision / Jon Feingersh Photography Inc (clb); DigitalVision / Jessie Casson (cb); The Image Bank / Glasshouse Images (bc); Moment / Oscar Wong (br). Getty Images / iStock: E+ / enigma_images (tr); E+ / Pekic (cla). 5 Getty Images: Stone / Catherine Delahaye. 6 Getty Images: Moment / Oscar Wong. 8-9 Getty Images / iStock: E+ / AJ_Watt. 13 Getty Images: Cavan Images (cr). 15 Getty Images / iStock: E+ / JohnnyGreig. 18 Getty Images: Westend61. 23 Shutterstock.com: ImageBROKER.com (bl). 28 Getty Images: Moment / Emilija Manevska (bc). 34 Dreamstime.com: Pojoslaw (bc). 35 Getty Images / iStock: E+ / Stefan Tomic. 39 Getty Images / iStock: E+ / Anchiy (c). 40 Getty Images: Frank Herholdt (c). 41 Corbis: Cameron (cra). 42 Getty Images: Photodisc / Daniel Tardif. 44 Getty Images / iStock: E+ / lostinbids (bl, bc, br). 47 Getty Images: Anthony Bradshaw (c). 49 Getty Images: Collection Mix: Subjects / Guerilla (cra). Getty Images / iStock: E+ / FatCamera (ca). 55 Alamy Images: Peter Usbeck (br). Getty Images: Louie Psihoyos (tr). 57 Getty Images: Moment / d3sign (fbl, bl, bc). 58 Getty Images / iStock: E+ / CocoSan (bc); E+ / FatCamera (fbl). 59 Getty Images / iStock: Vetta / SelectStock (bl). Photolibrary: Philippe Dannic (tc). 60 Getty Images: Ian Hooton / Spl (br). Photolibrary: Gyssels (bc). 61 Dreamstime.com: Polina Zubko (cr). Science Photo Library: Dr P. Marazzi (bc). 63 Mother & Baby Picture Library: Ruth Jenkinson (br). 69 Dreamstime.com: Pojoslaw (br). 75 Getty Images / iStock: E+ / DonnaDiavolo (br). 81 Alamy Stock Photo: Jennie Hart (cl). 82 Getty Images / iStock: E+ / FatCamera. 83 Dorling Kindersley: Antonia Deutsch (cr). 90 Getty Images / iStock: E+ / enigma_images. 96 Dreamstime.com: Thitaree Mahawong. 97 Getty Images / iStock: E+ / Isbjorn. 100 Getty Images: Moment / skaman306. 101 Getty Images: DigitalVision / Kohei Hara. 102 Getty Images / iStock: E+ / pixdeluxe. 103 Getty Images / iStock: Westend61. 105 Getty Images / iStock: E+ / damircudic. 106 Getty Images: Moment / Karl Tapales. 107 Alamy Stock Photo: Addictive Stock Creatives (cr). 110 Getty Images: Westend61. 111 Corbis: Sean Justice (cra). 114 Getty Images / iStock: E+ / FatCamera. 117 Getty Images: Image Source / Manuela Larissegger. 122 Getty Images: Westend61. 129 Getty Images / iStock: E+ / Anchiy (cra); Prostock-Studio (ca). 130 Getty Images: Tetra images / Blend Images - JGI / Tom Grill. 135 Getty Images: Corbis Documentary / Andria Patino. 136 Getty Images: Tetra images / Inti St Clair. 138 Getty Images: Maskot.

140 Getty Images / iStock: E+ / lechatnoir. 142 Corbis: Fabrik Studios / Index Stock (cra). 146 Getty Images: Moment / Kevin Liu (c). 152 Getty Images / iStock: PeopleImages. 156 Getty Images / iStock: E+ / hsyncoban. 160 Getty Images: Moment Open / Kevin Liu. 161 Alamy Stock Photo: Cultura Creative RF / Sporrer / Rupp. 164 Getty Images / iStock: E+ / FG Trade. 166 Getty Images / iStock: E+ / AJ_Watt. 167 Getty Images: IndiaPix / IndiaPicture. 170 Getty Images: Jozef Polc / 500px. 173 Getty Images / iStock: E+ / SDI Productions (cl). 175 Getty Images / iStock: E+ / urbazon. 178 Getty Images: Stone / Catherine Delahaye. 181 Getty Images / iStock: E+ / SolStock. 183 Getty Images: Moment / Oscar Wong. 185 Getty Images / iStock: MonthiraYodtiwong (cra). 187 Getty Images: Westend61. 189 Alamy Stock Photo: Irina Sapozhnikova. 195 Getty Images / iStock: E+ / FreshSplash. 201 Corbis: Lisa B. (bl). 202 Getty Images: Moment / Images by Jazmyn Luo. 203 Getty Images / iStock: E+ / mgstudyo. 207 Getty Images: Moment / Davide Casarini. 210 Getty Images: DigitalVision / Jon Feingersh Photography Inc. 213 Getty Images: DigitalVision / MoMo Productions. 215 Getty Images / iStock: petrunjela. 218 Getty Images: Photodisc / Mitch Diamond. 225 Getty Images: Moment / d3sign. 231 Getty Images: The Image Bank / Cecile Lavabre. 232 Getty Images / iStock: E+ / Miodrag Ignjatovic. 234 Getty Images: Moment / Yasser Chalid. 240 Getty Images: DigitalVision / Willie B. Thomas. 241 Getty Images / iStock: E+ / SolStock. 242 Getty Images: Moment / Oscar Wong. 246 Getty Images / iStock: E+ / FatCamera. 248 Mother & Baby Picture Library: Ian Hooton (bl). 254 Getty Images / iStock: E+ / Onfokus. 256 Getty Images: Moment / Catherine Falls Commercial. 259 Getty Images: Westend61. 260 Getty Images: DigitalVision / Oliver Rossi. 261 Getty Images / iStock: E+ / PixelsEffect. 263 Getty Images: Westend61. 265 Getty Images: Stone / Catherine Delahaye. 266 Getty Images / iStock: E+ / SolStock. 267 Getty Images / iStock: E+ / SolStock. 269 Getty Images: Moment / Oscar Wong (c, cr). 271 Getty Images / iStock: E+ / Pekic. 273 Getty Images / iStock: romrodinka. 277 Getty Images: Moment / Oscar Wong. 279 Corbis: Image Source (bl). 280 Getty Images: Brand X Pictures / BFG Images. 289 Getty Images: Moment / Laura Olivas. 295 Getty Images: Moment / Oscar Wong (cra). 297 Getty Images: Cavan Images. 298 Getty Images: Moment / Tanja Ivanova. 301 Getty Images: DigitalVision / Jessie Casson. 303 Getty Images / iStock: Tatiana Dyuvbanova (cr). 307 Getty Images: The Image Bank / Glasshouse Images. 308 Getty Images: Fabrice LEROUGE (cla). 312 Getty Images: Tetra images / Jamie Grill. 314 Getty Images / iStock: E+ / SolStock. 316 Getty Images / iStock: E+ / Drs Producoes. 317 Getty Images / iStock: E+ / Tempura. 320 Getty Images: Jose Luis Pelaez, Inc. / Blend Images (cla). 327 Alamy Images: moodboard (br). 330 Getty Images: Tetra images / Jessica Peterson. 331 Corbis: Brigitte Sporrer (cra). 335 Getty Images / iStock: E+ / SolStock. 342 Getty Images: Westend61. 347 Getty Images: Stone / Bjarte Rettedal. 348 Getty Images / iStock: Andrey Zhuravlev. 349 Getty Images: Stone / Tony Anderson. 352 Getty Images: Moment / Layland Masuda. 354 Getty Images: DigitalVision / Solskin (cra). Getty Images: David M. Zuber (bc). 357 Alamy Images: Ian nolan (ca). 359 Getty Images: Moment / Oscar Wong. 362 Getty Images / iStock: E+ / Pekic. 364 Getty Images / iStock: E+ / SDI Productions. 367 Dorling Kindersley: dave king (bc). 368 Mother & Baby Picture Library: Ian Hooton (c). 370 Science Photo Library: Dr P. Marazzi (bc). 372 Getty Images: DigitalVision / Justin Paget. 373 Science Photo Library: Chris Knapton (bc). 374 Getty Images: Brand X Pictures / Science Photo Library—IAN HOOTON. (bl). Science Photo Library: (c). 375 Science Photo Library: Dr H. C. Robinson (bl). 376 Getty Images: Ruth Jenkinson / Spl (br). 378 Meningitis Trust www.meningitis-trust.org: (bl).

Cover images: Front: Getty Images: DigitalVision / Jose Luis Pelaez Inc fbr, Stone / Jade Albert Studio, Inc. bl; Getty Images / iStock: Digital Vision / Photodisc br, Tom Merton / OJO Images fbl

All other images © Dorling Kindersley

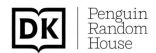

DK | Penguin Random House

DK UK
Senior Editor Sophie Blackman
Senior Acquisitions Editor Becky Alexander
Senior Designer Glenda Fisher
Senior US Editor Megan Douglass
Picture Researchers Jo Chukualim, Amy Moss
Jacket Designer Glenda Fisher
Production Editor David Almond
Senior Production Controller Stephanie McConnell
Assistant Editor Jasmin Lennie
Editorial Manager Ruth O'Rourke
Art Director Maxine Pedliham
Publishing Director Katie Cowan

Consultants Aiwyne Foo, Helen Moore, Holly Markham
US Consultant Gwynette Marschall, MD
Editors Judy Barratt, Nicola Deschamps
Designer Hannah Moore

DK INDIA
Editor Ankita Gupta
DTP Designers Umesh Singh Rawat, Anurag Trivedi
DTP Coordinator Pushpak Tyagi
Senior Picture Researcher Aditya Katyal
Assistant Picture Research Administrator Manpreet Kaur
Pre-production Manager Balwant Singh
Creative Head Malavika Talukder

THE DAY-BY-DAY BABY BOOK

DK UK
Senior Editors Victoria Heyworth-Dunne, Amanda Lebentz
Senior Designers Nicola Rodway, Pamela Shiels
Editorial Assistant Kathryn Meeker
Senior Production Editor Clare McLean
Production Controller Seyhan Esen
Creative Technical Support Sonia Charbonnier
New Photography Vanessa Davies
Art Direction for Photography Emma Forge
Managing Editor Penny Smith
Managing Art Editor Marianne Markham
Publishing Manager Anna Davidson
Publisher Peggy Vance

DK INDIA
Senior Editor Alicia Ingty
Editors Janashree Singha, Himanshi Sharma
Art Editor Ira Sharma
Assistant Art Editor Ridhi Khanna
Managing Editor Glenda Fernandes
Managing Art Editor Navidita Thapa
DTP Manager Sunil Sharma
DTP Designers Anurag Trivedi, Satish Chandra Gaur

This American Edition, 2023
Based on content first published in 2012 in
The Day-by-Day Baby Book by
Published in the United States by DK Publishing
1745 Broadway, 20th Floor, New York, NY 10019

Copyright © 2012, 2023 Dorling Kindersley Limited
DK, a Division of Penguin Random House LLC
23 24 25 26 27 10 9 8 7 6 5 4 3 2 1
001–336985–Dec/2023

A catalog record for this book is available from the Library of Congress.
ISBN: 978-0-7440-8641-6

Printed and bound in China.

www.dk.com

Publisher notes

The publisher would like to thank Naorem Anuja for editorial support, Kathy Steer for the proofread, and Ruth Ellis for the index.

Neither the publisher nor the author is engaged in rendering professional advice or services to the individual reader. The ideas, procedures, and suggestions contained in this book are not intended as a substitute for consulting with your physician. All matters regarding your health require medical supervision. Neither the author nor the publisher shall be liable or responsible for any loss or damage allegedly arising from any information or suggestion in this book.

Gender identities

DK recognizes all gender identities, and acknowledges that the sex someone was assigned at birth based on their sexual organs may not align with their own gender identity. People may self-identify as any gender or no gender (including, but not limited to, that of a cis or trans woman, of a cis or trans man, or of a nonbinary person).

As gender language, and its use in our society evolves, the scientific and medical communities continue to reassess their own phrasing. Most of the studies referred to in this book use "women" to describe people whose sex was assigned as female at birth, and "men" to describe people whose sex was assigned as male at birth.

MIX
Paper | Supporting responsible forestry
FSC™ C018179

This book was made with Forest Stewardship Council™ certified paper—one small step in DK's commitment to a sustainable future. For more information go to www.dk.com/our-green-pledge

12/5/23